PTSD and Mild Traumatic Brain Injury

PTSD and Mild Traumatic Brain Injury

EDITED BY

Jennifer J. Vasterling
Richard A. Bryant
Terence M. Keane

THE GUILFORD PRESS
New York   London

©2012 by The Guilford Press
A Division of Guilford Publications, Inc.
72 Spring Street, New York, NY 10012
www.guilford.com

Printed in the United States of America

This book is printed on acid-free paper.

Last digit is print number: 9   8   7   6   5   4   3   2   1

The authors have checked with sources believed to be reliable in their efforts to
provide information that is complete and generally in accord with the standards
of practice that are accepted at the time of publication. However, in view of the
possibility of human error or changes in behavioral, mental health, or medical
sciences, neither the authors, nor the editors and publisher, nor any other party
who has been involved in the preparation or publication of this work warrants
that the information contained herein is in every respect accurate or complete,
and they are not responsible for any errors or omissions or the results obtained
from the use of such information. Readers are encouraged to confirm the
information contained in this book with other sources.

Library of Congress Cataloging-in-Publication Data is available
from the publisher.

ISBN 978-1-4625-0338-4

About the Editors

Jennifer J. Vasterling, PhD, is Chief of Psychology at the VA Boston Healthcare System. She is also a clinical neuropsychologist, an active researcher in the VA National Center for PTSD, and Professor of Psychiatry at Boston University School of Medicine. Dr. Vasterling is a recipient of the Award for Outstanding Contributions to the Science of Trauma Psychology from the American Psychological Association (Division 56, Division of Trauma Psychology). She is an authority on the neuropsychological features of PTSD and is known for her work examining the cognitive and emotional changes that accompany war-zone deployment.

Richard A. Bryant, PhD, is Scientia Professor of Psychology at the University of New South Wales. He is also an Australian Research Council Laureate Fellow and Director of the Traumatic Stress Clinic at Westmead Hospital in Sydney. Dr. Bryant is a recipient of honors including the Distinguished Contribution to Psychological Science Award from the Australian Psychological Society and the Robert S. Laufer Award for Outstanding Scientific Achievement from the International Society for Traumatic Stress Studies (ISTSS). His work focuses on the intersection of PTSD and traumatic brain injury, the assessment and treatment of acute trauma reactions, and the cognitive and biological mechanisms underpinning traumatic stress.

Terence M. Keane, PhD, is Director and Associate Chief of Staff for Research and Development at the VA National Center for PTSD, Behavioral Sciences Division, VA Boston Healthcare System. He is also Assistant Dean for Research and Professor and Vice-Chairman of Psychiatry at Boston University School of Medicine. Dr. Keane is a recipient of the Lifetime Achievement Award from the ISTSS, among numerous other awards. He developed many of the most widely used PTSD assessment measures and is an authority on the cognitive-behavioral treatment of PTSD.

Contributors

Jomana Amara, PhD, Defense Resource Management Institute, Naval Postgraduate School, Monterey, California

Melissa M. Amick, PhD, Translational Research Center for Traumatic Brain Injury and Stress Disorders, VA Boston Healthcare System; Department of Psychiatry, Boston University School of Medicine, Boston, Massachusetts

Erin D. Bigler, PhD, Department of Psychology and Neuroscience Center, Brigham Young University, Provo, Utah

Richard A. Bryant, PhD, School of Psychology, University of New South Wales, Sydney, Australia

Carl A. Castro, PhD, United States Army Medical Research and Materiel Command, Fort Detrick, Maryland

Sara L. Dolan, PhD, Department of Psychology and Neuroscience, Baylor University, Waco, Texas

Jon D. Elhai, PhD, Department of Psychology, University of Toledo, Toledo, Ohio

Frank A. Fee, PhD, private practice, Houston, Texas

Catherine B. Fortier, PhD, Translational Research Center for Traumatic Brain Injury and Stress Disorders, VA Boston Healthcare System, and Department of Psychiatry, Harvard Medical School, Boston, Massachusetts

Mark W. Gilbertson, PhD, Manchester VA Medical Center, Manchester, New Hampshire; Department of Psychiatry, Boston University School of Medicine, Boston, Massachusetts

Leslie M. Guidotti Breting, PhD, Department of Psychiatry and Behavioral Sciences, NorthShore University HealthSystem, Evanston, Illinois

Ann Hendricks, PhD, Health Care Financing and Economics, VA Boston Healthcare System, and Department of Health Policy and Management, Boston University School of Public Health, Boston, Massachusetts

Jennifer Highley, NP, Department of Behavioral Health, USA MEDDAC, West Point, New York; Columbia University School of Nursing, New York, New York

Grant L. Iverson, PhD, Department of Psychiatry, University of British Columbia, Vancouver, British Columbia, Canada; Defense and Veterans Brain Injury Center, Walter Reed Army Medical Center, Washington, DC

Katherine M. Iverson, PhD, National Center for PTSD, VA Boston Healthcare System, and Department of Psychiatry, Boston University School of Medicine, Boston, Massachusetts

Danny Kaloupek, PhD, National Center for PTSD, VA Boston Healthcare System; Department of Psychiatry, Boston University School of Medicine, Boston, Massachusetts

Terence M. Keane, PhD, National Center for PTSD, VA Boston Healthcare System; Department of Psychiatry and Department of Psychology, Boston University, Boston, Massachusetts

Rachel Kimerling, PhD, National Center for PTSD and Center for Health Care Evaluations, Washington, DC; VA Palo Alto Healthcare System, Palo Alto, California

Maxine Krengel, PhD, VA Boston Healthcare System; Department of Psychiatry, Boston University School of Medicine, Boston, Massachusetts

Henry L. Lew, MD, PhD, Defense and Veterans Brain Injury Center, Department of Defense, Richmond, Virginia; University of Hawaii at Manoa, Honolulu, Hawaii

Brett T. Litz, PhD, VA Boston Healthcare System; Department of Psychiatry, and Department of Psychology, Boston University, Boston, Massachusetts

Brian P. Marx, PhD, VA National Center for PTSD, VA Boston Healthcare System, and Department of Psychiatry, Boston University School of Medicine, Boston, Massachusetts

William L. Maxwell, PhD, Department of Anatomy, University of Glasgow, Glasgow, Scotland

Lisa M. Najavits, PhD, VA Boston Healthcare System, and Department of Psychiatry, Boston University School of Medicine, Boston, Massachusetts

John D. Otis, VA Boston Healthcare System, and Department of Psychiatry and Department of Psychology, Boston University, Boston, Massachusetts

Jasmeet Pannu Hayes, PhD, National Center for PTSD, VA Boston Healthcare System, and Department of Psychiatry, Boston University School of Medicine, Boston, Massachusetts

Jennie Ponsford, PhD, MAPsS, School of Psychology and Psychiatry, Monash University; Monash–Epworth Rehabilitation Research Centre, Epworth Hospital; and National Trauma Research Institute, Alfred Hospital, Melbourne, Australia

Jerry J. Sweet, PhD, Department of Psychiatry and Behavioral Sciences, NorthShore University HealthSystem, Evanston, Illinois

Carlos Tun, MD, Physical Medicine and Rehabilitation Service, VA Boston Healthcare System, and Department of Physical Medicine and Rehabilitation, Harvard Medical School, Boston, Massachusetts

Erin W. Ulloa, PhD, Behavioral Health Lab, Philadelphia VA Medical Center, Philadelphia, Pennsylvania

Rodney D. Vanderploeg, PhD, ABPP-CN, Department of Mental Health and Behavioral Sciences, HSR&D/RR&D Center of Excellence: Maximizing Rehabilitation Outcomes; Defense and Veterans Brain Injury Center, James A. Haley Veterans Hospital; and Department of Psychiatry and Neurosciences and Department of Psychology, University South Florida, Tampa, Florida

Jennifer J. Vasterling, PhD, Psychology Service and VA National Center for PTSD, VA Boston Healthcare System; and Department of Psychiatry, Boston University School of Medicine, Boston, Massachusetts

Mieke Verfaellie, PhD, Memory Disorders Research Center, VA Boston Healthcare System, and Department of Psychiatry, Boston University School of Medicine, Boston, Massachusetts

Contents

xi

INTRODUCTION

Understanding the Interface of Traumatic Stress and Mild Traumatic Brain Injury

Background and Conceptual Framework

Jennifer J. Vasterling, Richard A. Bryant, and Terence M. Keane

The recent wars in Afghanistan and Iraq highlight the need for paying increased attention to stress-related psychological disorders, traumatic brain injury (TBI), and the intersection between these conditions. Stress-related disorders, such as posttraumatic stress disorder (PTSD), and TBI are often considered "invisible injuries" because they are not as readily observable to others as a broken leg, scar, or amputation may be, yet they may impart significant disruption to life and impose functional disability. Within the broad categories of stress-related disorders and TBI, PTSD and mild TBI (mTBI) have emerged as particular concerns—both in their own right and as conditions that occur concomitantly in a large number of people. Although recent wars have focused attention on PTSD and mTBI in an unprecedented way, the issues surrounding the causes, effects, and management of these interacting conditions are relevant to both civilian and military contexts.

U.S. population-based surveys estimate the prevalence of PTSD in the general community to be at 7–8% (Kessler, Sonnega, Bromet, Hughes, & Nelson, 1995), although rates of PTSD climb in higher risk groups such as people exposed to community violence (e.g., Silva et al., 2000; Zinzow et

3

al., 2009) or those serving in the military (e.g., Dohwenrend et al., 2006; Kulka et al., 1990). TBI likewise affects many people. Over 1.1 million people with TBI seek care annually in U.S. emergency rooms, with the majority of these TBIs classified as mild (Corrigan, Selassie, & Orman, 2010). As striking as these emergency room figures are, they may underestimate the occurrence of milder TBIs, given that many people will not seek emergency services if their loss of consciousness is brief and their symptoms are transient.

The prevalence rates of PTSD and mTBI in American service members returning from Operation Enduring Freedom (OEF) and Operation Iraqi Freedom (OIF) have been reported to be as high as 13.8% and 19.5%, respectively (Tanielian & Jaycox, 2008), although rates of both PTSD and TBI among military personnel deployed from international forces were reported to be lower (Fear et al., 2010; Rona et al., 2011). As various chapters of this volume suggest, the prevalence of PTSD and mTBI in service members returning from OEF and OIF is difficult to capture (Carlson et al., 2011). Variance in estimates is likely attributable to limitations to real-time documentation of war-zone injuries and events, and differences in sampling strategies and time frames. The challenges in estimating prevalence also highlight the ambiguity surrounding the operational definitions of PTSD and mTBI, and how they are assessed. These issues are critical for all practitioners, regardless of the civilian or military context in which they work, and are addressed across many chapters of this volume.

In addition to the occurrence of each condition when considered alone, PTSD and mTBI frequently co-occur. For example, among those veterans in a RAND study reporting TBI, 33.8% also screened positive for PTSD. A study of 2,525 deployed U.S. Army infantry soldiers likewise showed high rates of PTSD–mTBI comorbidity (Hoge et al., 2008). In the U.S. Army study, 44% of soldiers reporting TBI with any alteration of consciousness also screened positive for PTSD, and 27% of soldiers reporting TBI with outright loss of consciousness screened positive for PTSD. In some treatment contexts serving combat veterans the comorbidity may occur even more frequently (Lew et al., 2009).

There are also a number of civilian contexts that may lead to both PTSD and mTBI. Motor vehicle accidents, domestic violence, and other types of assaults, for example, all confer risk of both PTSD and TBI. The commonality of these injury contexts is that the events that result in brain injury are often also psychologically traumatic. Further, in some contexts (e.g., combat, domestic violence), even if the specific event leading to a TBI does not precipitate PTSD, the TBI occurs in a context of persistent and repeated exposure to extreme psychological stress and/or life threat. This volume takes into consideration a range of contexts that might lead to the development of comorbid PTSD and mTBI.

Definitions

Although PTSD can accompany a TBI of any severity level, we focus in this volume on milder TBIs for two primary reasons. First, mTBI is among the most prevalent of TBIs and is seemingly more likely to be associated with PTSD than moderate and more severe TBI (Zatzick et al., 2010). Thus, many clinicians more commonly confront the PTSD–TBI comorbidity at the milder end of the TBI spectrum. Second, there is significant controversy regarding health care policy and best clinical practices for patients presenting with PTSD and mTBI (Hoge, Goldberg, & Castro, 2009). Because the milder forms of TBI may be the least well understood of all TBIs, it is mTBI that drives the sometimes polarizing policy and conceptual debates that currently permeate the field and leave clinicians searching for answers (Sayer et al., 2009).

As several chapters in this volume highlight, ambiguous definitions surrounding mTBI and related constructs add to the confusion. "Mild TBI" represents a relatively broad range of injury attributes and outcomes. Most definitions of TBI, including those espoused by multi-agency consensus conferences (Menon, Schwab, Wright, & Maas, 2010), the World Health Organization (Ruff et al., 2009), the Centers for Disease Control and Prevention (National Center for Injury Prevention and Control, 2003), and the American Congress of Rehabilitation Medicine (1993) require two basic components: (1) at least a transient disruption in brain function and/or other evidence of brain injury and (2) the precipitant of an external force to the head. Operational definitions set upper severity limits for mTBI, the most common of which are (1) loss of consciousness (LOC) not to exceed 30 minutes and (2) posttraumatic amnesia (PTA) (i.e., the duration of time in which the formation of new memories is impaired following the injury) not to exceed 24 hours. The term "concussion" is often used interchangeably with mTBI and has been recommended as a less stigmatizing term as compared to "TBI" (Hoge et al., 2009), but as Bigler and Maxwell (Chapter 2, this volume) point out, not all experts agree that the two terms are synonymous.

Further contributing to potential misunderstanding, the brain injury may be confused with its functional sequelae, which are often labeled as postconcussive symptoms or postconcussive syndrome (PCS). Some commentators argue that TBI should be considered a chronic disorder that extends beyond the initial injury (Masel & DeWitt, 2010) and that the original injury is rarely a discrete, time-limited event. However, as described by Bigler and Maxwell (Chapter 2, this volume), evidence is just now emerging regarding the potential chronicity of the actual pathophysiology of milder injuries. The implications of this evidence also suggest that TBI severity is continuous as a construct, rather than reflecting discrete categories.

Thus, the term "mild TBI," especially when referring to an enduring disorder, may imply different meanings to different researchers and clinicians.
Clear definitions of mTBI are needed to improve clinical care, standardize
research, and facilitate better demarcations between mTBI and its comorbid disorders.

Definitions of PTSD are somewhat more straightforward but are likely
to show some continued evolution as formal taxonomic systems are revised.
Although revision of PTSD criteria are currently under consideration for
the next edition of the *Diagnostic and Statistical Manual of Mental Disorders* (DSM) (Friedman, Resick, Bryant, & Brewin, 2011), authors throughout this volume adopt the current criteria for PTSD delineated in the text
revision of the fourth edition of the DSM (DSM-IV-TR; American Psychiatric Association, 2000). Like TBI, in thinking about PTSD, it is important
to distinguish between the initial traumatic event, one that might or might
not lead to PTSD, and the symptoms and functional impairment that can
result from psychological trauma exposure. Finally, it is relevant that PTSD
symptoms occur on a continuum and do not necessarily remain static in
time in terms of their presence, severity, or functional impact.

PTSD and mTBI: A Conceptual Framework

As displayed in Figure 1.1, we view the potential causal pathways between
psychological trauma/PTSD and mTBI/postconcussive symptoms as complex, leaving open the possibilities of bidirectional influences. Not mutually
exclusive, PTSD and mTBI (and associated postconcussive symptoms) may
also occur independently as a result of a common event or context that
increases the risk of both psychological trauma exposure and brain injury.
Figure 1 provides a combat example, but the same relationships would hold
true of moving vehicle, industrial, or occupational accidents; interpersonal
assaults; and other circumstances that are both psychologically traumatic
and confer risk of brain injury. Although not depicted in the figure, the
clinical presentation of the comorbidity is also complicated by other factors such as orthopedic injury, pain conditions, substance abuse and dependence, and other mental health disorders, such as depression.

In keeping with this framework, we constructed this volume to address
the complexities of caring for patients with comorbid PTSD and mTBI,
rather than limiting discussion to an oversimplified dichotomy surrounding
the question of whether postconcussive symptoms are primarily "neurological" or "psychiatric" in nature. The clinical presentation of the comorbidity is indeed complex, with PTSD and mTBI characterized by overlapping
symptom presentations, neural substrates, and functional consequences. It
is important to remember that sophisticated research into the mechanisms

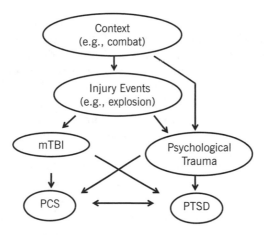

FIGURE 1.1. Hypothesized relationships among context, injury events, mild traumatic brain injury (mTBI), psychological trauma, postconcussive symptoms (PCS), and posttraumatic stress disorder (PTSD).

of mTBI is in its infancy, and there is much we simply do not yet understand about the effects of mild brain injuries. We also recognize that each of these conditions is also commonly associated with other psychiatric disorders including depression and substance abuse, and other physical comorbidities such as chronic pain. Our emphasis centers on how best to recognize this comorbidity and its associated clinical problems, how best to structure interventions for various aspects of the presentation, and which factors might be worthwhile to consider from the perspective of health care delivery systems. More specifically, we attempt in this volume to address the following four questions:

1. To what extent and via what mechanisms do PTSD and mTBI potentially complicate each other?
2. Which other factors complicate recovery from PTSD and mTBI?
3. What do we know about treatment of patients with comorbid PTSD/mTBI?
4. How should care of patients with PTSD and mTBI be optimally structured?

Organization of the Volume

The first section of the volume describes the mechanisms underlying PTSD and mTBI, the clinical presentation and potential courses of each condition, and mechanisms by which the two conditions may complicate each other. Bigler and Maxwell (Chapter 2) define mTBI and describe the scale of the problem with epidemiological data. The thrust of the chapter, however, is on understanding the mechanisms of neural injury, the potential course of physiological recovery, and how neuroimaging may be used to learn more about the smaller subset of mTBI survivors who do not recover quickly from the injury and continue to express symptoms and display marked functional impairment. Iverson (Chapter 3) presents a biopsychosocial model of mTBI, emphasizing the role that psychosocial and other contextual factors may contribute in addition to underlying pathophysiology in impeding recovery from brain injury. Hayes and Gilbertson (Chapter 4) describe the clinical presentation of PTSD and the psychosocial, environmental, and neural factors that alter risk of its development and maintenance. In their chapter, Hayes and Gilbertson additionally discuss the neurobiological and neuropsychological correlates of PTSD, including areas of overlap with TBI. Finally, Verfaellie, Amick, and Vasterling (Chapter 5) draw more broadly from the literature on non-TBI sources of neurocognitive variation to consider TBI-related neurocognitive mechanisms that may heighten risk of PTSD or affect the course and expression of PTSD.

The second section of the volume recognizes that PTSD and TBI do not occur in a vacuum and that associated conditions may interfere with recovery from them. Although there are many factors that may complicate recovery from both mTBI and PTSD, we focus on two of the most common and potentially debilitating of such associated conditions: chronic pain and substance abuse. Otis, Fortier, and Keane (Chapter 6) highlight the frequency in which chronic pain occurs with PTSD and mTBI and describe the complexities of the clinical presentation in patients with PTSD, mTBI, and pain disorders. They further discuss treatment options, drawing from an existing integrated intervention for PTSD and chronic pain. Similarly, Najavits, Highley, Dolan, and Fee (Chapter 7) discuss patterns of substance use predating and following PTSD and TBI and how the trimorbidity of substance use disorders, PTSD, and TBI, may complicate treatments. Najavits and her colleagues draw from established interventions designed to address PTSD and substance use to make recommendations for treatment of the trimorbidity.

The third section of the book addresses the clinical management of comorbid PTSD and mTBI. Because of the complexities of assessing PTSD and mTBI, especially when they are comorbid, we devote two chapters to assessment. In the first, Ulloa, Marx, Vanderploeg, and Vasterling (Chapter 8) focus on assessment of PTSD and mTBI when considered alone and in combination. In the second, Elhai, Sweet, Guidotti Breting, and Kaloupek (Chapter 9) consider the special circumstances of evaluations that are performed in litigation, compensation/disability evaluations, and other contexts that pose threats to the validity of the assessment process. The next two chapters discuss psychosocial treatment interventions for PTSD and mTBI. Ponsford (Chapter 10) focuses on cognitive rehabilitation therapy for mTBI. Bryant and Litz (Chapter 11) discuss cognitive-behavioral interventions for PTSD, including how they might be best structured when mTBI factors into the clinical presentation. The final two chapters of the volume center on the context in which care is delivered to patients with PTSD and mTBI. Bryant, Castro, and Iverson (Chapter 12) consider military mTBI in particular as a special context and describe clinical considerations relevant to the military environment and combat-related TBIs. Finally, Hendricks, Krengel, Iverson, Kimerling, Tun, Amara, and Lew (Chapter 13) adopt a health economics approach to consider factors that could potentially guide allocation of clinical resources in contexts in which such resources are limited. Although Hendricks et al. use Veterans Health Administration data to illustrate the costs associated with treatment, many of the factors discussed can be more broadly generalized to other health care contexts.

We conclude with a synthesis of the information presented throughout, returning to the questions posed above. Through this volume, we hope to spark continued discussion of the complexities of providing care to patients with PTSD and mTBI using some of the differing perspectives on the topic to move toward rational, well-considered approaches to service delivery. In doing so, we anticipate that the work contained within this volume will have broad appeal to the diverse set of professionals from mental health, rehabilitation, and neuroscience fields that care for, and through empirical research, try to better understand these patients with the complex comorbidity of PTSD and mTBI.

References

American Congress of Rehabilitation Medicine Head Injury Interdisciplinary Special Interest Group. (1993). Definition of mild traumatic brain injury. *Journal of Head Trauma Rehabilitation, 8*, 86–87.

American Psychiatric Association. (2000). *Diagnostic and statistical manual of mental disorders* (4th ed., text rev.). Washington, DC: Author.

Carlson, K. F., Kehle, S. M., Meis, L. A., Greer, N., Macdonald, R., Rutks, I., et al. (2011). Prevalence, assessment, and treatment of mild traumatic brain injury and posttraumatic stress disorder: A systematic review of the evidence. *Journal of Head Trauma Rehabilitation, 26*, 103–115.

Corrigan, J. D., Selassie, A. W., & Orman, J. A. (2010). The epidemiology of traumatic brain injury. *Journal of Head Trauma Rehabilitation, 25*(2), 72–80.

Dohrenwend, B., Turner, J., Turse, N., Adams, B., Koenen, K., & Marshall, R. (2006). The psychological risks of Vietnam for US veterans: A revisit with new data and methods. *Science, 313*(5789), 979–982.

Fear, N. T., Jones, M., Murphy, D., Hull, L., Iversen, A. C., Coker, B., et al. (2010). What are the consequences of deployment to Iraq and Afghanistan on the mental health of the UK armed forces?: A cohort study. *Lancet, 375,* 1783–1797.

Friedman, M. J., Resick, P. A., Bryant, R. A., & Brewin, C. R. (2011). Considering PTSD for DSM-5. *Depression and Anxiety.* (Online prepublication).

Hoge, C. W., Goldberg, H. M., & Castro, C. A. (2009) Care of war veterans with mild traumatic brain injury: Flawed perspectives. *New England Journal of Medicine, 360,* 1588–1591.

Hoge, C. W., McGurk, D., Thomas, J. L., Cox, A. L., Engel, C. C., & Castro, C. A. (2008). Mild traumatic brain injury in U.S. soldiers returning from Iraq. *New England Journal of Medicine, 358,* 453–463.

Kessler, R. C., Sonnega, A., Bromet, E., Hughes, M., & Nelson, C. B. (1995). Posttraumatic stress disorder in the National Comorbidity Survey. *Archives of General Psychiatry, 52*(12), 1048–1060.

Kulka, R., Schlenger, W., Fairbank, J., Hough, R., Jordan, B., Marmar, C., et al. (1990). *Trauma and the Vietnam War generation.* New York: Brunner/Mazel.

Lew, H., Otis, J. D., Tun, C., Kerns, R. D., Clark, M. E., & Cifu, D. X. (2009). Prevalence of chronic pain, posttraumatic stress disorder and persistent postconcussive symptoms in OEF/OIF Veterans: The Polytrauma Clinical Triad. *Journal of Rehabilitation, Research and Development, 46,* 697–702.

Masel, B. E., & DeWitt, D. S. (2010). Traumatic brain injury: A disease process, not an event. *Journal of Neurotrauma, 27,* 1529–1540.

Menon, D. K., Schwab, K., Wright, D. W., & Maas, A. I. (2010). Position statement: Definition of traumatic brain injury. *Archives of Physical Medicine and Rehabilitation, 91*(11), 1637–1640.

National Center for Injury Prevention and Control. (2003). *Report to Congress on mild traumatic brain injury in the United States: Steps to prevent a serious public health problem.* Atlanta, GA: Centers for Disease Control and Injury Prevention.

Rona, R. J., Jones, M., Fear, N. T., Hull, L., Murphy, D., Machell, L., et al. (2011, April 25). Mild traumatic brain injury in UK military personnel returning from Afghanistan and Iraq: Cohort and cross-sectional analyses. *Journal of Head Trauma Rehabilitation.* (Online prepublication)

Ruff, R. M., Iverson, G. L., Barth, J. T., Bush, S. S., Broshek, D. K., & NAN Policy and Planning Committee. (2009). Recommendations for diagnosing a mild traumatic brain injury: A National Academy of Neuropsychology education paper. *Archives of Clinical Neuropsychology, 24,* 3–10.

Sayer, N. A., Rettmann, N. A., Carlson, K. E., Bernardy, N., Sigford, B .J., Hamblen, J. L., et al. (2009). Veterans with history of mild traumatic brain injury and posttraumatic stress disorder: Challenges from provider perspective. *Journal of Rehabilitation Research and Development, 46,* 703–716.

Silva, R. R., Alpert, M., Munoz, D. M., Singh, S., Matzner, F., & Dummit, S. (2000). Stress and vulnerability to posttraumatic stress disorder in children and adolescents. *American Journal of Psychiatry, 157,* 1229–1235.

Tanielian, T., & Jaycox, L. H. (2008). *Invisible wounds of war: Psychological and cognitive injuries, their consequences, and services to assist recovery.* Santa Monica, CA: RAND Corporation.

Zatzick, D. F., Rivara, F. P., Jurkovich, G. J., Hoge, C. W., Wang, J., Fan, M. Y., et al. (2010). Multisite investigation of traumatic brain injuries, posttraumatic stress disorder, and self-reported health and cognitive impairments. *Archives of General Psychiatry, 67,* 1291–1300.

Zinzow, H. M., Ruggiero, K. J., Resnick, H., Hanson, R., Smith, D., Saunders, B., et al. (2009). Prevalence and mental health consequences of witnessed parental and community violence in a national sample of adolescents. *Journal of Child Psychology and Psychiatry, 50,* 441–450.

PART II

CLINICAL PRESENTATIONS AND MECHANISMS

CHAPTER 2

Understanding Mild Traumatic Brain Injury

Neuropathology and Neuroimaging

Erin D. Bigler and William L. Maxwell

Traumatic brain injury (TBI)[1] is a common occurrence for which emergency department (ED) records in the United States show over 1.1 million visits annually (Corrigan, Selassie, & Orman, 2010). Eighty-five percent of all TBIs evaluated in the ED are considered to be mild TBIs (mTBIs). About 200,000 cases of mTBI evaluated in the ED occur from sports and recreational activities (Centers for Disease Control and Prevention, 2007). However, the true incidence of mTBI is considered to be much higher because many mTBI cases are never evaluated in the ED, medically assessed, or treated (Bazarian et al., 2005). For example, Ryu, Feinstein, Colantonio, Streiner, and Dawson (2009) examined ED records in addition to clinic and

---

[1] Brain injury nomenclature can be confusing. The term "head injury" is often used to imply brain injury, but of course there can be trauma to the head that never produces any injury to the brain. For the purposes of this chapter, TBI signifies a traumatic injury to the brain as a consequence of an impact injury and/or from the influences of rapid, violent acceleration/deceleration to the head that affect the brain. In this sense TBI is a spectrum of head injury. The label "concussion" is a term that connotes the mildest form of head injury and is typically used to indicate an injury where loss of consciousness, if present at all, is brief, with minimal to no posttraumatic amnesia and negative computed tomography, if clinical neuroimaging is even done. On a continuum, concussion represents the mildest form of TBI followed by mild, moderate, and severe.

family practice records within a health care provider system and observed a 653/100,000 TBI rate, the majority of which were mTBIs. Accordingly, mTBI represents one of the most common of all injuries, with an estimated 57 million people having sustained an mTBI worldwide (Messe et al., 2010).

Fortunately, the majority of mTBIs produce only transient changes in neurological status that spontaneously resolve. Some recent, well-designed, large-scale prospective studies indicate that those with symptoms persisting for 1 year or more after an mTBI may be as low as 2.3% in pediatric cases (Barlow et al., 2010) but as high as ~30% in adults (Rickels, von Wild, & Wenzlaff, 2010; Whitnall, McMillan, Murray, & Teasdale, 2006; Zumstein et al., 2010), particularly when acute computed tomography (CT) shows microhemorrhage(s), contusion, or edema (Smits et al., 2008). The difference in the frequency of persisting symptoms between children and adults with mTBI likely relates to the mechanism of injury and the developmental stage of the central nervous system at the time of injury. mTBIs from motor vehicle accidents (MVAs) and violent assaults occur with a higher frequency in adults (Thurman, Coronado, & Selassie, 2007), whereas mTBIs occurring in children are more likely to occur from falls or being hit by an object (Ommaya, Goldsmith, & Thibault, 2002). Also, size/weight and body configuration differences between children and adults influence the potential for mTBI following an impact injury (Arbogast et al., 2009; Bussone & Duma, 2010; Danelson et al., 2008). After age 60, falls become a major cause of mTBIs.

The recovery norm following an mTBI is that within minutes to hours or days postinjury the majority of individuals will become asymptomatic, returning to preinjury levels of function (Williams, Potter, & Ryland, 2010; Wilson, 1990). With rapid recovery to the norm, the assumed neurological effects of mTBI-related trauma are thought to be mostly transient biochemical and physiological changes, which are briefly discussed below. However, the focus of this chapter is on the minority of mTBI patients who may experience more permanent sequelae. Given the epidemiological rates of mTBI described above, if even a small percentage experience persisting symptoms, mTBI represents a major worldwide health concern (Vaishnavi, Rao, & Fann, 2009; Yeates, 2010).

By the very nature of war, natural disasters, and terroristic acts, TBI has become a common occurrence associated with such events. Indeed, mTBI in the recent wars in Iraq and Afghanistan has been labeled as the "signature injury" of these conflicts (Hayward, 2008). Modern conflicts not only involve the typical mechanisms for head injury (e.g., direct assault or blunt force trauma, MVAs, falls, being struck by a projectile) but also blast injuries (Moore & Jaffee, 2010). All of the common methods of sustaining a TBI involve some direct trauma or translational force to the brain and/ or the deforming action of rapid acceleration/deceleration (Biasca & Maxwell, 2007). In blast injury, the propagation of the blast wave across the head produces brain deformation within the cranium without a physical object striking the head (Alley, Schimizze, & Son, 2010; Risling et al., 2010).

Modern warfare and the use of explosives in terrorist attacks have resulted in an exponential increase in individuals exposed to blast injuries and the likelihood of experiencing mTBI (DeKosky, Ikonomovic, & Gandy, 2010; Rosenfeld & Ford, 2010). Two major blast-related terrorist events in the United States have been extensively studied with regards to brain injury: the September 11 World Trade Center attacks (Rutland-Brown et al., 2007) and the 1995 Oklahoma City bombing (Walilko et al., 2009). Terrorist acts have become a worldwide problem for which the incidence of head injuries may be as high as 30% among those who survive (Bhatoe, 2008). In addition to important issues related to diagnosing the presence of a brain injury in the blast-exposed individual, such individuals will often experience the co-occurrence of a posttraumatic stress disorder (PTSD; Zatzick et al., 2010). While this chapter focuses on the neuropathology and neuroimaging of mTBI, it is important to note that significant overlap exists between the brain regions most vulnerable to mTBI and those regions that underlie PTSD (Bigler, 2008; Stein & McAllister, 2009).

This chapter provides a basic overview of the pathophysiological effects of mTBI, mechanisms of acute injury, and the circumstances where more permanent neuropathological sequelae may occur. The theme for this review is that much of the basic neuropathology of mTBI occurs as a disconnection, either physiologically, structurally, or a combination caused by axonal injury. Understanding the mechanisms of neuronal injury, in particular axonal injury, in mTBI assists in defining the neurocognitive and neurobehavioral sequelae of the injury. The other theme of this chapter is that neuroimaging techniques have reached a level of sophistication and sensitivity to detect subtle pathology associated with mTBI that heretofore has only been inferred but has not been detected (Kou et al., 2010; Niogi & Mukherjee, 2010; Van Boven et al., 2009), including blast-related mTBI (Kou et al., 2010; Matthews et al., 2010; Peskind et al., 2010).

Terminology and definitional statements as to severity of injury have always been a problem in brain injury classification. In this chapter, the term "mTBI" refers to events meeting the injury criteria from either the American Congress of Rehabilitation Medicine (1993) guidelines (see Table 2.1) or the closely related World Health Organization (WHO) guidelines (see Carroll, Cassidy, Holm, Kraus, & Coronado, 2004; Carroll, Cassidy, Peloso, et al., 2004). For this review, the term "concussion," drawn from

TABLE 2.1. American Congress of Rehabilitation Medicine (1993) Definition of mTBI

Traumatically induced, physiological disruption of brain function, manifested by at least one of the following:
- Any period of loss of consciousness
- Any loss of memory for events immediately before or after the accident
- Any alteration in mental state at the time of the accident
- Focal neurologic deficits that may or may not be transient

And all three of the following criteria characterize the severity of the injury:
- Loss of consciousness for 30 minutes or less
- Glasgow Coma Scale (GCS) score of 13 or more after 30 minutes
- Posttraumatic amnesia (PTA) lasting for not more than 24 hours

sports medicine (in which some of the mildest brain injuries occur) will be used, albeit sparingly because it implies only the mildest form of mTBI (see Table 2.2). Also, recently the International and Interagency Initiative toward Common Data Elements for Research on Traumatic Brain Injury and Psychological Health offered this position statement on the TBI definition from the Demographics and Clinical Assessment Working Group: "TBI is defined as an alteration in brain function, or other evidence of brain pathology, caused by an external force" (Menon, Schwab, Wright, & Maas, 2010, p. 1637).

TABLE 2.2. Third International Conference on Concussion (McCrory et al., 2009) Definition of Concussion

A complex pathophysiological process affecting the brain, induced by traumatic biomechanical forces.

Common features that incorporate constructs that may be utilized in defining the nature of a concussive head injury include:
- Concussion may be caused either by a direct blow to the head, face, or neck or a blow elsewhere on the body with an "impulsive" force transmitted to the head.
- Concussion typically results in the rapid onset of short-lived impairment of neurologic function that resolves spontaneously.
- Concussion may result in neuropathological changes but the acute clinical symptoms largely reflect a functional disturbance rather than a structural injury.
- Concussion results in a graded set of clinical symptoms that may or may not involve loss of consciousness. Resolution of the clinical and cognitive symptoms typically follows a sequential course. In a small percentage of cases, however, postconcussive symptoms may be prolonged.
- No abnormality on standard structural neuroimaging studies is seen in concussion.

The Injury

The neuropathology of mTBI has been extensively reviewed by Biasca and Maxwell (2007). An almost unlimited number of potential mechanisms of injury exist that can produce an mTBI. Biomechanical impact to the head in the form of blunt trauma sufficient to produce a concussion deforms brain tissue beyond normal tolerance limits, stretching axons and disrupting cellular function, as shown in the schematic in Plate 2.1 (from Ropper & Gorson, 2007). This illustration also shows brain regions most likely to sustain the greatest deformation in mTBI, which include the upper brainstem and its neurons associated with the reticular activating system (RAS); the thalamus and its neurons that participate in the diffuse thalamic projection system (DTPS); the hypothalamic–pituitary–adrenocortical axis (HPA), inferior frontal lobe, and frontal polar region; the medial temporal lobe and polar regions (not shown in this illustration); the corpus callosum; and the corticospinal tract, with the thalamus and fornix suspended beneath the corpus callosum connecting the hippocampus. More will be said about each of these areas.

Neuropathology of mTBI

From a neuropathological perspective, Graham and Lantos (2002) make the following statement: "axonal damage is the most important single factor contributing to the severity of brain damage and to the outcome in any patient who sustains a blunt head injury"(p. 867). This supports the hypothesis that all TBIs reside on a continuum of injury where the central factor determining severity is how transient or permanent the degree of axonal injury. Biasca and Maxwell (2007), Bigler and Maxwell (in press), and Saatman, Serbst, and Burkhardt (2009) provide detailed reviews of the basic neuropathology of TBI. Briefly, trauma-induced biomechanical and biochemical changes to the axon membrane (axolemma) and underlying protein scaffolding and neurofilaments that configure the internal structure of the axon via activation of calpains (calcium-sensitive neutral proteases) represent the basic mechanisms that result in neural damage from TBI (Buki & Povlishock, 2006; Maxwell, Povlishock, & Graham, 1997; Saatman et al., 2009). The microenvironment where the pathological consequences play out is often challenging to conceptualize. This pathology may only be visualized by means of transmission electron microscopy because most myelinated nerve fibers in the central nervous system (CNS) are between 1 and 3 micrometers (microns, or μm, 1/100th to 1/30th of the thickness of a human scalp hair) (Maxwell, Watt, Graham, & Gennarelli, 1993). But it is the surrounding outer membrane of the axon, the axolemma, where the truly delicate nature of neural structure resides. The axolemma is but a few nanometers (a billionth of a meter) thick, yet is critical for all aspects of ion permeability and gating in neural transmission.

The major understanding of TBI micropathology has been largely derived from the extensive experimental TBI animal model literature and in humans with moderate-to-severe TBI who succumb to their injuries. However, a few postmortem mTBI studies have been published (Blumbergs et al., 1994, 1995; Oppenheimer, 1968) that demonstrate typical trauma-induced axonal pathology in mTBI as shown in Plate 2.3.

In severe head injuries, at the moment of impact, severe biomechanical shear/strain is placed upon the central white matter of the brain, typically rendering an immediate deep coma, possibly because of instantaneous fragmentation or shearing of the axolemma at foci along the length of injured axons, and almost immediate chemical degradation of the structural integrity of the axonal cytoskeleton. These abrupt and immediate effects typically occur in less than 1 hour. This is referred to as *primary* axotomy (Maxwell et al., 1993). But it cannot be overemphasized that *primary axotomy* will *not* have occurred in a patient diagnosed with mTBI. In mTBI, rather than an axon undergoing mechanical shearing at the time of insult, axons are briefly, in a matter of milliseconds, exposed to mechanical tensile loading over a very short time period which damages the axolemma, causing it to become leaky to sodium and calcium ions (Wang et al., 2009), which, if not quickly corrected by the injured cell, results in a cascade of other cellular events that, over a period of at least 4–6 hours (Maxwell et al., 1997), results in the axon undergoing fragmentation, which is referred to as *secondary axotomy*. Examples of differing stages of secondary axotomy are shown in Plate 2.3 occurring within 18 hours of mTBI.

Although Oppenheimer (1968) first demonstrated in an autopsied case of mTBI the presence of axonal degeneration similar to that observed in more severe TBI (see Peerless & Rewcastle, 1967; Strich, 1956), he also observed small hemorrhages, or petechia. When blood degrades it is marked by the presence of hemosiderin, a protein by-product that stains the brain and becomes a biomarker of prior hemorrhage. Capillaries are as delicate and subject to the same shear/strain action in the brain as are axons. Capillaries are between 7 and 10μm in diameter, just large enough to allow a single erythrocyte to pass one by one as it delivers oxygen to the billions of neural cells that make up the brain. When a capillary wall is breeched, blood escapes into the surrounding parenchyma, where natural degradation of hemorrhagic debris occurs. Bigler (2004) has shown the presence of hemosiderin in an mTBI case that was autopsied, who had no clinically significant findings on conventional imaging. Hemosiderin deposits can be detected by certain magnetic resonance imaging (MRI) techniques when accumulations approximate a cubic millimeter or larger, as shown in Plate 2.2. In mTBI the

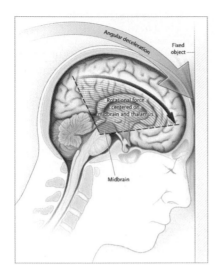

PLATE 2.1. Hypothetical biomechanics that produce concussion. The pathophysiological basis for sustaining a concussion is thought to result from rapid rotational motion of the cerebral hemispheres in the anterior–posterior plane, around the fulcrum of the fixed-in-place upper brainstem. The green reflects the upper brainstem, in particular the midbrain region which houses important ascending pathways of the reticular activating system involved in consciousness. Note the zone of rotational forces includes the thalamus and hypothalamus, fornix, corpus callosum, and cingulate gyrus. The zones of greatest cortical impact, and therefore the greatest deformation of surface areas of the cerebral cortex, occur in the frontal region, especially the frontal polar and orbitofrontal regions depicted in red. The temporal lobe, not seen in this illustration, which would be on the lateral surface from this view, has a similar involvement where the temporal polar, ventral, and medial aspects of the temporal lobe are most vulnerable to deformation. Note also that the pituitary and the delicate region that connects the pituitary to the hypothalamus, the infundibulum, are particularly in the plane for deformation forces. From Ropper and Gorson (2007). Copyright 2007 by the Massachusetts Medical Society. Reprinted by permission.

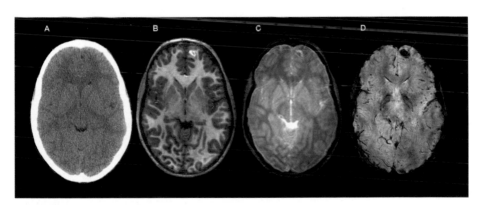

PLATE 2.2. Negative day-of-injury CT is shown in A in an adolescent who sustained an mTBI. Comparison of (A) axial CT scan, (B) axial T1-weighted MRI, (C) axial magnetization transfer imaging (MTI), and (D) susceptibility-weighted imaging (SWI) shown at the same level of prefrontal region to demonstrate the utility of SWI and MTR in detecting lesions that may be more difficult to detect on conventional imaging. CT was performed on the day of injury and the other three imaging modalities were acquired 1 week after this 12-year-old male sustained a mTBI complicated by a small left frontal hemorrhagic lesion (see red arrows in B, C, and D). The subject manifested residual memory deficit and slowed processing of information on cognitive testing performed at the same time as the MRI, MTI, and SWI. SWI (D) shows a left frontal hemorrhagic shear injury that is more extensive than the lesion seen on MRI (B) and that is not evident at all on CT (A) at this level. MTI shows a lack of MT effect (higher signal intensity at the arrow), corresponding to a lower magnetization transfer ratio value reflecting left frontal white matter injury. A case used with permission from Jill Hunter, MD, Elisabeth A. Wilde, PhD, and Harvey S. Levin, PhD. From Bigler and Maxwell (in press). Reprinted with permission from Springer Science & Business Media.

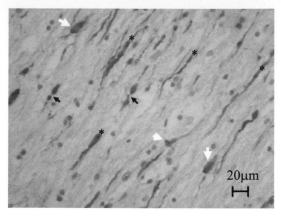

PLATE 2.3. A medium-power light micrograph of part of a central white matter tract from a patient who suffered mTBI with complications and died from respiratory failure as a result of thoracic injuries 18 hours after entry to hospital. The field is part of a paraffin section labeled for β-amyloid precursor protein, a marker for axonal injury. The irregular, orange profiles represent axons within which focal loss of fast axonal transport has resulted in abnormal accumulation of the amyloid protein. The purple circles are the nuclei of glial supporting cells and are probably mostly oligodendrocytes. Within this field are a range of types of abnormal axons which represent different stages in the pathological cascade culminating in secondary axotomy. Injured axons form "axonal swellings"(*) on either side of the focus of loss of axonal transport. Axonal swellings continue to increase in diameter as a result of continued anterograde and retrograde axonal transport and a constriction occurs (black arrow) at some point within the axonal swelling. The axon undergoes secondary axotomy thereat and separates into fragments. The regions of increased axonal caliber are then at the ends of the fragments and are referred to as "axonal degeneration bulbs" (white arrow). The axonal fragment now separated from the neuronal cell body then degenerates. From Bigler and Maxwell (in press). Reprinted with permission from Springer Science & Business Media.

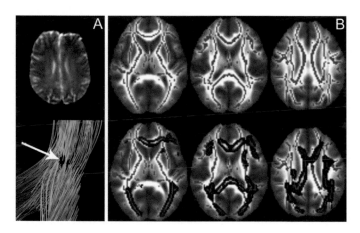

PLATE 2.4. (A) Conventional neuroimaging revealed no abnormalities in this 49-year-old patient with mild TBI who was imaged 16 months after the initial trauma. However, DTI analysis showed abnormalities in the left frontal white matter (red spot, top axial view) where DTI analysis of the tracts (bottom left) in the frontal forceps region of the frontal lobe shows tract discontinuities (arrow). These are probably focal areas of white matter degradation. From Rutgers et al. (2008). Copyright 2008 by the American Society of Neuroradiology. Reprinted by permission. (B) The top image shows the results of tract-based spatial statistical analyses (TBSS) of DTI data in an mTBI study of patients with good outcome (no persisting symptoms) compared to controls with the underlying white matter tract "skeleton" shown in green. Note that the top row shows no areas of difference in those patients with mTBI with good outcome and controls. However, the bottom row compares the poor outcome mTBI subjects to controls showing wide-spread differences involving long coursing white matter tracts and the corpus callosum. Clusters were significant at $p < .05$, corrected for multiple comparisons. From Messe et al. (2011). Copyright 2011 by John Wiley & Sons, Inc. Reprinted by permission.

presence of MRI-identified hemosiderin is considered a distinct marker of brain injury and likely axonal damage (Gean & Fischbein, 2010).

If sufficient neuronal damage occurs to cause cell death following TBI, the aggregate accumulation of neuronal loss will show up as brain atrophy. Based on quantitative MRI analyses, reductions in brain volume following mTBI also have been reported in some patients (Govind et al., 2010; Govindaraju et al., 2004; Levine et al., 2008; MacKenzie et al., 2002), with the degree of atrophic change related to the severity of injury (Levine et al., 2008; MacKenzie et al., 2002). Regional atrophic changes have also been reported (Messe et al., 2011). Likewise, the burden of microhemorrhages in mTBI relates to neuropsychological outcome (de Guise et al., 2010; Scheid, Walther, Guthke, Preul, & von Cramon, 2006).

Neurometabolic Cascade

The acute effects of sports concussion followed by restoration of function and return to baseline generally can be explained by physiological alterations induced by cellular deformation. The reversibility of the effects of concussion has received considerable attention, both in human and animal research. For example, Giza and Hovda (2001) introduced a model they describe as the "neurometabolic cascade" of concussion about a decade ago and updated it in 2011 (Barkhoudarian, Hovda, & Giza, 2011). The transient nature of a neurometabolic cascade provides an explanatory framework for why the majority of mTBI cases have a favorable outcome.

Magnetic resonance spectroscopy (MRS) represents a functional neuroimaging technique where indices of energy metabolism, such as N-acetylaspartate (NAA) levels, can be examined. Vagnozzi et al. (2010) examined athletes who sustained concussion, had negative conventional MRI, but then underwent MRS at 3, 15, 22, and 30 days postinjury. NAA levels reflected initial pathological changes that normalized over time. Talavage et al. (2010), using functional MRI (fMRI) to assess concussed athletes, also demonstrated prolonged activation anomalies beyond the time frame in which cognitive functions normalized. In nonathlete mTBI patients, mostly injured in MVAs, Yeo et al. (2011) also observed a prolonged return to normalization pattern in MRS findings in mTBI. A very important point of these and others where physiological markers of mTBI have been used (see Heitger et al., 2009; Makdissi et al., 2010; McCrea, Prichep, Powell, Chabot, & Barr, 2010; Slobounov et al., 2010) is that traditional neuropsychological measures often appear to return to baseline *before* physiological restoration occurs. As such, being "asymptomatic" by neuropsychological standards does not mean that underlying pathophysiological abnormalities are not present (McCrea et al., 2010) and may require linking cognitive assessment with functional neuroimaging (see Pardini et al., 2010).

Part of the neurometabolic cascade is thought to initiate a neuroinflammatory response to injury (Downes & Crack, 2010). DTI studies within 24 hours to a few days post-mTBI have shown changes in white matter integrity suggestive of neuroinflammation (Bazarian et al., 2007; Chu et al., 2010; Wilde et al., 2008; Wu et al., 2010). What is particularly interesting and informative is that these studies observe neuroinflammatory responses in white matter regions that would be predicted from the mTBI acceleration/deceleration model in Plate 2.1. How acute neuroinflammation may continue to affect neurocognitive function and whether it may be a predictor of some outcome is unknown at this time. Metting and colleagues demonstrated that day of injury CT perfusion findings related to outcome 6 months later as well as to the degree of PTA (Metting, Rödiger, de Jong, Stewart, Kremer, & van der Naalt, 2010; Metting, Rödiger, Stewart, Oudkerk, De Keyser, & van der Naalt, 2009). CT perfusion represents an index of blood flow. Once a TBI neurometabolic cascade is initiated, blood flow may be altered by a number of neuroinflammatory vascular and brain parenchymal reactions, including subtle edema. While the Metting et al. findings indicate the potential for acute metabolic disruption to predict long-term outcome, others like Mayer et al. (2010) have shown that in some patients with mTBI a presumed neuroinflammatory response persists at least months postinjury, leading some to speculate on the role of neuroinflammation in persistent neurocognitive and neurobehavioral sequelae of mTBI (Whitney, Eidem, Peng, Huang, & Zheng, 2009).

Boxing has long been known to potentially result in an encephalopathy (Nowak, Smith, & Reyes, 2009) and is the sports-related concussion that was first studied clinically and histologically (Jordan, 1992). Recently, Orrison et al. (2009) examined boxers and extreme sport combatants and showed a high level of subtle clinical MRI findings, including atrophic changes. Particular interest has been focused on athletes with a history of concussion who develop neuropsychiatric symptoms (Chen, Johnston, Petrides, & Ptito, 2008). McKee et al. (2009, 2010) have undertaken postmortem examinations in contact-sport athletes who have died from nonneurological reasons but display postmortem neuropathological degenerative changes including the detection of β-amyloid labeled axons even in young athletes. Indeed the issue of mTBI and later-in-life dementia has been raised (Gavett, Stern, Cantu, Nowinski, & McKee, 2010).

The Biomechanics of mTBI

As the definitions listed in Table 2.1 indicate, TBI occurs because biomechanical forces rapidly and forcibly shift brain parenchyma from its original position, moorings, and configuration, with particular adverse effects on the axon. Since the axon mediates passage of information from the neuronal cell body to its terminal field, damage or disruption of axon integrity fundamentally affects neural function. "Traumatic axonal injury" or TAI is a consistent feature of human TBI (Buki & Povlishock, 2006). The term "diffuse axonal injury" (DAI) has also been used, but DAI has more specific meaning for the acute neuropathological effects of axonal injury in humans (Biasca & Maxwell, 2007; Graham & Lantos, 2002) and should only be applied to human patients. Axons within the CNS are usually myelinated, with a fat rich sleeve or envelope surrounding each individual axon, which gives the pale or white color to so-called CNS white matter. Myelinated axons tend to shear or be damaged if the mechanical strain is applied rapidly over ~ 20 milliseconds or less. As already shown, Plate 2.1 diagrammatically illustrates where some of the greatest axonal deformation and strain forces occur in the brain. Importantly, although Plate 2.1 implies a single motion, actually with any TBI the brain parenchyma is *not* exposed to a single episode of mechanical strain, but to a series of smaller and smaller strains in opposite directions until movement of the brain is damped after acceleration and or deceleration. This results in many diverse directional strains occurring within milliseconds. All types of brain injuries can be modeled biomechanically (Sabet, Christoforou, Zatlin, Genin, & Bayly, 2008), including blast injury (Desmoulin & Dionne, 2009). From these types of studies it is apparent that nerve fibers passing obliquely through the cerebral hemispheres may be exposed to different rates of mechanical loading at one point in their course to other points. This also explains, in part, why with any given injury some axons may experience traumatic injury whereas others do not.

Returning to Plate 2.1, of particular relevance to mTBI is that the strains that occur within the brain particularly affect long-coursing white matter networks of the brain. Many of these tracts are critical for speed of neural processing required for attention and working memory (Vincent, Kahn, Snyder, Raichle, & Buckner, 2008), disruption of which occurs following TBI (Nakamura, Hillary, & Biswal, 2009). Likewise, complex neural networks especially between the HPA, frontal, temporal, and limbic areas regulate mood, motivation, drive, and associated behaviors—all of which can be affected in mTBI.

Experimental TBI models demonstrate strain effects to the deep white matter within the cerebral hemispheres and corpus callosum along with deformation of the striatum and hippocampus, with the amount of pathology related to severity of impact (Hamberger, Viano, Saljo, & Bolouri, 2009). Viano et al. (2005) demonstrate particular lateral movement/distortion of the fornix, probably uniquely affected in humans because it is partly suspended in the cerebrospinal fluid between the two lateral ventricles and the third ventricle in its descent to the mammillary bodies. This makes the fornix particularly vulnerable to lateral movement and stretch and may be a major factor in human mTBI and its injury in mTBI has been documented (Yallampalli et al., in press).

Neuroimaging of mTBI

Neuroimaging findings of mTBI vary whether the patient is examined in the acute, subacute, or chronic stage postinjury and, of course, which type of neuroimaging technique is used. From a strict medical management standpoint, the first neuroimaging method performed on the mTBI patient is a CT scan because it can be performed relatively quickly and is well suited for detecting neurosurgical lesions that could be life-threatening. However, a negative CT scan should not be interpreted as an "absence" of brain pathology from trauma because x-ray beam technology is limited in detecting subtle pathology.

CT is only positive in ~20% or less of mTBI cases, typically identifying abnormalities in the form of small hemorrhages (petechia), subtle edema, contusions, subarachnoid hemorrhages, and skull fractures (Smits et al., 2008). Few mTBI patients have more serious pathology that requires neurosurgical intervention, but life-threatening hemorrhagic lesions and edema do occur in mTBI (McCrory, Berkovic, & Cordner, 2000). In the past, a distinction was made where any positive intracranial CT abnormality in mTBI indicated a "complicated mTBI," and this remains a useful distinction for initial medical management. However, as demonstrated in Plate 2.3, it is now a rather meaningless distinction for cognitive and behavioral outcome from mTBI in the light of advanced neuroimaging methods using magnetic resonance imaging (MRI) technologies that are several fold more sensitive in detecting traumatic abnormalities (Bigler & Maxwell, in press).

Both positron emission tomography (PET) and single photon emission computed tomography (SPECT) imaging studies indicate metabolic changes, particularly in the polar and medial temporal lobe and the polar and inferior frontal lobar regions, following mTBI (Gowda et al., 2006; Lewine et al., 2007; Umile, Sandel, Alavi, Terry, & Plotkin, 2002). Physiological disruption of the medial temporal and inferior frontal regions likely relates to the universality of changes in memory seen during the acute phase of mTBI. Likewise, any persisting involvement of these regions or their connections likely relates to changes in memory, emotional, and executive functions that may accompany mTBI, both acutely as well as chronically.

Because petechial hemorrhages (small hemorrhages caused by broken vessels) that occur in mTBI can be best detected by MRI, as shown in Plate 2.2, this has become a marker of traumatic axonal injury (TAI) in mTBI

(Aiken & Gean, 2010). Often TBI-related petechial hemorrhages occur at the gray–white matter margin, deep within the central white matter and/or within the corpus callosum.

In the chronic stage, diffusion tensor imaging (DTI) is now the neuroimaging method that likely best assesses white matter integrity in mTBI (Kou et al., 2010; Newcombe et al., 2011; Niogi & Mukherjee, 2010), where DTI findings potentially represent a biomarker of mTBI (Bigler & Bazarian, 2010). DTI has the capability of demonstrating more subtle white matter abnormalities and discontinuities in tracts as shown in Plate 2.4.

Plate 2.4 also summarizes the work of Meese and colleagues (2011), who compared mTBI patients who had "good" outcome, indicating no residual symptoms, to mTBI patients who had "poor" outcome, indicating persistence of symptoms following mTBI. Significant DTI differences were observed in the poor-outcome mTBI patients, most notable in long-coursing pathways connecting the frontal lobe with the rest of the brain, anterior thalamic radiations, and corpus callosum as shown in Plate 2.4. Also notable was that in comparison to the healthy controls, the patients with mTBI showed some reductions in gray matter cortical volume, consistent with TBI being associated with cell body loss as well (Maxwell, MacKinnon, Stewart, & Graham, 2010). The generalized nature of some of the DTI-documented white matter changes in mTBI have been substantiated by several investigations (Newcombe et al., 2011; Smits et al., 2011).

While chronic-stage DTI studies of mTBI likely reflect the degradation of axon integrity that begins with the neuropathological features shown in Plate 2.3, within hours to days postinjury DTI may also indicate neuroinflammatory reactions within the white matter, as previously discussed (Bazarian et al., 2007; Chu et al., 2010; Mayer et al., 2010; Wilde et al., 2008; Wu et al., 2010).

How Neuroimaging Findings Relate to Neurocognitive and Neurobehavioral Sequelae of mTBI

The controversies over mTBI and related sequelae represent centuries-old debates (Evans, 2010; Jacobson, 1995). For mTBI critics in the past, with no consistent radiographic findings, issues of secondary gain and compensation neurosis and pre- or coexisting psychiatric disorders (in particular depression and somatoform disorders) have been the perennial explanatory arguments against a neurobiological explanation of mTBI. However, well-designed investigations that have controlled for factors such as secondary gain, litigation, and psychiatric diagnosis have demonstrated less efficient memory, diminished executive ability, and problematic emotional changes in patients with mTBI (Geary, Kraus, Pliskin, & Little, 2010; Heitger et al., 2009; Konrad et al., 2010; Little et al., 2010). Little et al. (2010) and Geary et al. (2010) show how subtle pathology disrupting frontal and thalamic pathways in the brain related to deficits in memory and executive function in patients with mTBI. As new neuroimaging methods identify underlying pathology associated with mTBI, it is likely that an improved understanding of how neuropathological changes can be objectively identified and relate to neurobehavioral sequelae in some patients with mTBI will emerge.

The first DTI study that systematically examined patients with mTBI did not occur until 2005 (Inglese et al., 2005). This means that prior to DTI, *all* mTBI studies lacked an accurate biomarker of mTBI. Now, in addition to DTI, neuroimaging methods like MRS and fMRI also have a role in identifying potential pathological changes associated with mTBI (see reviews by Belanger, Vanderploeg, Curtiss, & Warden, 2007; Bigler & Maxwell, 2011; Jantzen, 2010; Niogi & Mukherjee, 2010). These studies reinforce the evidence that the selectivity of white matter damage and disrupted connectivity may be the key to understanding mTBI. From this approach, it is not so much about where or how large a lesion may be, but how a lesion disrupts functional connectivity. When underlying neuropathology persists, viewing mTBI within a disconnection framework also helps explain the diversity of mTBI symptoms as there are almost an unlimited number of pathways and connections within the brain that could be affected, and therefore no two injuries associated with mTBI would be identical or produce identical symptoms.

Silver, McAllister, and Arciniegas (2009) summarized the neuropsychiatric sequelae of mTBI to include problems with "cognition (attention, concentration, executive functioning, memory, and speed of information processing); psychiatric symptoms (personality changes, affective disorders, anxiety disorders, psychosis, sleep disorders, aggression, and irritability), and physical problems, such as headache, chronic pain, vision impairment, dizziness, and, rarely, epilepsy" (p. 656). Most of these symptoms have substantial subjectivity to them, making them difficult to empirically investigate. However, neuroimaging provides potential biomarkers to more completely investigate how these commonplace subjective symptoms relate to underlying neurobiology and neuropathology. For example, well-designed investigations have shown the frequency of fatigue symptoms in mTBI (Bay & de-Leon, 2010; Norrie et al., 2010; Zumstein et al., 2010), with neuroimaging studies demonstrating how relevant brain regions like ventromedial frontal and HPA damage in TBI may lead to fatigue (Bavisetty et al., 2008; Pardini, Krueger, Raymont, & Grafman, 2010). Problems with drive and motivation are also commonplace symptoms of patients with mTBI (Gasquoine, 1997; McAllister & Arciniegas, 2002), often ascribed to pathology associated with frontal lobe damage as demonstrated by neuroimaging studies (Koenigs & Grafman, 2009; Levin & Kraus, 1994) and the complex neuropsychiatric sequelae that may attend mTBI (Vaishnavi et al., 2009).

mTBI and PTSD: Overlapping Neuroanatomy

Interesting parallels exist between brain regions thought to relate to the major sequelae associated with mTBI and those related to the expression of PTSD (Van Boven et al., 2009; Vasterling, Verfaellie, & Sullivan, 2009). In PTSD, the critical brain regions involve the amygdala, HPA, and other frontotemporolimbic regions that participate in the induction, expression, and maintenance of these symptoms (Jovanovic & Ressler, 2010; Lanius et al., 2010; Yehuda, 2002). Returning to Plate 2.1 and much of the discussion above, frontotemporolimbic areas and their interconnectiveness are key to understanding the effects of mTBI. A number of commentators have explored the anatomical overlap between mTBI and PTSD (McAllister & Stein, 2010; Rosenfeld & Ford, 2010; Thurmond et al., 2010). Indeed, Daniels et al. (2010) discuss PTSD as alterations in functional connectivity of these systems, which is the same discussion made in this chapter that underlies mTBI. Furthermore, there may be common neurotrophic factors within these brain regions common to both mTBI and PTSD that have neuropathological consequences that mediate the comorbid association between mTBI and PTSD (Kaplan, Vasterling, & Vedak, 2010).

Summary and Conclusions

TBI deforms neural cells beyond their normal tolerance limits in which the severity of injury depends on the amount and degree of deformation. The majority of patients who sustain an mTBI experience a good outcome associated with transient physiological effects in which neurological, neurocognitive, and neurobehavioral consequences are short-lived, quickly returning to preinjury baseline levels. Once homeostasis is returned, recovery ensues. However, more permanent neuropathological consequences may occur in mTBI when cellular deformation, particular involving the axon, results in cell damage or cell death. Damaged axons diminish or disrupt the functional connectivity of the brain and slow processing. The location and degree of underlying axonal damage may relate to the type and persistence of symptoms following an mTBI. Long-coursing and interhemispheric white matter tracts are most likely affected by mTBI and likely underlie many of the common mTBI symptoms when they persist. When neuropathological effects underlie persistent symptoms following an mTBI, disruptions of white matter tracts within frontotemporolimbic regions are likely associated with the majority of neurobehavioral and neurocognitive features of mTBI and probably play a role in PTSD as well.

References

Aiken, A. H., & Gean, A. D. (2010). Imaging of head trauma. *Seminars in Roentgenology, 45*(2), 63–79.

Alley, M. D., Schimizze, B. R., & Son, S. F. (2010). Experimental modeling of explosive blast-related traumatic brain injuries. *Neuroimage, 54*(Suppl. 1), S45–S54.

American Congress of Rehabilitation Medicine Head Injury Interdisciplinary Special Interest Group. (1993). Definition of mild traumatic brain injury. *Journal of Head Trauma Rehabilitation, 8,* 86–87.

Arbogast, K. B., Balasubramanian, S., Seacrist, T., Maltese, M. R., Garcia-Espana, J. F., Hopely, T., et al. (2009). Comparison of kinematic responses of the head and spine for children and adults in low-speed frontal sled tests. *Stapp Car Crash Journal, 53,* 329–372.

Barkhoudarian, G., Hovda, D. A., & Giza, C. C. (2011). The molecular pathophysiology of concussive brain injury. *Clinics in Sports Medicine, 30*(1), 33–48.

Barlow, K. M., Crawford, S., Stevenson, A., Sandhu, S. S., Belanger, F., & Dewey, D. (2010). Epidemiology of postconcussion syndrome in pediatric mild traumatic brain injury. *Pediatrics, 126*(2), e374–e381.

Bavisetty, S., McArthur, D. L., Dusick, J. R., Wang, C., Cohan, P., Boscardin, W. J., et al. (2008). Chronic hypopituitarism after traumatic brain injury: Risk assessment and relationship to outcome. *Neurosurgery, 62*(5), 1080–1093.

Bay, E., & de-Leon, M. B. (2010, December 16). Chronic stress and fatigue-related quality of life after mild to moderate traumatic brain injury. *Journal of Head Trauma Rehabilitation.* (Online prepublication)

Bazarian, J. J., McClung, J., Shah, M. N., Cheng, Y. T., Flesher, W., & Kraus, J. (2005). Mild traumatic brain injury in the United States, 1998–2000. *Brain Injury, 19*(2), 85–91.

Bazarian, J. J., Zhong, J., Blyth, B., Zhu, T., Kavcic, V., & Peterson, D. (2007). Diffusion tensor imaging detects clinically important axonal damage after mild traumatic brain injury: A pilot study. *Journal of Neurotrauma, 24*(9), 1447–1459.

Belanger, H. G., Vanderploeg, R. D., Curtiss, G., & Warden, D. L. (2007). Recent neuroimaging techniques in mild traumatic brain injury. *Journal of Neuropsychiatry and Clinical Neurosciences, 19*(1), 5–20.

Bhatoe, H. S. (2008). Blast injury and the neurosurgeon. *Indian Journal of Neurotrauma, 5*(1), 3–6.

Biasca, N., & Maxwell, W. L. (2007). Minor traumatic brain injury in sports: A review in order to prevent neurological sequelae. *Progress in Brain Research, 161,* 263–291.

Bigler, E. D. (2004). Neuropsychological results and neuropathological findings at autopsy in a case of mild traumatic brain injury. *Journal of the International Neuropsychological Society, 10*(5), 794–806.

Bigler, E. D. (2008). Neuropsychology and clinical neuroscience of persistent post-concussive syndrome. *Journal of the International Neuropsychological Society, 14*(1), 1–22.

Bigler, E. D., & Bazarian, J. J. (2010). Diffusion tensor imaging: A biomarker for mild traumatic brain injury? *Neurology, 74*(8), 626–627.

Bigler, E. D., & Maxwell, W. L. (in press). Neuropathology and neuroimaging of mild traumatic brain injury. *Brain Imaging and Behavior.*

Blumbergs, P. C., Scott, G., Manavis, J., Wainwright, H., Simpson, D. A., & McLean, A. J. (1994). Staining of amyloid precursor protein to study axonal damage in mild head injury. *Lancet, 344*(8929), 1055–1056.

Blumbergs, P. C., Scott, G., Manavis, J., Wainwright, H., Simpson, D. A., & McLean, A. J. (1995). Topography of axonal injury as defined by amyloid precursor protein and the sector scoring method in mild and severe closed head injury. *Journal of Neurotrauma, 12*(4), 565–572.

Buki, A., & Povlishock, J. T. (2006). All roads lead to disconnection?—Traumatic axonal injury revisited. *Acta Neurochirurgica, 148*(2), 181–193.

Bussone, W. R., & Duma, S. M. (2010). The effect of gender and body size on angular accelerations of the head observed during everyday activities—Biomed 2010. *Biomedical Sciences Instrumentation, 46,* 166–171.

Carroll, L. J., Cassidy, J. D., Holm, L., Kraus, J., & Coronado, V. G. (2004). Methodological issues and research recommendations for mild traumatic brain injury: The WHO Collaborating Centre Task Force on Mild Traumatic Brain Injury. *Journal of Rehabilitation Medicine, 43*(Suppl.), 113–125.

Carroll, L. J., Cassidy, J. D., Peloso, P. M., Borg, J., von Holst, H., Holm, L., et al. (2004). Prognosis for mild traumatic brain injury: Results of the WHO Collaborating Centre Task Force on Mild Traumatic Brain Injury. *Journal of Rehabilitation Medicine, 43*(Suppl.), 84–105.

Centers for Disease Control and Prevention (2007). Nonfatal traumatic brain injuries from sports and recreation activities—United States, 2001–2005. *Morbidity and Mortality Weekly Report, 56*(29), 733–737.

Chen, J. K., Johnston, K. M., Petrides, M., & Ptito, A. (2008). Neural substrates of symptoms of depression following concussion in male athletes with persisting postconcussion symptoms. *Archives of General Psychiatry, 65*(1), 81–89.

Chu, Z., Wilde, E. A., Hunter, J. V., McCauley, S. R., Bigler, E. D., Troyanskaya, M., et al. (2010). Voxel-based analysis of diffusion tensor imaging in mild traumatic brain injury in adolescents. *American Journal of Neuroradiology, 31*(2), 340–346.

Corrigan, J. D., Selassie, A. W., & Orman, J. A. (2010). The epidemiology of traumatic brain injury. *Journal of Head Trauma Rehabilitation, 25*(2), 72–80.

Danelson, K. A., Yu, M., Gayzik, F. S., Geer, C. P., Slice, D. E., & Stitzel, J. D. (2008). Geometric scaling factors for the pediatric brainstem. *Biomedical Sciences Instrumentation, 44,* 153–158.

Daniels, J. K., McFarlane, A. C., Bluhm, R. L., Moores, K. A., Clark, C. R., Shaw, M. E., et al. (2010). Switching between executive and default mode networks in posttraumatic stress disorder: Alterations in functional connectivity. *Journal of Psychiatry and Neuroscience, 35*(4), 258–266.

de Guise, E., Lepage, J. F., Tinawi, S., LeBlanc, J., Dagher, J., Lamoureux, J., et al. (2010). Comprehensive clinical picture of patients with complicated vs. uncomplicated mild traumatic brain injury. *Clinical Neuropsychologist, 24*(7), 1113–1130.

DeKosky, S. T., Ikonomovic, M. D., & Gandy, S. (2010). Traumatic brain injury—Football, warfare, and long-term effects. *New England Journal of Medicine, 363*(14), 1293–1296.

Desmoulin, G. T., & Dionne, J. P. (2009). Blast-induced neurotrauma: Surrogate use, loading mechanisms, and cellular responses. *Journal of Trauma, 67*(5), 1113–1122.

Downes, C. E., & Crack, P. J. (2010). Neural injury following stroke: Are Toll-like receptors the link between the immune system and the CNS? *British Journal of Pharmacology, 160*(8), 1872–1888.

Evans, R. W. (2010). Persistent post-traumatic headache, postconcussion syndrome, and whiplash injuries: The evidence for a non-traumatic basis with an historical review. *Headache, 50*(4), 716–724.

Gasquoine, P. G. (1997). Postconcussion symptoms. *Neuropsychology Review, 7*(2), 77–85.

Gavett, B. E., Stern, R. A., Cantu, R. C., Nowinski, C. J., & McKee, A. C. (2010). Mild traumatic brain injury: A risk factor for neurodegeneration. *Alzheimers Research and Therapy, 2*(3), 18. Available at *http://alzres.com/content/2/18.*

Gean, A. D., & Fischbein, N. J. (2010). Head trauma. *Neuroimaging Clinics of North America, 20*(4), 527–556.

Geary, E. K., Kraus, M. F., Pliskin, N. H., & Little, D. M. (2010). Verbal learning differences in chronic mild traumatic brain injury. *Journal of the International Neuropsychology Society, 16*(3), 506–516.

Giza, C. C., & Hovda, D. A. (2001). The neurometabolic cascade of concussion. *Journal of Athletic Training, 36*(3), 228–235.

Govind, V., Gold, S., Kaliannan, K., Saigal, G., Falcone, S., Arheart, K. L., et al. (2010). Whole-brain proton MR spectroscopic imaging of mild-to-moderate traumatic brain injury and correlation with neuropsychological deficits. *Journal of Neurotrauma, 27*(3), 483–496.

Govindaraju, V., Gauger, G. E., Manley, G. T., Ebel, A., Meeker, M., & Maudsley, A. A. (2004). Volumetric proton spectroscopic imaging of mild traumatic brain injury. *American Journal of Neuroradiology, 25*(5), 730–737.

Gowda, N. K., Agrawal, D., Bal, C., Chandrashekar, N., Tripati, M., Bandopadhyaya, G. P., et al. (2006). Technetium Tc-99m ethyl cysteinate dimer brain single-photon emission CT in mild traumatic brain injury: A prospective study. *American Journal of Neuroradiology, 27*(2), 447–451.

Graham, D. I., & Lantos, P. L. (2002). *Greenfield's neuropathology* (7th ed.). London: Arnold.

Hamberger, A., Viano, D. C., Saljo, A., & Bolouri, H. (2009). Concussion in professional football: Morphology of brain injuries in the NFL concussion model—part 16. *Neurosurgery, 64*(6), 1174–1182.

Hayward, P. (2008). Traumatic brain injury: The signature of modern conflicts. *Lancet Neurology, 7*(3), 200–201.

Heitger, M. H., Jones, R. D., Macleod, A. D., Snell, D. L., Frampton, C. M., & Anderson, T. J. (2009). Impaired eye movements in post-concussion syndrome indicate suboptimal brain function beyond the influence of depression, malingering or intellectual ability. *Brain, 132*(Pt. 10), 2850–2870.

Inglese, M., Makani, S., Johnson, G., Cohen, B. A., Silver, J. A., Gonen, O., et al. (2005). Diffuse axonal injury in mild traumatic brain injury: A diffusion tensor imaging study. *Journal of Neurosurgery, 103*(2), 298–303.

Jacobson, R. R. (1995). The post-concussional syndrome: Physiogenesis, psychogenesis and malingering. An integrative model. *Journal of Psychosomatic Research, 39*(6), 675–693.

Jantzen, K. J. (2010). Functional magnetic resonance imaging of mild traumatic brain injury. *Journal of Head Trauma Rehabilitation, 25*(4), 256–266.

Jordan, B. D. (1992). *Medical aspects of boxing.* Boca Raton, FL: CRC Press.

Jovanovic, T., & Ressler, K. J. (2010). How the neurocircuitry and genetics of fear inhibition may inform our understanding of PTSD. *American Journal of Psychiatry, 167*(6), 648–662.

Kaplan, G. B., Vasterling, J. J., & Vedak, P. C. (2010). Brain-derived neurotrophic factor in traumatic brain injury, post-traumatic stress disorder, and their comorbid conditions: Role in pathogenesis and treatment. *Behavioural Pharmacology, 21*(5–6), 427–437.

Koenigs, M., & Grafman, J. (2009). The functional neuroanatomy of depression: Distinct roles for ventromedial and dorsolateral prefrontal cortex. *Behavioural Brain Research, 201*(2), 239–243.

Konrad, C., Geburek, A. J., Rist, F., Blumenroth, H., Fischer, B., Husstedt, I., et al. (2010). Long-term cognitive and emotional consequences of mild traumatic brain injury. *Psychological Medicine, 22*, 1–15.

Kou, Z., Wu, Z., Tong, K. A., Holshouser, B., Benson, R. R., Hu, J., et al. (2010). The role of advanced MR imaging findings as biomarkers of traumatic brain injury. *Journal of Head Trauma Rehabilitation, 25*(4), 267–282.

Lanius, R. A., Vermetten, E., Loewenstein, R. J., Brand, B., Schmahl, C., Bremner, J. D., et al. (2010). Emotion modulation in PTSD: Clinical and neurobiological evidence for a dissociative subtype. *American Journal of Psychiatry, 167*(6), 640–647.

Levin, H., & Kraus, M. F. (1994). The frontal lobes and traumatic brain injury. *Journal of Neuropsychiatry and Clinical Neurosciences, 6*(4), 443–454.

Levine, B., Kovacevic, N., Nica, E. I., Cheung, G., Gao, F., Schwartz, M. L., et al. (2008). The Toronto traumatic brain injury study: Injury severity and quantified MRI. *Neurology, 70*(10), 771–778.

Lewine, J. D., Davis, J. T., Bigler, E. D., Thoma, R., Hill, D., Funke, M., et al. (2007). Objective documentation of traumatic brain injury subsequent to mild head trauma: Multimodal brain imaging with MEG, SPECT, and MRI. *Journal of Head Trauma Rehabilitation, 22*(3), 141–155.

Little, D. M., Kraus, M. F., Joseph, J., Geary, E. K., Susmaras, T., Zhou, X. J., et al. (2010). Thalamic integrity underlies executive dysfunction in traumatic brain injury. *Neurology, 74*(7), 558–564.

MacKenzie, J. D., Siddiqi, F., Babb, J. S., Bagley, L. J., Mannon, L. J., Sinson, G. P., et al. (2002). Brain atrophy in mild or moderate traumatic brain injury: A longitudinal quantitative analysis. *American Journal of Neuroradiology, 23*(9), 1509–1515.

Makdissi, M., Darby, D., Maruff, P., Ugoni, A., Brukner, P., & McCrory, P. R. (2010). Natural history of concussion in sport: Markers of severity and implications for management. *American Journal of Sports Medicine, 38*(3), 464–471.

Matthews, S. C., Strigo, I. A., Simmons, A. N., O'Connell, R. M., Reinhardt, L. E., & Moseley, S. A. (2010). A multimodal imaging study in U.S. veterans of Operations Iraqi and Enduring Freedom with and without major depression after blast-related concussion. *Neuroimage, 54*(Suppl. 1), S69–S75.

Maxwell, W. L., MacKinnon, M. A., Stewart, J. E., & Graham, D. I. (2010). Stereology of cerebral cortex after traumatic brain injury matched to the Glasgow outcome score. *Brain, 133*(Pt. 1), 139–160.

Maxwell, W. L., Povlishock, J. T., & Graham, D. L. (1997). A mechanistic analysis of nondisruptive axonal injury: A review. *Journal of Neurotrauma, 14*(7), 419–440.

Maxwell, W. L., Watt, C., Graham, D. I., & Gennarelli, T. A. (1993). Ultrastructural evidence of axonal shearing as a result of lateral acceleration of the head in non-human primates. *Acta Neuropathologica, 86*(2), 136–144.

Mayer, A. R., Ling, J., Mannell, M. V., Gasparovic, C., Phillips, J. P., Doezema, D., et al. (2010). A prospective diffusion tensor imaging study in mild traumatic brain injury. *Neurology, 74*(8), 643–650.

McAllister, T. W., & Arciniegas, D. (2002). Evaluation and treatment of postconcussive symptoms. *NeuroRehabilitation, 17*(4), 265–283.

McAllister, T. W., & Stein, M. B. (2010). Effects of psychological and biomechanical trauma on brain and behavior. *Annals of the New York Academy of Sciences, 1208*, 46–57.

McCrea, M., Prichep, L., Powell, M. R., Chabot, R., & Barr, W. B. (2010). Acute effects and recovery after sport-related concussion: A neurocognitive and quantitative brain electrical activity study. *Journal of Head Trauma Rehabilitation, 25*(4), 283–292.

McCrory, P. R., Berkovic, S. F., & Cordner, S. M. (2000). Deaths due to brain injury among footballers in Victoria, 1968–1999. *Medical Journal of Australia, 172*(5), 217–219.

McCrory, P. R., Meeuwisse, W., Johnston, K., Dvorak, J., Aubry, M., Molloy, M., et al. (2009). Consensus Statement on Concussion in Sport: The 3rd International Conference on Concussion in Sport held in Zurich, November 2008. [Consensus Development Conference.] *British Journal of Sports Medicine, 43*(Suppl. 1), i76–i90.

McKee, A. C., Cantu, R. C., Nowinski, C. J., Hedley-Whyte, E. T., Gavett, B. E., Budson, A. E., et al. (2009). Chronic traumatic encephalopathy in athletes: Progressive tauopathy after repetitive head injury. *Journal of Neuropathology and Experimental Neurology, 68*(7), 709–735.

McKee, A. C., Gavett, B. E., Stern, R. A., Nowinski, C. J., Cantu, R. C., Kowall, N. W., et al. (2010). TDP-43 proteinopathy and motor neuron disease in chronic traumatic encephalopathy. *Journal of Neuropathology and Experimental Neurology, 69*(9), 918–929.

Menon, D. K., Schwab, K., Wright, D. W., & Maas, A. I. (2010). Position statement: Definition of traumatic brain injury. *Archives of Physical Medicine and Rehabilitation, 91*(11), 1637–1640.

Messe, A., Caplain, S., Paradot, G., Garrigue, D., Mineo, J. F., Soto Ares, G., et al. (2011). Diffusion tensor imaging and white matter lesions at the subacute stage in mild traumatic brain injury with persistent neurobehavioral impairment. *Human Brain Mapping, 32*(6), 999–1011.

Metting, Z., Rödiger, L. A., Stewart, R. E., Oudkerk, M., De Keyser, J., & van der Naalt, J. (2009). Perfusion computed tomography in the acute phase of mild head injury: Regional dysfunction and prognostic value. *Annals of Neurology, 66*(6), 809–816.

Metting, Z., Rödiger, L. A., de Jong, B. M., Stewart, R. E., Kremer, B. P., & van der Naalt, J. (2010). Acute cerebral perfusion CT abnormalities associated with posttraumatic amnesia in mild head injury. *Journal of Neurotrauma, 27*(12), 2183–2189.

Moore, D. F., & Jaffee, M. S. (2010). Military traumatic brain injury and blast. *NeuroRehabilitation, 26*(3), 179–181.

Nakamura, T., Hillary, F. G., & Biswal, B. B. (2009). Resting network plasticity following brain injury. *PLoS One, 4*(12), e8220.

Newcombe, V., Chatfield, D., Outtrim, J., Vowler, S., Manktelow, A., Cross, J., et al. (2011). Mapping traumatic axonal injury using diffusion tensor imaging: Correlations with functional outcome. *PloS One, 6*(5), e19214.

Niogi, S. N., & Mukherjee, P. (2010). Diffusion tensor imaging of mild traumatic brain injury. *Journal of Head Trauma Rehabilitation, 25*(4), 241–255.

Norrie, J., Heitger, M., Leathem, J., Anderson, T., Jones, R., & Flett, R. (2010). Mild traumatic brain injury and fatigue: A prospective longitudinal study. *Brain Injury, 24*(13–14), 1528–1538.

Nowak, L. A., Smith, G. G., & Reyes, P. F. (2009). Dementia in a retired world boxing champion: Case report and literature review. *Clinical Neuropathology, 28*(4), 275–280.

Ommaya, A. K., Goldsmith, W., & Thibault, L. (2002). Biomechanics and neuropathology of adult and paediatric head injury. *British Journal of Neurosurgery, 16*(3), 220–242.

Oppenheimer, D. R. (1968). Microscopic lesions in the brain following head injury. *Journal of Neurology, Neurosurgery, and Psychiatry, 31*(4), 299–306.

Orrison, W. W., Hanson, E. H., Alamo, T., Watson, D., Sharma, M., Perkins, T. G., et al. (2009). Traumatic brain injury: A review and high-field MRI findings in 100 unarmed combatants using a literature-based checklist approach. *Journal of Neurotrauma, 26*(5), 689–701.

Pardini, J. E., Pardini, D. A., Becker, J. T., Dunfee, K. L., Eddy, W. F., Lovell, M. R., et al. (2010). Postconcussive symptoms are associated with compensatory cortical recruitment during a working memory task. *Neurosurgery, 67*(4), 1020–1027.

Pardini, M., Krueger, F., Raymont, V., & Grafman, J. (2010). Ventromedial prefrontal cortex modulates fatigue after penetrating traumatic brain injury. *Neurology, 74*(9), 749–754.

Peerless, S. J., & Rewcastle, N. B. (1967). Shear injuries of the brain. *Canadian Medical Association Journal, 96*(10), 577–582.

Peskind, E. R., Petrie, E. C., Cross, D. J., Pagulayan, K., McCraw, K., Hoff, D., et al. (2010). Cerebrocerebellar hypometabolism associated with repetitive blast exposure mild traumatic brain injury in 12 Iraq war veterans with persistent post-concussive symptoms. *Neuroimage, 54*(Suppl. 1), S76–S82.

Rickels, E., von Wild, K., & Wenzlaff, P. (2010). Head injury in Germany: A population-based prospective study on epidemiology, causes, treatment and outcome of all degrees of head-injury severity in two distinct areas. *Brain Injury, 24*(12), 1491–1504.

Risling, M., Plantman, S., Angeria, M., Rostami, E., Bellander, B. M., Kirkegaard, M., et al. (2010). Mechanisms of blast induced brain injuries, experimental studies in rats. *Neuroimage, 54*(Suppl. 1), S89–S97.

Ropper, A. H., & Gorson, K. C. (2007). Clinical practice: Concussion. *New England Journal of Medicine, 356*(2), 166–172.

Rosenfeld, J. V., & Ford, N. L. (2010). Bomb blast, mild traumatic brain injury and psychiatric morbidity: A review. *Injury, 41*(5), 437–443.

Rutgers, D. R., Toulgoat, F., Cazejust, J., Fillard, P., Lasjaunais, P., & Ducreux, D. (2008). White matter abnormalities in mild traumatic brain injury: A diffusion sensor imaging study. *American Journal of Neuroradiology, 29,* 514–519.

Rutland-Brown, W., Langlois, J. A., Nicaj, L., Thomas, R. G. Jr., Wilt, S. A., & Bazarian, J. J. (2007). Traumatic brain injuries after mass-casualty incidents: Lessons from the 11 September 2001 World Trade Center attacks. *Prehospital and Disaster Medicine, 22*(3), 157–164.

Ryu, W. H., Feinstein, A., Colantonio, A., Streiner, D. L., & Dawson, D. R. (2009). Early identification and incidence of mild TBI in Ontario. *Canadian Journal of Neurological Sciences, 36*(4), 429–435.

Saatman, K. E., Serbst, G., & Burkhardt, M. F. (2009). Axonal damage due to traumatic brain injury. In A. Lajtha, N. Banik, & S. K. Ray (Eds.), *Handbook of neurochemistry and molecular neurobiology* (pp. 344–356). New York: Springer.

Sabet, A. A., Christoforou, E., Zatlin, B., Genin, G. M., & Bayly, P. V. (2008). Deformation of the human brain induced by mild angular head acceleration. *Journal of Biomechanics, 41*(2), 307–315.

Scheid, R., Walther, K., Guthke, T., Preul, C., & von Cramon, D. Y. (2006). Cognitive sequelae of diffuse axonal injury. *Archives of Neurology, 63*(3), 418–424.

Silver, J. M., McAllister, T. W., & Arciniegas, D. B. (2009). Depression and cognitive complaints following mild traumatic brain injury. *American Journal of Psychiatry, 166*(6), 653–661.

Slobounov, S. M., Zhang, K., Pennell, D., Ray, W., Johnson, B., & Sebastianelli, W. (2010). Functional abnormalities in normally appearing athletes following mild traumatic brain injury: A functional MRI study. *Experimental Brain Research, 202*(2), 341–354.

Smits, M., Houston, G. C., Dippel, D. W., Wielopolski, P. A., Vernooij, M. W., Koudstaal, P. J., et al. (2011). Microstructural brain injury in post-concussion syndrome after minor head injury. *Neuroradiology, 53*(8), 553–563.

Smits, M., Hunink, M. G., van Rijssel, D. A., Dekker, H. M., Vos, P. E., Kool, D. R., et al. (2008). Outcome after complicated minor head injury. *American Journal of Neuroradiology, 29*(3), 506–513.

Stein, M. B., & McAllister, T. W. (2009). Exploring the convergence of posttraumatic stress disorder and mild traumatic brain injury. *American Journal of Psychiatry, 166*(7), 768–776.

Strich, S. J. (1956). Diffuse degeneration of the cerebral white matter in severe dementia following head injury. *Journal of Neurology, Neurosurgery, and Psychiatry, 19*(3), 163–185.

Talavage, T. M., Nauman, E., Breedlove, E. L., Yoruk, U., Dye, A. E., Morigaki, K., et al. (2010, October 10). Functionally-detected cognitive impairment in high school football players without clinically-diagnosed concussion. *Journal of Neurotrauma.* (Online prepublication)

Thurman, D. J., Coronado, V., & Selassie, A. (2007). *The epidemiology of TBI: Implications for public health.* New York: Demos.

Thurmond, V. A., Hicks, R., Gleason, T., Miller, A. C., Szuflita, N., Orman, J., et al. (2010). Advancing integrated research in psychological health and traumatic brain injury: Common data elements. *Archives of Physical Medicine and Rehabilitation, 91*(11), 1633–1636.

Umile, E. M., Sandel, M. E., Alavi, A., Terry, C. M., & Plotkin, R. C. (2002). Dynamic imaging in mild traumatic brain injury: Support for the theory of medial temporal vulnerability. *Archives of Physical Medicine and Rehabilitation, 83*(11), 1506–1513.

Vagnozzi, R., Signoretti, S., Cristofori, L., Alessandrini, F., Floris, R., Isgro, E., et al. (2010). Assessment of metabolic brain damage and recovery following mild traumatic brain injury: A multicentre, proton magnetic resonance spectroscopic study in concussed patients. *Brain, 133*(11), 3232–3242.

Vaishnavi, S., Rao, V., & Fann, J. R. (2009). Neuropsychiatric problems after traumatic brain injury: Unraveling the silent epidemic. *Psychosomatics, 50*(3), 198–205.

Van Boven, R. W., Harrington, G. S., Hackney, D. B., Ebel, A., Gauger, G., Bremner, J. D., et al. (2009). Advances in neuroimaging of traumatic brain injury and posttraumatic stress disorder. *Journal of Rehabilitation Research and Development, 46*(6), 717–757.

Vasterling, J. J., Verfaellie, M., & Sullivan, K. D. (2009). Mild traumatic brain injury and posttraumatic stress disorder in returning veterans: Perspectives from cognitive neuroscience. *Clinical Psychology Review, 29*(8), 674–684.

Viano, D. C., Casson, I. R., Pellman, E. J., Zhang, L., King, A. I., & Yang, K. H. (2005). Concussion in professional football: Brain responses by finite element analysis: Part 9. *Neurosurgery, 57*(5), 891–916.

Vincent, J. L., Kahn, I., Snyder, A. Z., Raichle, M. E., & Buckner, R. L. (2008). Evidence for a frontoparietal control system revealed by intrinsic functional connectivity. *Journal of Neurophysiology, 100*(6), 3328–3342.

Walilko, T., North, C., Young, L. A., Lux, W. E., Warden, D. L., Jaffee, M. S., et al. (2009). Head injury as a PTSD predictor among Oklahoma City bombing survivors. *Journal of Trauma, 67*(6), 1311–1319.

Wang, J. A., Lin, W., Morris, T., Banderali, U., Juranka, P. F., & Morris, C. E. (2009). Membrane trauma and Na+ leak from Nav1.6 channels. *American Journal of Physiology–Cell Physiology, 297*(4), C823–834.

Whitnall, L., McMillan, T. M., Murray, G. D., & Teasdale, G. M. (2006).

Disability in young people and adults after head injury: 5–7 year follow up of a prospective cohort study. *Journal of Neurology, Neurosurgery, and Psychiatry, 77*(5), 640–645.

Whitney, N. P., Eidem, T. M., Peng, H., Huang, Y., & Zheng, J. C. (2009). Inflammation mediates varying effects in neurogenesis: Relevance to the pathogenesis of brain injury and neurodegenerative disorders. *Journal of Neurochemistry, 108*(6), 1343–1359.

Wilde, E. A., McCauley, S. R., Hunter, J. V., Bigler, E. D., Chu, Z., Wang, Z. J., et al. (2008). Diffusion tensor imaging of acute mild traumatic brain injury in adolescents. *Neurology, 70*(12), 948–955.

Williams, W. H., Potter, S., & Ryland, H. (2010). Mild traumatic brain injury and postconcussion syndrome: A neuropsychological perspective. *Journal of Neurology, Neurosurgery, and Psychiatry, 81*, 1116–1122.

Wilson, J. T. (1990). The relationship between neuropsychological function and brain damage detected by neuroimaging after closed head injury. *Brain Injury, 4*(4), 349–363.

Wu, T. C., Wilde, E. A., Bigler, E. D., Yallampalli, R., McCauley, S. R., Troyanskaya, M., et al. (2010). Evaluating the relationship between memory functioning and cingulum bundles in acute mild traumatic brain injury using diffusion tensor imaging. *Journal of Neurotrauma, 27*(2), 303–307.

Yallampalli, R., Wilde, E. A., Bigler, E. D., McCauley, S. R., Hanten, G., Troyanskaya, M., et al. (in press). Acute white matter differences in the fornix following mild traumatic brain injury using diffusion tensor imaging. *Journal of Neuroimaging*.

Yeates, K. O. (2010). Mild traumatic brain injury and postconcussive symptoms in children and adolescents. *Journal of the International Neuropsychological Society, 16*(6), 953–960.

Yehuda, R. (2002). Post-traumatic stress disorder. *New England Journal of Medicine, 346*(2), 108–114.

Yeo, R., Gasparovic, C., Merideth, F. L., Ruhl, D. A., Doezema, D., & Mayer, A. (2011). A longitudinal proton magnetic resonance spectroscopy study of mild traumatic brain injury. *Journal of Neurotrauma, 28*(1), 1–11.

Zatzick, D. F., Rivara, F. P., Jurkovich, G. J., Hoge, C. W., Wang, J., Fan, M. Y., et al. (2010). Multisite investigation of traumatic brain injuries, posttraumatic stress disorder, and self-reported health and cognitive impairments. *Archives of General Psychiatry, 67*(12), 1291–1300.

Zumstein, M. A., Moser, M., Mottini, M., Ott, S. R., Sadowski-Cron, C., Radanov, B. P., et al. (2010). Long-term outcome in patients with mild traumatic brain injury: A prospective observational study. *Journal of Trauma*. (Online publication.)

CHAPTER 3

A Biopsychosocial Conceptualization of Poor Outcome from Mild Traumatic Brain Injury

Grant L. Iverson

The Biopsychosocial Model

Poor outcome following mild traumatic brain injury (mTBI) defies parsimonious explanation. Without question, some patients have poor outcome from this injury. A binary polarized view on the cause of poor outcome, be it pathophysiogenesis or psychogenesis, is outdated, simplistic, inadequate, and inconsistent with the body of diverse accumulated evidence over the past 30 years. The crux of the problem with understanding poor outcome is that there are numerous studies that provide clarity and persuasive evidence on *specific issues*—but when those issues are aggregated, then clarity and persuasiveness diminish dramatically. This diverse range of evidence is discussed in this chapter, leading to the ultimate conclusion that the only reasonable approach to understanding poor outcome from mTBI is a biopsychosocial perspective. This perspective, by necessity, embraces a multifactorial, interwoven, biopsychosocial conceptualization of poor outcome from this injury that is the antithesis of parsimony.

A biopsychosocial conceptualization of poor outcome from mTBI is presented in Figure 3.1. It has long been appreciated that preinjury medical, neurological, psychiatric, and personality factors can influence outcome from a mild injury to the brain. For example, Symonds (1937) wrote: "The symptom picture depends not only upon the kind of injury, but upon the

37

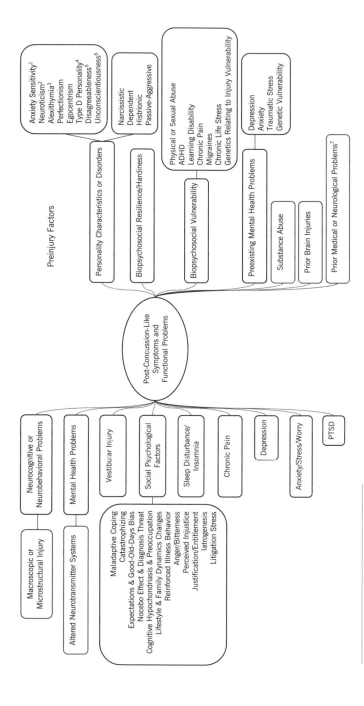

FIGURE 3.1. A biopsychosocial conceptualization of poor outcome from mTBI. Copyright 2011 by Grant L. Iverson. Reprinted by permission.

[1] Anxiety Sensitivity: A trait comprised of physical, psychological, and social preoccupations and concerns, is characterized by fear of anxiety-related bodily sensations.
[2] Neuroticism: A personality trait characterized by a strong tendency to experience negative emotions such as anxiety, depression, anger, and self-consciousness. Individuals with this trait have considerable difficulty coping with stress.
[3] Alexithymia: A cluster of traits characterized by difficulty identifying feelings, difficulty describing feelings to others, externally oriented thinking, and limited capacity for imaginal thinking.
[4] Type D Personality: A personality trait characterized by antagonism, skepticism, and egocentrism.
[5] Disagreeableness: This personality pattern is characterized by two stable personality traits: negative affectivity and social inhibition.
[6] Unconscientiousness: A personality trait characterized by reduced self-discipline and ambition, disorganization, and a more lackadaisical approach to life.
[7] For example, hypertension, heart disease, cardiac surgery, diabetes, thyroid problems, and small vessel ischemic disease.

kind of brain." On the right side of the figure, a diverse range of preinjury biopsychosocial characteristics are presented. These include personality characteristics, mental health problems, and previous brain injuries.

Resilience and vulnerability, although interrelated, should not be considered opposite ends of a single psychological or biopsychosocial dimension. Resilience is comprised of a diverse set of psychological, social, and biological factors that confer some degree of protection from poor outcome following mTBI (e.g., positive coping style, high self-efficacy, hardiness, positive emotions and optimism, humor, social and occupational support, genetics, serotonin transport and binding, norepinephrine biosynthesis and availability, dopaminergic brain reward systems, sympathetic nervous system regulation, neuropeptides, hypothalamic–pituitary–adrenal axis, cortisol, and other stress hormones) (Feder, Nestler, & Charney, 2009; Hoge, Austin, & Pollack, 2007; Southwick, Vythilingam, & Charney, 2005). From a psychological perspective, resilience is an intrinsic characteristic underlying a person's ability to successfully adapt to acute stress and more chronic forms of adversity. Possible underpinnings of resilience include (1) facing fears; (2) adaptive coping; (3) optimism and positive emotions; (4) cognitive reappraisal, positive reframing, and acceptance; (5) social competence and social support; and (6) purpose in life, a moral compass, and meaning and spirituality (Feder et al., 2009). Hardiness has been conceptualized as a personality characteristic consisting of three psychological attitudes and beliefs: commitment, challenge, and control. Through commitment, a person turns events into something meaningful and important. Control refers to the belief that one can influence the course of events. Challenge refers to a belief system in which wisdom and growth are gained from difficult experiences.

Vulnerability is sometimes conceptualized as a superordinate composition of individual risk factors. Vulnerability to depression, for example, is believed to arise from the *cumulative impact* (Kendler, Thornton, & Gardner, 2000, 2001; Monroe & Harkness, 2005) of genetics (Binder & Nemeroff, 2009; Hauger, Risbrough, Oakley, Olivares-Reyes, & Dautzenberg, 2009; McGuffin et al., 2005; Sullivan, Neale, & Kendler, 2000), adverse events in childhood (Bradley et al., 2008; Gatt et al., 2009; Heim et al., 2009; Heim, Newport, Mletzko, Miller, & Nemeroff, 2008), and ongoing life stressors (Farmer & McGuffin, 2003; Friis, Wittchen, Pfister, & Lieb, 2002; Kendler, Hettema, Butera, Gardner, & Prescott, 2003; Kendler, Karkowski, & Prescott, 1999). Obviously, there is no reason to believe that people who have sustained an mTBI would be immune to these preinjury and co-occurring factors in Figure 3.1 that contribute to both resilience and vulnerability. These preinjury factors can influence the initial presentation, acute outcome, course, and long-term outcome from injury. These distal preinjury factors can interact with a diverse range of proximal co-occurring factors creating tremendous complexity in disentangling the cause of post-concussion-like symptoms long after an mTBI.

On the left side of Figure 3.1, numerous physiological, psychological, psychiatric, social psychological, and contextual factors that can influence how the course and long-term outcome from injury are portrayed. Most of these factors are reviewed in this chapter.

Definitional Issues

There is no universally accepted definition of mTBI. The injury is classified based on the initial severity indicators, not outcome. The three primary severity indicators are duration of unconsciousness, Glasgow Coma Scale (GCS) scores in the first 30 minutes postinjury, and duration of posttraumatic amnesia (PTA). A common, but not universally accepted, classification system for TBI is provided in Table 3.1. A definition of mTBI, provided by the World Health Organization (WHO) Collaborating Centre Task Force on Mild Traumatic Brain Injury, is reprinted below.

> mTBI is an acute brain injury resulting from mechanical energy to the head from external physical forces. Operational criteria for clinical identification include: (i) 1 or more of the following: confusion or disorientation, loss of consciousness for 30 minutes or less, post-traumatic amnesia for less than 24 hours, and/or other transient neurological abnormalities such as focal signs, seizure, and intracranial lesion not requiring surgery; (ii) Glasgow Coma Scale score of 13–15 after 30 minutes post-injury or later upon presentation for healthcare. These manifestations of mTBI must not be due to drugs, alcohol, medications, caused by other injuries or treatment for other injuries (e.g. systemic injuries, facial injuries or intubation), caused by other problems (e.g. psychological trauma, language barrier or coexisting medical conditions) or caused by penetrating

TABLE 3.1. Common Classification System for TBI

Classification	Duration of unconsciousness	Glasgow Coma Scale	Posttraumatic amnesia
Mild	< 30 minutes	13–15[a]	< 24 hours
Moderate	30 minutes–24 hours	9–12	1–7 days
Severe	> 24 hours	3–8	> 7 days

Note. This is not a universally agreed-upon classification system.
[a]Defined as the lowest GCS score obtained 30 minutes or more postinjury.

craniocerebral injury. (Carroll, Cassidy, Holm, Kraus, & Coronado, 2004, p. 115)

This definition is very similar to the definition developed by the Mild Traumatic Brain Injury Committee of the Head Injury Interdisciplinary Special Interest Group of the American Congress of Rehabilitation Medicine (1993). It is also similar to the conceptual definition of mTBI offered by the Centers for Disease Control and Prevention (CDC) working group (2003). The WHO workgroup definition has been endorsed as reasonable for use in clinical practice and research (Ruff, Iverson, Barth, Bush, & Broshek, 2009).

What is immediately apparent is that the definition of mTBI is extraordinarily broad, encompassing blows to the head resulting in transient alterations in mental status to high velocity forces resulting in vigorous displacement of the brain within the cranial vault leading to stretching of white matter tracts, widespread cellular dysfunction, and macroscopic structural brain damage. The mainstream definition of mTBI is so broad that it encompasses individuals who appear to recover functionally within the first 24 hours and individuals with injuries abutting the moderate TBI classification range who have some degree of permanent change in their functioning. As such, without question, mTBIs are not created equally.

Is mTBI Associated with Permanent Brain Damage?

The answer to this simple question is partially known, with confidence, but far from fully understood. There is a subtype of mTBI called "complicated" mTBI. Complicated mTBI, in the original definition (Williams, Levin, & Eisenberg, 1990), was differentiated from uncomplicated mTBI by the presence of (1) a depressed skull fracture, and/or (2) a trauma-related intracranial abnormality (e.g., hemorrhage, contusion, or edema). Provided that the duration of unconsciousness, GCS, and duration of PTA are all in the "mild" severity range, most mainstream definitions of mTBI include "complicated" injuries in the definition. Numerous studies suggest that complicated mTBIs are associated with worse outcome than uncomplicated mTBIs (Iverson, 2006a; Lange, Iverson, & Franzen, 2009; Temkin, Machamer, & Dikmen, 2003; van der Naalt, Hew, van Zomeren, Sluiter, & Minderhoud, 1999; Williams et al., 1990; Wilson, Hadley, Scott, & Harper, 1996), but not all studies have reached this conclusion (Hofman et al., 2001; Hughes et al., 2004; McCauley, Boake, Levin, Contant, & Song, 2001), and the magnitude of the difference has been relatively modest in some studies.

Recently, the U.S. Department of Defense has conceptualized complicated mTBI as "moderate" TBI.

Returning to the question of whether mTBI is associated with permanent brain damage (i.e., macrostructural or microstructural)—the answer is yes for some people. Is mTBI associated with macroscopic brain damage in most or all people?—The answer is no. Is mTBI associated with microstructural white matter changes?—Again, yes for some people. We do not know, however, what percentage of mTBI cases show clear evidence of microstructural white matter changes. As seen in Figure 3.2, white matter is pervasive and potentially vulnerable to mechanical forces. Diffusion tensor imaging (DTI) is an MRI technique that examines the integrity of white matter in the brain at a microstructural level by measuring the directionality and magnitude of water diffusion in white matter. As reviewed in more detail by Bigler and Maxwell (Chapter 2, this volume), researchers have reported differences between groups of patients who have sustained mTBIs versus healthy control subjects on DTI within the first 3 months postinjury (Inglese, Bomsztyk, et al., 2005a; Kumar et al., 2009; Rutgers et al., 2008) and in small groups of patients with chronic problems seen long after their injury (Inglese, Makani, et al., 2005b; Kraus et al., 2007; Lipton et al., 2008; Lipton et al., 2009). In a recent review, Maller and colleagues (2010) noted that microstructural changes in white matter have been identified in frontal–temporal regions, the corpus callosum, and the internal capsule in TBI studies.

For some people the injury appears to represent cellular dysfunction that may or may not lead to permanent cellular damage. In the milder forms of this injury, cellular damage, if present, might be difficult to accurately

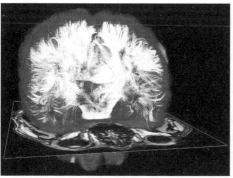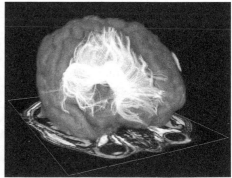

FIGURE 3.2. White matter tracts in the brain and isolated corpus callosum: DTI tractography. Images provided by Burkhard Mädler, PhD, University of Bonn-Medical Center, Cologne Area, Germany.

detect with modern technology for many years to come. Moreover, this possible cellular damage will be difficult to distinguish from preexisting or unrelated cellular damage associated with many other medical problems, psychiatric problems, neurological conditions, substance misuse, or environmental toxins. This will be an ongoing challenge for imaging and neuroscience researchers.

If the brain is temporarily or permanently damaged following an mTBI, does that mean that the person will have obvious and permanent changes in functioning? Fortunately, the natural history of recovery from mTBI is reasonably well understood, most people follow a fairly predictable course, and prognosis is generally favorable. This is discussed in the next section.

Acute Outcome

Our knowledge of the acute pathophysiology of human mTBI is limited due to heavy reliance on animal experimentation, but our knowledge of acute functional outcome is well developed and based on a body of evidence with human subjects. There have been numerous studies, for example, with concussed athletes. A concussion is associated with, and presumably causes, acute and significant changes in physical, psychological, behavioral, and cognitive functioning in some, but not all, injured athletes. Examples of physical symptoms include headaches, disturbed balance, perceived dizziness, hyperacusis, photosensitivity, nausea, and sleep disturbance (insomnia or hypersomnia). These physical, psychological, and cognitive (e.g., concentration and memory difficulty) symptoms are at their worst in the first 72 hours postinjury and rapidly resolve in the majority of athletes over the course of 2 to 30 days. Although the outcome is favorable, the *acute* pathophysiology and functional impairment should not be underestimated or considered benign. This is illustrated in Figure 3.3. These aggregated effect sizes, expressed in pooled and weighted standard deviation units, were derived from meta-analytic reviews of the literature. It is clear from the figure that the acute effects of mTBI are diverse and severe—but fortunately the injury is typically associated with a favorable outcome.

Neuropsychological Outcome

mTBI has an adverse effect on cognition. This has been established, repeatedly, in studies with athletes and civilian trauma patients. As seen in Figure 3.3, the adverse effect of injury on cognition, is pronounced in the initial days postinjury and appears to resolve, in group studies, by 1 to 3 months

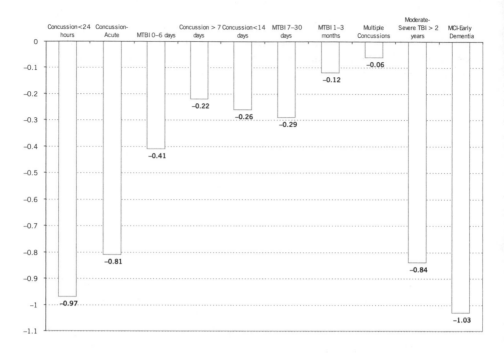

FIGURE 3.3. Meta-analytic effect sizes: Adverse effects on neuropsychological functioning. Effect sizes typically are expressed in pooled, weighted standard deviation units. However, across studies, there are some minor variations in the methods of calculation. For this figure, the overall effect on cognitive or neuropsychological functioning is reported. Effect sizes less than 0.3 should be considered very small and difficult to detect in individual patients because the patient and control groups largely overlap. Sport-related concussion < 24 hours and > 7 days from Belanger and Vanderploeg (2005); concussion-acute and concussion < 14 days from Broglio and Puetz (2008); MTBI 0–6 days, 7–30 days, 1–3 months, moderate–severe > 24 months, all in Schretlen and Shapiro (2003); multiple concussions (Belanger, Spiegel, & Vanderploeg, 2010); and mild cognitive impairment (MCI) or early dementia based on memory testing (Bäckman, Jones, Berger, Laukka, & Small, 2005). From Iverson (2011). Copyright 2010 by Springer Publishing Company. Reprinted by permission.

postinjury (sooner for athletes) (Belanger, Curtiss, Demery, Lebowitz, & Vanderploeg, 2005; Belanger & Vanderploeg, 2005; Binder, 1997; McCrea et al., 2009; Schretlen & Shapiro, 2003). Therefore, for the vast majority of people the vast majority of the time, cognitive deficits should not be present after 6–12 months.

This does not mean, of course, that all patients who sustain an mTBI experience a full and swift recovery of their cognitive functioning. There could be individuals with poor neuropsychological outcome, embedded in past group studies, that get obscured by group statistical analyses (Iverson, 2010). It is possible, although this has not been demonstrated definitively and scientifically, that a small minority of people who sustain mTBIs, especially complicated mTBIs, have some degree of permanent brain damage that is directly causing some degree of permanent impairment in cognition. The problem with establishing brain injury as the sole or primary cause of cognitive diminishment or impairment long after an mTBI is that (1) the literature suggests that this is a low-prevalence condition; (2) it is well established in medicine that low-prevalence conditions can be difficult to identify accurately; (3) numerous preexisting and comorbid physical conditions, medical problems, and emotional problems are associated with cognitive problems (i.e., "all roads lead to cognitive difficulty"); and (4) neuropsychological test results can be influenced by genetic, developmental, medical, emotional, situational, and motivational factors. As such, the identification and quantification of cognitive problems, and the attribution of causation for these problems, often relies more heavily on clinical judgment than empirical evidence.

Conceptualizing the Postconcussion Syndrome

The fourth edition of the *Diagnostic and Statistical Manual of Mental Disorders* (DSM-IV; American Psychiatric Association, 1994) and the 10th edition of the *International Classification of Diseases* (ICD-10; World Health Organization, 1992) include diagnostic criteria for postconcussion syndrome (PCS), although the DSM-IV does not recognize PCS as a mental disorder and instead addends research criteria. As can be seen in Tables 3.2 and 3.3, there are several differences between the two diagnostic systems. The three biggest differences are that (1) ICD-10 requires symptoms to be present for more than 1 month and DSM-IV requires symptoms to be present for more than 3 months; (2) DSM-IV, but not ICD-10, requires objective evidence of impairment in attention or memory on neuropsychological testing; and (3) DSM-IV, but not ICD-10, requires evidence of impairment in social and/or occupational functioning. These core differences account for why it is more common to meet diagnostic criteria according to ICD-10 versus DSM-IV (Boake et al., 2004; McCauley et al., 2005).

After decades of research, PCS has not been widely accepted as a true neurological, psychiatric, neuropsychiatric, medical, or psychological disorder. Most experienced clinicians and researchers agree that there is a subgroup of people who report ongoing symptoms and problems long after an mTBI. The confusion, disagreement, and lack of consensus relates to what is causing and maintaining the symptoms and problems.

TABLE 3.2. ICD-10 Definition of Postconcussional Syndrome

In 1992, the World Health Organization included research criteria for "postconcussional syndrome" in the ICD-10 (World Health Organization, 1992). According to these criteria, a person must have a history of "head trauma with a loss of consciousness" preceding the onset of symptoms by *a period of up to 4 weeks* and have at least *three of six* symptom categories listed below.

1. Headaches, dizziness, general malaise, excessive fatigue, or noise intolerance
2. Irritability, emotional lability, depression, or anxiety
3. Subjective complaints of concentration or memory difficulty
4. Insomnia
5. Reduced tolerance to alcohol
6. Preoccupation with these symptoms and fear of permanent brain damage

> The syndrome occurs following head trauma (usually sufficiently severe to result in loss of consciousness) and includes a number of disparate symptoms such as headache, dizziness (usually lacking the features of true vertigo), fatigue, irritability, difficulty in concentrating and performing mental tasks, impairment of memory, insomnia, and reduced tolerance to stress, emotional excitement, or alcohol. These symptoms may be accompanied by feelings of depression or anxiety, resulting from some loss of self-esteem and fear of permanent brain damage. Such feelings enhance the original symptoms and a vicious circle results. Some patients become hypochondriacal, embark on a search for diagnosis and cure, and may adopt a permanent sick role. The etiology of these symptoms is not always clear, and both organic and psychological factors have been proposed to account for them. The nosological status of this condition is thus somewhat uncertain. There is little doubt, however, that this syndrome is common and distressing to the patient. Diagnostic Guidelines: At least three of the features described above should be present for a definite diagnosis. Careful evaluation with laboratory techniques (electroencephalography, brain stem evoked potentials, brain imaging, oculonystagmography) may yield objective evidence to substantiate the symptoms but results are often negative. The complaints are not necessarily associated with compensation motives. (World Health Organization, 1992, section F07.2)

TABLE 3.3. DSM-IV Definition of Postconcussional Disorder

The DSM-IV has "research criteria" for the "postconcussional disorder." According to these criteria, the individual with a history of head trauma must show *objective evidence* on neuropsychological testing of declines in cognitive functioning, such as attention, concentration, learning, or memory. The person must also report three or more subjective symptoms, present for at least 3 months, from the list below.

1. Becoming fatigued easily
2. Disordered sleep
3. Headache
4. Vertigo or dizziness
5. Irritability or aggression on little or no provocation
6. Anxiety, depression, or affective liability
7. Changes in personality (e.g., social or sexual inappropriateness)
8. Apathy or lack of spontaneity

Nonspecificity Conundrum

It is now well understood that PCS is a nonspecific cluster of symptoms that can be mimicked by a number of preexisting or comorbid conditions. Moreover, healthy adults report very similar symptoms because headaches, sleep difficulty, irritability, and memory failures are relatively common in daily life (Gouvier, Uddo-Crane, & Brown, 1988; Iverson & Lange, 2003; Machulda, Bergquist, Ito, & Chew, 1998; Mittenberg, DiGiulio, Perrin, & Bass, 1992; Sawchyn, Brulot, & Strauss, 2000; Trahan, Ross, & Trahan, 2001; Wong, Regennitter, & Barrios, 1994). In fact, Iverson and Lange (2003) reported that 72–79% of healthy adults reported experiencing, *at mild or greater severity*, three or more symptoms comprising PCS according to the criteria in DSM-IV or ICD-10. Based on reporting symptoms as *moderate to severe*, a significant minority of subjects met DSM-IV (14.6%) or ICD-10 (12.5%) self-report criteria for PCS. Thus, in this study the prevalence of PCS in healthy uninjured adults was comparable to or greater than the estimated prevalence of the syndrome in people with a history of mTBI.

Post-concussion-like symptoms are very common in clinical groups. Researchers have reported high rates of these symptoms in outpatients seen for psychological treatment (Fox, Lees-Haley, Ernest, & Dolezal-Wood, 1995), outpatients with minor medical problems (Lees-Haley & Brown, 1993), personal injury litigants (Dunn, Lees-Haley, Brown, Williams, & English, 1995; Lees-Haley & Brown, 1993), and individuals with post-traumatic stress disorder (PTSD) (Foa, Cashman, Jaycox, & Perry, 1997), orthopedic injuries (Mickeviciene et al., 2004), chronic pain (Gasquoine, 2000; Iverson & McCracken, 1997; Radanov, Dvorak, & Valach, 1992; Smith-Seemiller, Fow, Kant, & Franzen, 2003), and whiplash (Sullivan, Hall, Bartolacci, Sullivan, & Adams, 2002). As described by Otis, Fortier, and Keane (Chapter 6, this volume), chronic pain can also mimic PCS (Gasquoine, 2000; Iverson & McCracken, 1997; Smith-Seemiller et al., 2003).

Anxiety Disorders and Somatic Preoccupation

According to the ICD-10 diagnostic criteria for PCS, symptoms following an mTBI "may be accompanied by feelings of depression or anxiety, resulting from some loss of self-esteem and fear of permanent brain damage. Such feelings enhance the original symptoms and a vicious circle results. Some patients become hypochondriacal, embark on a search for diagnosis and cure, and may adopt a permanent sick role" (World Health Organization, 1992, section F07.2). Clinicians working with symptomatic patients are acutely aware that anxiety, and fear of permanent brain damage, can be prominent psychological features. Moreover, exacerbation of preinjury anxiety problems in people who sustain an mTBI is commonly seen in clinical settings.

Anxiety-related problems and disorders can underlie post-concussion-like symptoms. Anxiety disorders diagnosed in people who have sustained brain injuries include generalized anxiety disorder, panic disorder, obsessive–compulsive disorder, specific phobias (e.g., driving), and PTSD (Warden & Labbate, 2005). Symptoms of stress and anxiety occur frequently in patients who are symptomatic beyond a few weeks postinjury. In a prospective study, Ponsford and colleagues (2000) reported that patients who were symptomatic at 3 months postinjury were likely to have high levels of stress and anxiety. In addition, patients with PTSD often report the same symptoms as patients who have sustained mTBIs. For example, in a sample of 128 patients with PTSD, 89% reported irritability, 56% reported memory problems, 92% reported concentration problems, and 90% reported difficulty sleeping (Foa et al., 1997). Therefore, PTSD might underlie post-concussion-like symptom reporting in some people.

Depression

Depression is probably the most challenging diagnostic consideration in regards to poor outcome from mTBI. In fact, for many years I have wondered if the "postconcussion syndrome," as manifested long after injury, is predominantly a depressive disorder (i.e., the syndrome is a depressive condition, with or without marked sadness, in most people). In neuropsychiatry, there is concern that TBIs alter brain physiology, and/or create a psychological burden, precipitating the development of depression. Researchers have reported that people who sustain a TBI are at increased risk for developing depression (Kreutzer, Seel, & Gourley, 2001; Seel et al., 2003), with prevalence rates varying widely (e.g., from 11 to 77%) (e.g., Jorge, Robinson, Starkstein, & Arndt, 1993; Silver, Kramer, Greenwald, & Weissman, 2001; Varney, Martzke, & Roberts, 1987). Rates of depression in the first 3 months following mTBI have ranged from 12 to 44% across studies (Goldstein, Levin, Goldman, Clark, & Altonen, 2001; Horner et al., 2005; Levin et al., 2001; Levin et al., 2005; McCauley et al., 2001; Mooney & Speed, 2001; Parker & Rosenblum, 1996). Causation of depression following TBI of any severity is complex and not well understood.

Researchers have reported that people who suffer TBIs of all severities have higher rates of *preinjury* psychiatric disorders (Bombardier et al., 2010; Chamelian & Feinstein, 2004; Federoff et al., 1992; Hibbard et al., 2004; Jorge et al., 1993), such as depression and substance abuse. It is established in the literature that the number of prior episodes of depression is predictive of the likelihood of developing a future episode of depression. For example, at least 60% of people who have a single episode of major depressive disorder will likely have a second episode, 70% of those who have had two prior episodes will likely have a third, and 90% of those who have had three prior episodes will likely have a fourth (American Psychiatric Association, 2000, p. 372). Therefore, patients with a history of depression, especially those with multiple prior episodes, should be at increased risk for developing depression following brain injury, bodily injury, or significant life stress. Moreover, they would be at increased risk for developing depression, at some point postinjury, but for reasons unrelated to the injury.

It is methodologically and conceptually challenging to study depression following TBI because there is some overlap in the symptoms of depression and that of moderate-to-severe brain injury (e.g., concentration problems, memory problems, irritability, amotivation/apathy, and fatigue), and there is dramatic overlap between the symptoms of depression and those of PCS. This was demonstrated most persuasively in a study involving 64 physician-diagnosed inpatients or outpatients with depression who had independently confirmed diagnoses on the Structured Clinical Interview for DSM-IV (Iverson, 2006b). These research participants completed the British Columbia Postconcussion Symptom Inventory, a 16-item measure designed to assess the frequency and severity of symptoms based on ICD-10 criteria for PCS. Approximately 90% of patients with depression met liberal self-report criteria (i.e., symptoms endorsed as "mild" were included) for a PCS and more than 50% met very conservative symptom criteria for the diagnosis (i.e., all symptoms had to be reported as "moderate–severe").

In summary, depression is a heterogeneous condition. It is theoretically plausible that depression can arise (1) directly or indirectly from the neurobiological consequences of the brain injury; (2) as a psychological reaction to deficits and problems associated with having a brain injury; (3) as a comorbid condition with an anxiety disorder, such as PTSD, chronic pain, and/or insomnia; or (4) a combination of these factors. Of course, depression can also arise *de novo*, incidentally, sometime postinjury—such as in response to life stressors that are unrelated or peripherally related to the original injury. It can also arise as part of a preexisting chronic relapsing and remitting condition.

Expectations, Misattribution, and the Accuracy of Symptom Reporting

The challenge for the clinician is to determine whether self-reported, nonspecific symptoms, long after an injury, are related, partially related, or unrelated to the original injury. In most cases, this can be daunting. Symptom reporting can range from very precise, thorough, dispassionate, and highly accurate, to vague and incomplete. Researchers have reported that symptom reporting can be affected by personality characteristics such as narcissistic, avoidant, dependent, and borderline personality traits (Evered, Ruff, Baldo, & Isomura, 2003; Greiffenstein & Baker, 2001; Hibbard et al., 2000; Kay, Newman, Cavallo, Ezrachi, & Resnick, 1992). Symptoms and problems can be minimized and underreported by people who are stoic. Symptoms can also be amplified, exaggerated, and overreported by people with histrionic or hypochondriacal personality characteristics. Patients sometimes report past, mostly resolved symptoms, as if they were still a significant problem (i.e., false imputation), and some people exaggerate or fabricate symptoms and problems for financial gain.

A number of social psychological factors can influence a person's perception and reporting of symptoms. The "nocebo effect" is a psychological phenomenon by which a person develops symptom expectations after experiencing a negative event, such as serious illness or injury. As such, the expectation of symptoms associated with injury can cause or magnify the perception of these symptoms. This has been conceptualized as "expectation as etiology" in regards to symptom reporting following head trauma (Ferguson, Mittenberg, Barone, & Schneider, 1999; Gunstad & Suhr, 2001; Mittenberg et al., 1992). When a person *expects* to have symptoms, and *worries* about having symptoms, this can magnify the experience of symptoms and ascribe an emotional valence to them, which can further magnify the symptoms and reinforce the belief system that they are all caused by brain damage (not due in whole or in part to misattributions). In other words, symptoms such as fatigue, difficulty concentrating, or having memory failures—all common in daily life—can be magnified by an emotional reaction to them and by misattributing them to brain damage.

People who sustain mTBIs and are slow to recover might experience biased and inaccurate recall of how they felt and functioned *prior* to injury. They might overestimate their cognitive functioning and underestimate how often they experienced fatigue, irritability, headaches, difficulty concentrating, and memory lapses. This biased recall creates a greater distinction between pre- and postinjury functioning, reinforcing a belief system that the person has greater symptoms and deficits relative to the past than is actually the case. Researchers have termed this social psychological phenomenon the "good old days" bias (Gunstad & Suhr, 2001). In some studies, patients with back injuries, general trauma victims, and patients who have sustained mTBIs appear to overestimate the actual degree of change that has taken place postinjury, in part by retrospectively recalling fewer preinjury symptoms than are typically reported in healthy adults (Davis, 2002; Gunstad & Suhr, 2001, 2004; Hilsabeck, Gouvier, & Bolter, 1998;

Mittenberg et al., 1992). In two recent studies, individuals who were seen in early intervention programs for mTBI retrospectively recalled having fewer symptoms in their daily life prior to their injuries than are typically reported by the general public (Iverson, Lange, Brooks, & Rennison, 2010; Lange, Iverson, & Rose, 2010). In a study of workers' compensation claimants, the good old days bias was much more pronounced in workers who failed effort testing than those who passed effort testing (Iverson, Lange, et al., 2010). This, of course, raises the possibility that for some people recall bias might simply represent deliberate misrepresentation to create the impression of greater impairment or disability than is actually the case (see Elhai, Sweet, Guidotti, Breting, & Kaloupek, Chapter 9, this volume for an in-depth discussion of symptom validity).

Contextual and Methodological Factors

The context of the injury and evaluation may also determine how a patient presents clinically, at times making it difficult to discern the patient's actual functioning from the patient's depiction of his or her functioning. For example, as summarized by Elhai et al. (Chapter 9, this volume), evaluations conducted for workers compensation, personal injury litigation, civilian disability insurance, or military service-connected disability can be seriously confounded by exaggeration of symptoms and poor effort on cognitive testing. Moreover, patients often endorse more symptoms on psychological tests and questionnaires than during a clinical interview (Iverson, Brooks, Ashton, & Lange, 2010). There are several possible reasons for this, including the dynamics of the doctor–patient relationship, the thoroughness of a clinician approach to the interview, questionnaires serving to prompt a patient about a diverse range of symptoms that are not covered in the interview, and possible overendorsement tendencies on questionnaires. Thus, both the context of the evaluation and the methodology employed by the clinician can influence the probability of diagnosis.

Conclusions

mTBIs are heterogeneous. The injury falls on a broad spectrum of pathophysiology, from very mild neurometabolic changes in the brain with rapid recovery to permanent problems due to structural brain damage. Most definitions of mTBI include "complicated" injuries (injuries characterized by a depressed skull fracture, intracranial abnormality, or both). In other words, the mTBI spectrum is so broad that it encompasses injuries involving feeling temporarily dazed and being asymptomatic in a few hours to injuries involving loss of consciousness for 5 minutes, PTA for 12 hours, and a contusion visible on the day-of-injury CT scan.

Neuropsychological outcome from mTBI is reasonably well understood. Mild TBI has an enormous adverse effect on balance, cognitive functioning, and symptoms (e.g., headaches, photosensitivity, and perceived dizziness) in the first 24 hours postinjury. There is considerable evidence that neurocognitive deficits typically are not seen in athletes after 1–4 weeks and in trauma patients after 1–3 months in prospective group studies.

Anxiety, depression, and somatic preoccupation are relatively common following mTBI. Symptoms of anxiety and depression can mimic the PCS because many of the symptoms are nearly identical in these conditions. In fact, the "PCS," as manifested long after injury, might be a depressive disorder in many people (i.e., the syndrome is a depressive condition, with or without marked sadness). The etiology of the *persistent* PCS has never been agreed upon, and the validity of this diagnosis as a true syndrome or disorder continues to be questioned. The syndrome is a nonspecific cluster of symptoms that can be mimicked by a number of preexisting or comorbid conditions. A TBI-induced syndrome, theoretically, also can occur in tandem with these preexisting or comorbid conditions. Therefore, it is imperative for clinicians to systematically evaluate the possible contribution of many preexisting factors, differential diagnoses, comorbidities, and social-psychological factors that may *cause or maintain* self-reported symptoms after this injury (Figure 3.1). An injury to the head or brain is not necessary (and often not sufficient) to produce the constellation of symptoms and problems that comprise this syndrome.

Unfortunately, confusion, disagreement, and lack of consensus regarding poor outcome from mTBI fuels controversy, advocacy, disbelief, and frustration among patients, clinicians, third parties, and researchers. This can lead, unfortunately, to patients not receiving adequate treatment and rehabilitation services. Many of the treatment and rehabilitation approaches that are effective for traumatic stress, depression, and chronic pain can be adapted for use with individuals who have symptoms and problems that are believed to be partially or largely related to an mTBI. If we focus on treating what is treatable, we will reduce suffering and improve functioning in those who have poor outcome following this injury.

In reality, a tremendous amount is known about poor outcome following mTBI. What is known reinforces the idea that seeking a simplistic explanation regarding poor outcome is unrealistic and untenable. Poor outcome following mTBI has always been, and will continue to be, a source of interest, challenge, and frustration for patients, families, clinicians, researchers, insurance companies, trial lawyers, and governments. Occam's razor suggests that the simplest explanation is usually the best explanation. Parsimony pervades the foundations of science and medicine. Parsimonious scientific evidence established through good methodology and replication is usually considered persuasive. However, poor outcome following mTBI defies parsimonious explanation. The only reasonable approach to understanding poor outcome from mTBI is a biopsychosocial perspective. This perspective, by necessity, embraces a multifactorial, interwoven, biopsychosocial conceptualization of poor outcome from this injury.

Author Note

The views expressed in this chapter are those of the author and do not reflect the official policy of the Department of Defense or the United States Government.

References

American Psychiatric Association. (1994). *Diagnostic and statistical manual of mental disorders* (4th ed.). Washington, DC: Author.

American Psychiatric Association. (2000). *Diagnostic and statistical manual of mental disorders* (4th ed., text rev.). Washington, DC: Author.

Bäckman, L., Jones, S., Berger, A. K., Laukka, E. J., & Small, B. J. (2005). Cognitive impairment in preclinical Alzheimer's disease: A meta-analysis. *Neuropsychology, 19*(4), 520–531.

Belanger, H. G., Curtiss, G., Demery, J. A., Lebowitz, B. K., & Vanderploeg, R. D. (2005). Factors moderating neuropsychological outcomes following mild traumatic brain injury: A meta-analysis. *Journal of the International Neuropsychological Society, 11*(3), 215–227.

Belanger, H. G., Spiegel, E., & Vanderploeg, R. D. (2010). Neuropsychological performance following a history of multiple self-reported concussions: A meta-analysis. *Journal of the International Neuropsychological Society, 16*(2), 262–267.

Belanger, H. G., & Vanderploeg, R. D. (2005). The neuropsychological impact of sports-related concussion: A meta-analysis. *Journal of the International Neuropsychological Society, 11*(4), 345–357.

Binder, E. B., & Nemeroff, C. B. (2009). The CRF system, stress, depression and anxiety—Insights from human genetic studies. *Molecular Psychiatry.*

Binder, L. M. (1997). A review of mild head trauma: Part II. Clinical implications. *Journal of Clinical and Experimental Neuropsychology, 19*(3), 432–457.

Boake, C., McCauley, S. R., Levin, H. S., Contant, C. F., Song, J. X., Brown, S. A., et al. (2004). Limited agreement between criteria-based diagnoses of postconcussional syndrome. *Journal of Neuropsychiatry and Clinical Neurosciences, 16*(4), 493–499.

Bombardier, C. H., Fann, J. R., Temkin, N. R., Esselman, P. C., Barber, J., & Dikmen, S. S. (2010). Rates of major depressive disorder and clinical outcomes following traumatic brain injury. *Journal of the American Medical Association, 303*(19), 1938–1945.

Bradley, R. G., Binder, E. B., Epstein, M. P., Tang, Y., Nair, H. P., Liu, W., et al. (2008). Influence of child abuse on adult depression: Moderation by the corticotropin-releasing hormone receptor gene. *Archives of General Psychiatry, 65*(2), 190–200.

Broglio, S. P., & Puetz, T. W. (2008). The effect of sport concussion on neurocognitive function, self-report symptoms and postural control: A meta-analysis. *Sports Medicine, 38*(1), 53–67.

Carroll, L. J., Cassidy, J. D., Holm, L., Kraus, J., & Coronado, V. G. (2004). Methodological issues and research recommendations for mild traumatic brain injury: The WHO Collaborating Centre Task Force on Mild Traumatic Brain Injury. *Journal of Rehabilitation Medicine, 43*, 113–125.

Chamelian, L., & Feinstein, A. (2004). Outcome after mild to moderate traumatic brain injury: The role of dizziness. *Archives of Physical Medicine and Rehabilitation, 85*(10), 1662–1666.

Davis, C. H. (2002). Self-perception in mild traumatic brain injury. *American Journal of Physical Medicine and Rehabilitation, 81*(8), 609–621.

Dunn, J. T., Lees-Haley, P. R., Brown, R. S., Williams, C. W., & English, L. T. (1995). Neurotoxic complaint base rates of personal injury claimants: Implications for neuropsychological assessment. *Journal of Clinical Psychology, 51*(4), 577–584.

Evered, L., Ruff, R., Baldo, J., & Isomura, A. (2003). Emotional risk factors and postconcussional disorder. *Assessment, 10*(4), 420–427.

Farmer, A. E., & McGuffin, P. (2003). Humiliation, loss and other types of life events and difficulties: A comparison of depressed subjects, healthy controls and their siblings. *Psychological Medicine, 33*(7), 1169–1175.

Feder, A., Nestler, E. J., & Charney, D. S. (2009). Psychobiology and molecular genetics of resilience. *Nature Reviews, Neuroscience, 10*(6), 446–457.

Federoff, J. P., Starkstein, S. E., Forrester, A. W., Geisler, F. H., Jorge, R. E., Arndt, S., et al. (1992). Depression in patients with acute traumatic brain injury. *American Journal of Psychiatry, 149*, 918–923.

Ferguson, R. J., Mittenberg, W., Barone, D. F., & Schneider, B. (1999). Postconcussion syndrome following sports-related head injury: Expectation as etiology. *Neuropsychology, 13*(4), 582–589.

Foa, E. B., Cashman, L., Jaycox, L., & Perry, K. (1997). The validation of a self-report measure of posttraumatic stress disorder: The Posttraumatic Diagnostic Scale. *Psychological Assessment, 9*(4), 445–451.

Fox, D. D., Lees-Haley, P. R., Ernest, K., & Dolezal-Wood, S. (1995). Postconcussive symptoms: Base rates and etiology in psychiatric patients. *Clinical Neuropsychologist, 9*, 89–92.

Friis, R. H., Wittchen, H. U., Pfister, H., & Lieb, R. (2002). Life events and changes in the course of depression in young adults. *European Psychiatry, 17*(5), 241–253.

Gasquoine, P. G. (2000). Postconcussional symptoms in chronic back pain. *Applied Neuropsychology, 7*(2), 83–89.

Gatt, J. M., Nemeroff, C. B., Dobson-Stone, C., Paul, R. H., Bryant, R. A., Schofield, P. R., et al. (2009). Interactions between BDNF Val66Met polymorphism and early life stress predict brain and arousal pathways to syndromal depression and anxiety. *Molecular Psychiatry, 14*(7), 681–695.

Goldstein, F. C., Levin, H. S., Goldman, W. P., Clark, A. N., & Altonen, T. K. (2001). Cognitive and neurobehavioral functioning after mild versus moderate traumatic brain injury in older adults. *Journal of the International Neuropsychological Society, 7*(3), 373–383.

Gouvier, W. D., Uddo-Crane, M., & Brown, L. M. (1988). Base rates of postconcussional symptoms. *Archives of Clinical Neuropsychology, 3,* 273–278.

Greiffenstein, F. M., & Baker, J. W. (2001). Comparison of premorbid and postinjury mmpi-2 profiles in late postconcussion claimants. *Clinical Neuropsychologist, 15*(2), 162–170.

Gunstad, J., & Suhr, J. A. (2001). "Expectation as etiology" versus "the good old days": Postconcussion syndrome symptom reporting in athletes, headache sufferers, and depressed individuals. *Journal of the International Neuropsychological Society, 7*(3), 323–333.

Gunstad, J., & Suhr, J. A. (2004). Cognitive factors in postconcussion syndrome symptom report. *Archives of Clinical Neuropsychology, 19*(3), 391–405.

Hauger, R. L., Risbrough, V., Oakley, R. H., Olivares-Reyes, J. A., & Dautzenberg, F. M. (2009). Role of CRF receptor signaling in stress vulnerability, anxiety, and depression. *Annals of the New York Academy of Sciences, 1179,* 120–143.

Heim, C., Bradley, B., Mletzko, T. C., Deveau, T. C., Musselman, D. L., Nemeroff, C. B., et al. (2009). Effect of childhood trauma on adult depression and neuroendocrine function: Sex-specific moderation by CRH receptor 1 gene. *Frontiers in Behavioral Neuroscience, 3,* 1–10.

Heim, C., Newport, D. J., Mletzko, T., Miller, A. H., & Nemeroff, C. B. (2008). The link between childhood trauma and depression: Insights from HPA axis studies in humans. *Psychoneuroendocrinology, 33*(6), 693–710.

Hibbard, M. R., Ashman, T. A., Spielman, L. A., Chun, D., Charatz, H. J., & Melvin, S. (2004). Relationship between depression and psychosocial functioning after traumatic brain injury. *Archives of Physical Medicine and Rehabilitation, 85*(4, Suppl. 2), S43–S53.

Hibbard, M. R., Bogdany, J., Uysal, S., Kepler, K., Silver, J. M., Gordon, W. A., et al. (2000). Axis II psychopathology in individuals with traumatic brain injury. *Brain Injury, 14*(1), 45–61.

Hilsabeck, R. C., Gouvier, W. D., & Bolter, J. F. (1998). Reconstructive memory bias in recall of neuropsychological symptomatology. *Journal of Clinical and Experimental Neuropsychology, 20*(3), 328–338.

Hofman, P. A., Stapert, S. Z., van Kroonenburgh, M. J., Jolles, J., de Kruijk, J., & Wilmink, J. T. (2001). MR imaging, single-photon emission CT, and neurocognitive performance after mild traumatic brain injury. *American Journal of Neuroradiology, 22*(3), 441–449.

Hoge, E. A., Austin, E. D., & Pollack, M. H. (2007). Resilience: Research evidence and conceptual considerations for posttraumatic stress disorder. *Depression and Anxiety, 24*(2), 139–152.

Horner, M. D., Ferguson, P. L., Selassie, A. W., Labbate, L. A., Kniele, K., &

Corrigan, J. D. (2005). Patterns of alcohol use 1 year after traumatic brain injury: A population-based, epidemiological study. *Journal of the International Neuropsychological Society, 11*(3), 322–330.

Hughes, D. G., Jackson, A., Mason, D. L., Berry, E., Hollis, S., & Yates, D. W. (2004). Abnormalities on magnetic resonance imaging seen acutely following mild traumatic brain injury: Correlation with neuropsychological tests and delayed recovery. *Neuroradiology, 46*(7), 550–558.

Inglese, M., Bomsztyk, E., Gonen, O., Mannon, L. J., Grossman, R. I., & Rusinek, H. (2005). Dilated perivascular spaces: Hallmarks of mild traumatic brain injury. *American Journal of Neuroradiology, 26*(4), 719–724.

Inglese, M., Makani, S., Johnson, G., Cohen, B. A., Silver, J. A., Gonen, O., et al. (2005). Diffuse axonal injury in mild traumatic brain injury: A diffusion tensor imaging study. *Journal of Neurosurgery, 103*(2), 298–303.

Iverson, G. L. (2006a). Complicated vs uncomplicated mild traumatic brain injury: Acute neuropsychological outcome. *Brain Injury, 20*(13–14), 1335–1344.

Iverson, G. L. (2006b). Misdiagnosis of persistent postconcussion syndrome in patients with depression. *Archives of Clinical Neuropsychology, 21*(4), 303–310.

Iverson, G. L. (2010). Mild traumatic brain injury meta-analyses can obscure individual differences. *Brain Injury, 24*(10), 1246–1255.

Iverson, G. L. (2011). Evidence-based neuropsychological assessment of sport-related concussion. In F. M. Webbe (Ed.), *Handbook of sport neuropsychology* (pp. 131–154). New York: Springer.

Iverson, G. L., Brooks, B. L., Ashton, V. L., & Lange, R. T. (2010). Interview vs. questionnaire symptom reporting in people with post-concussion syndrome. *Journal of Head Trauma Rehabilitation, 25*(1), 25–30.

Iverson, G. L., & Lange, R. T. (2003). Examination of "postconcussion-like" symptoms in a healthy sample. *Applied Neuropsychology, 10*(3), 137–144.

Iverson, G. L., Lange, R. T., Brooks, B. L., & Rennison, V. L. (2010). "Good old days" bias following mild traumatic brain injury. *Clinical Neuropsychologist, 24*(1), 17–37.

Iverson, G. L., & McCracken, L. M. (1997). "Postconcussive" symptoms in persons with chronic pain. *Brain Injury, 11*(11), 783–790.

Jorge, R. E., Robinson, R. G., Starkstein, S. E., & Arndt, S. V. (1993). Depression and anxiety following traumatic brain injury. *Journal of Neuropsychiatry and Clinical Neurosciences, 5*(4), 369–374.

Kay, T., Newman, B., Cavallo, M., Ezrachi, O., & Resnick, M. (1992). Toward a neuropsychological model of functional disability after mild traumatic brain injury. *Neuropsychology, 6*(4), 371–384.

Kendler, K. S., Hettema, J. M., Butera, F., Gardner, C. O., & Prescott, C. A. (2003). Life event dimensions of loss, humiliation, entrapment, and danger in the prediction of onsets of major depression and generalized anxiety. *Archives of General Psychiatry, 60*(8), 789–796.

Kendler, K. S., Karkowski, L. M., & Prescott, C. A. (1999). Causal relationship between stressful life events and the onset of major depression. *American Journal of Psychiatry, 156*(6), 837–841.

Kendler, K. S., Thornton, L. M., & Gardner, C. O. (2000). Stressful life events and previous episodes in the etiology of major depression in women: An evaluation of the "kindling" hypothesis. *American Journal of Psychiatry, 157*(8), 1243–1251.

Kendler, K. S., Thornton, L. M., & Gardner, C. O. (2001). Genetic risk, number of previous depressive episodes, and stressful life events in predicting onset of major depression. *American Journal of Psychiatry, 158*(4), 582–586.

Kraus, M. F., Susmaras, T., Caughlin, B. P., Walker, C. J., Sweeney, J. A., & Little, D. M. (2007). White matter integrity and cognition in chronic traumatic brain injury: A diffusion tensor imaging study. *Brain, 130*(Pt. 10), 2508–2519.

Kreutzer, J. S., Seel, R. T., & Gourley, E. (2001). The prevalence and symptom rates of depression after traumatic brain injury: A comprehensive examination. *Brain Injury, 15*(7), 563–576.

Kumar, R., Gupta, R. K., Husain, M., Chaudhry, C., Srivastava, A., Saksena, S., et al. (2009). Comparative evaluation of corpus callosum DTI metrics in acute mild and moderate traumatic brain injury: Its correlation with neuropsychometric tests. *Brain Injury, 23*(7), 675–685.

Lange, R. T., Iverson, G. L., & Franzen, M. D. (2009). Neuropsychological functioning following complicated vs. uncomplicated mild traumatic brain injury. *Brain Injury, 23*(2), 83–91.

Lange, R. T., Iverson, G. L., & Rose, A. (2010). Post-concussion symptom reporting and the "good-old-days" bias following mild traumatic brain injury. *Archives of Clinical Neuropsychology, 25*(5), 442–450.

Lees-Haley, P. R., & Brown, R. S. (1993). Neuropsychological complaint base rates of 170 personal injury claimants. *Archives of Clinical Neuropsychology, 8*(3), 203–209.

Levin, H. S., Brown, S. A., Song, J. X., McCauley, S. R., Boake, C., Contant, C. F., et al. (2001). Depression and posttraumatic stress disorder at three months after mild to moderate traumatic brain injury. *Journal of Clinical and Experimental Neuropsychology, 23*(6), 754–769.

Levin, H. S., McCauley, S. R., Josic, C. P., Boake, C., Brown, S. A., Goodman, H. S., et al. (2005). Predicting depression following mild traumatic brain injury. *Archives of General Psychiatry, 62*(5), 523–528.

Lipton, M. L., Gellella, E., Lo, C., Gold, T., Ardekani, B. A., Shifteh, K., et al. (2008). Multifocal white matter ultrastructural abnormalities in mild traumatic brain injury with cognitive disability: A voxel-wise analysis of diffusion tensor imaging. *Journal of Neurotrauma, 25*(11), 1335–1342.

Lipton, M. L., Gulko, E., Zimmerman, M. E., Friedman, B. W., Kim, M., Gellella, E., et al. (2009). Diffusion-tensor imaging implicates prefrontal axonal injury in executive function impairment following very mild traumatic brain injury. *Radiology, 252*(3), 816–824.

Machulda, M. M., Bergquist, T. F., Ito, V., & Chew, S. (1998). Relationship between stress, coping, and post concussion symptoms in a healthy adult population. *Archives of Clinical Neuropsychology, 13*, 415–424.

Maller, J. J., Thomson, R. H., Lewis, P. M., Rose, S. E., Pannek, K., & Fitzgerald, P. B. (2010). Traumatic brain injury, major depression, and diffusion tensor imaging: Making connections. *Brain Research Reviews, 64*(1), 213–240.

McCauley, S. R., Boake, C., Levin, H. S., Contant, C. F., & Song, J. X. (2001).

Postconcussional disorder following mild to moderate traumatic brain injury: Anxiety, depression, and social support as risk factors and comorbidities. *Journal of Clinical and Experimental Neuropsychology, 23*(6), 792–808.

McCauley, S. R., Boake, C., Pedroza, C., Brown, S. A., Levin, H. S., Goodman, H. S., et al. (2005). Postconcussional disorder: Are the DSM-IV criteria an improvement over the ICD-10? *Journal of Nervous and Mental Disease, 193*(8), 540–550.

McCrea, M., Iverson, G. L., McAllister, T. W., Hammeke, T. A., Powell, M. R., Barr, W. B., et al. (2009). An integrated review of recovery after mild traumatic brain injury (MTBI): Implications for clinical management. *Clinical Neuropsychologist, 23*(8), 1368–1390.

McGuffin, P., Knight, J., Breen, G., Brewster, S., Boyd, P. R., Craddock, N., et al. (2005). Whole genome linkage scan of recurrent depressive disorder from the depression network study. *Human Molecular Genetics, 14*(22), 3337–3345.

Mickeviciene, D., Schrader, H., Obelieniene, D., Surkiene, D., Kunickas, R., Stovner, L. J., et al. (2004). A controlled prospective inception cohort study on the post-concussion syndrome outside the medicolegal context. *European Journal of Neurology, 11*(6), 411–419.

Mild Traumatic Brain Injury Committee, A. C. o. R. M., Head Injury Interdisciplinary Special Interest Group. (1993). Definition of mild traumatic brain injury. *Journal of Head Trauma Rehabilitation, 8*(3), 86–87.

Mittenberg, W., DiGiulio, D. V., Perrin, S., & Bass, A. E. (1992). Symptoms following mild head injury: Expectation as aetiology. *Journal of Neurology, Neurosurgery and Psychiatry, 55*, 200–204.

Monroe, S. M., & Harkness, K. L. (2005). Life stress, the "kindling" hypothesis, and the recurrence of depression: Considerations from a life stress perspective. *Psychological Review, 112*(2), 417–445.

Mooney, G., & Speed, J. (2001). The association between mild traumatic brain injury and psychiatric conditions. *Brain Injury, 15*(10), 865–877.

National Center for Injury Prevention and Control. (2003). *Report to congress on mild traumatic brain injury in the United States: Steps to prevent a serious public health problem.* Atlanta, GA: Centers for Disease Control and Prevention.

Parker, R. S., & Rosenblum, A. (1996). IQ loss and emotional dysfunctions after mild head injury incurred in a motor vehicle accident. *Journal of Clinical Psychology, 52*(1), 32–43.

Ponsford, J., Willmott, C., Rothwell, A., Cameron, P., Kelly, A. M., Nelms, R., et al. (2000). Factors influencing outcome following mild traumatic brain injury in adults. *Journal of the International Neuropsychological Society, 6*(5), 568–579.

Radanov, B. P., Dvorak, J., & Valach, L. (1992). Cognitive deficits in patients after soft tissue injury of the cervical spine. *Spine, 17*(2), 127–131.

Ruff, R. M., Iverson, G. L., Barth, J. T., Bush, S. S., & Broshek, D. K. (2009). Recommendations for diagnosing a mild traumatic brain injury: A National Academy of Neuropsychology education paper. *Archives of Clinical Neuropsychology, 24*(1), 3–10.

Rutgers, D. R., Fillard, P., Paradot, G., Tadie, M., Lasjaunias, P., & Ducreux, D. (2008). Diffusion tensor imaging characteristics of the corpus callosum in mild, moderate, and severe traumatic brain injury. *American Journal of Neuroradiology, 29*(9), 1730–1735.

Sawchyn, J. M., Brulot, M. M., & Strauss, E. (2000). Note on the use of the Post-concussion Syndrome Checklist. *Archives of Clinical Neuropsychology, 15*, 1–8.

Schretlen, D. J., & Shapiro, A. M. (2003). A quantitative review of the effects of traumatic brain injury on cognitive functioning. *International Review of Psychiatry, 15*(4), 341–349.

Seel, R. T., Kreutzer, J. S., Rosenthal, M., Hammond, F. M., Corrigan, J. D., & Black, K. (2003). Depression after traumatic brain injury: A National Institute on Disability and Rehabilitation Research Model Systems multicenter investigation. *Archives of Physical Medicine and Rehabilitation, 84*(2), 177–184.

Silver, J. M., Kramer, R., Greenwald, S., & Weissman, M. (2001). The association between head injuries and psychiatric disorders: Findings from the New Haven NIMH Epidemiologic Catchment Area Study. *Brain Injury, 15*(11), 935–945.

Smith-Seemiller, L., Fow, N. R., Kant, R., & Franzen, M. D. (2003). Presence of post-concussion syndrome symptoms in patients with chronic pain vs. mild traumatic brain injury. *Brain Injury, 17*(3), 199–206.

Southwick, S. M., Vythilingam, M., & Charney, D. S. (2005). The psychobiology of depression and resilience to stress: Implications for prevention and treatment. *Annual Review of Clinical Psychology, 1*, 255–291.

Sullivan, M. J., Hall, E., Bartolacci, R., Sullivan, M. E., & Adams, H. (2002). Perceived cognitive deficits, emotional distress and disability following whiplash injury. *Pain Research and Management, 7*(3), 120–126.

Sullivan, P. F., Neale, M. C., & Kendler, K. S. (2000). Genetic epidemiology of major depression: Review and meta-analysis. *American Journal of Psychiatry, 157*(10), 1552–1562.

Symonds, C. P. (1937). The assessment of symptoms following head injury. *Guys Hospital Gazette, 51*, 461–468.

Temkin, N. R., Machamer, J. E., & Dikmen, S. S. (2003). Correlates of functional status 3–5 years after traumatic brain injury with CT abnormalities. *Journal of Neurotrauma, 20*(3), 229–241.

Trahan, D. E., Ross, C. E., & Trahan, S. L. (2001). Relationships among postconcussional-type symptoms, depression, and anxiety in neurologically normal young adults and victims of brain injury. *Archives of Clinical Neuropsychology, 16*, 435–445.

van der Naalt, J., Hew, J. M., van Zomeren, A. H., Sluiter, W. J., & Minderhoud, J. M. (1999). Computed tomography and magnetic resonance imaging in mild to moderate head injury: Early and late imaging related to outcome. *Annals of Neurology, 46*(1), 70–78.

Varney, N., Martzke, J., & Roberts, R. (1987). Major depression in patients with closed head injury. *Neuropsychology, 1*, 7–8.

Warden, D. L., & Labbate, L. A. (2005). Posttraumatic stress disorder and other anxiety disorders. In J. M. Silver., T. W. McAllister. & S. C. Yudofsky (Eds.), *Textbook of traumatic brain injury* (pp. 231–243). Arlington, VA: American Psychiatric Publishing.

Williams, D. H., Levin, H. S., & Eisenberg, H. M. (1990). Mild head injury classification. *Neurosurgery, 27*(3), 422–428.

Wilson, J. T. L., Hadley, D. M., Scott, L. C., & Harper, A. (1996). Neuropsychological significance of contusional lesions identified by MRI. In B. P. Uzzell & H. H. Stonnington (Eds.), *Recovery after traumatic brain injury* (pp. 29–50). Mahwah, NJ: Erlbaum.

Wong, J. L., Regennitter, R. P., & Barrios, F. (1994). Base rate and simulated symptoms of mild head injury among normals. *Archives of Clinical Neuropsychology, 9,* 411–425.

World Health Organization. (1992). *International statistical classification of diseases and related health problems—10th edition.* Geneva, Switzerland: Author.

CHAPTER 4

Understanding Posttraumatic Stress Disorder

Implications for Comorbid Posttraumatic Stress Disorder and Mild Traumatic Brain Injury

Jasmeet Pannu Hayes and Mark W. Gilbertson

Posttraumatic stress disorder (PTSD) can develop after exposure to terrifying and life-threatening events such as warfare, natural disasters, and physical and sexual assault. For individuals suffering from PTSD, memories of the traumatic event may begin to permeate all aspects of life despite attempts to avoid triggers and reminders of the trauma. Previously non-threatening stimuli become potential threats, inducing hyperarousal and hypervigilance. Traumatic memories may become inescapable and impair the individual's ability to maintain close relationships, enjoy pleasurable activities, and make plans for the future. With the rise in global terrorism and military actions underway in Iraq and Afghanistan, the societal impact of PTSD has received even greater attention. However, until recently, little attention had been paid to the public health impact of co-occurring PTSD and traumatic brain injury (TBI) despite the frequency with which traumatic events produce both conditions and the overlap in posttraumatic symptoms. Understanding the course of PTSD and the circumstances involved in developing the disorder may provide a solid knowledge base that will help to characterize signs and symptoms that do or do not overlap with TBI.

The primary goal of this chapter is to provide a broad overview of clinical and research PTSD findings, including the epidemiology of the disorder within the U.S. population, risk and protective factors, and signs and symptoms within the framework of neurobiological theories of PTSD development and maintenance. Finally, we offer concluding remarks that summarize the immense progress made over the last few decades in PTSD research and address potential future directions toward understanding PTSD in the upcoming decade, including how PTSD is best contextualized when mild TBI (mTBI) is also a clinical consideration.

Epidemiology of PTSD

Exposure to traumatic events is quite common in the United States. Between 50 and 60% of the adult U.S. population is exposed to at least one traumatic event at some point in their lifetime (Kessler, Sonnega, Bromet, Hughes, & Nelson, 1995) and in some urban areas, such as Detroit, exposure to traumatic events is substantially higher, at 90% (Breslau et al., 1998). In addition, exposure to multiple traumas is remarkably common. In the National Comorbidity Survey (NCS; Kessler et al., 1995), 56% of all men and 49% of all women who reported trauma exposure had been exposed to more than one traumatic event, while individuals reported exposure to five discrete traumatic events on average in the Detroit Area Survey of Trauma study. The prevalence rate of PTSD is estimated to be 7–8% in the general population (Kessler et al., 1995), although prevalence estimates have varied depending on the type of trauma exposure and demographic characteristics, as described in the subsequent section. For instance, prevalence rates are higher among individuals exposed to military combat. According to the National Vietnam Veterans Readjustment Survey (NVVRS), approximately 30% of male and 27% of female Vietnam-era veterans had lifetime PTSD, with 15% of men and 9% of women having current PTSD (Kulka et al., 1990). A recent reexamination of the NVVRS data utilizing more stringent criteria adjusted the overall lifetime prevalence rate downward to approximately 19% (Dohrenwend et al., 2006). Consistent with this finding, prevalence estimates from more recent wars suggest that between 12 and 20% of veterans of Operation Enduring Freedom (OEF) and Operation Iraqi Freedom (OIF) met diagnostic criteria for PTSD after their return home from combat (Hoge et al., 2004; Tanielian & Jaycox, 2008). In the general population, women tend to have higher prevalence rates of PTSD than men (10.4% compared with 5%, according to the NCS). Men and women are typically exposed to different types of traumas. Men more often report combat, witnessing someone being badly hurt or killed, and accidents as being their worst traumas, whereas women more often report rape, sexual molestation, and physical abuse as their most upsetting traumatic event (Kessler et al., 1995).

Traumatic events associated with PTSD are often also associated with TBI. The most common events that cause TBI are motor vehicle accidents, assaults, and falls (Bruns & Hauser, 2003), which frequently also lead to PTSD. Among military personnel fighting in the OEF/OIF conflicts, the prevalence rate of comorbid PTSD and TBI is estimated to be approximately 7% (Tanielian & Jaycox, 2008). With the preponderance of improvised explosive devices and other readily available explosive devices in the OEF/OIF conflicts, the prevalence rate of comorbid PTSD and TBI among returning military personnel is likely to rise. It is noteworthy that the physical and psychological symptoms associated with PTSD and TBI symptoms substantially overlap. Individuals with PTSD or TBI often report difficulty with concentration, irritability and anger, sleep disturbance, and fatigue (Stein & McAllister, 2009). As greater numbers of soldiers diagnosed with both PTSD and TBI seek medical treatment, it will become increasingly important for clinicians to assess for TBI within the context of a PTSD evaluation.

Clinical Definition of PTSD

In its current conceptualization, PTSD develops after direct exposure to a Criterion A1 event, defined as an extreme traumatic event that involves actual or threatened death, serious injury, or threat to one's physical integrity; witnessing an event that involves death, serious injury, or threat to the physical integrity of another person; or learning about the death or serious injury of a family member or close friend (DSM-IV-TR; American Psychiatric Association, 2000). In addition, the individual must have responded to the traumatic event with fear, helplessness, or horror (referred to as Criterion A2). The classic signs and symptoms of PTSD can be broadly divided into three symptom clusters. Symptom cluster B involves persistent recollections of the traumatic event, often in the form of distressing dreams and nightmares, intrusive memories of the event, and dissociative flashbacks. Cluster C symptoms involve persistent avoidance of people, places, and activities that serve as reminders of the traumatic event, as well as symptoms of emotional numbing, such as loss of interest in activities that were previously enjoyed, difficulty having a full range of emotions, and altered expectations of one's ability to lead a long, fulfilling life. Although the avoidance and numbing symptoms are placed within the same cluster, there is growing consensus that they may in fact represent two distinct constructs.

Recent studies examining the factor structure of PTSD have supported a four-factor model of PTSD symptoms in which the avoidance symptoms differentiate from the numbing symptoms (Asmundson et al., 2000; King, Leskin, King, & Weathers, 1998; McDonald et al., 2008). These findings may guide future adjustments to the PTSD diagnosis. Symptom cluster D involves symptoms of hyperarousal including difficulty with sleep, irritability and anger, poor concentration, hypervigilance, and exaggerated startle response. To meet criteria for PTSD, symptoms must also be present for more than 1 month (in contrast to acute stress disorder, in which symptoms resolve within 4 weeks of the trauma event), and cause significant distress or impairment in social and occupational functioning.

The typical course of PTSD begins with the development of symptoms within 6 months of the onset of the traumatic event, although delays in symptom occurrence can occur. Individuals who experience symptoms for greater than 3 months are diagnosed with chronic PTSD, which is associated with a host of poor health outcomes, including heart disease, obesity, alcohol abuse, and lowered perceptions of general health (Boscarino, 2008; Dobie et al., 2004; Hoge, Terhakopian, Castro, Messer, & Engel, 2007). A recent study showed that the risk of dementia among U.S. veterans with PTSD was nearly twice that of veterans without PTSD (Yaffe et al., 2010), underscoring the importance of treatment for chronic PTSD.

Importantly, a subset of individuals experience significant traumatic distress that may be of reduced severity. The term "subsyndromal" or "partial" PTSD refers to individuals who suffer from symptoms of PTSD but who do not meet all the criteria. Although defined in different ways, one characterization includes experiencing at least one symptom from each of the B, C, and D cluster symptoms (Stein, Walker, Hazen, & Forde, 1997). Recognizing subsyndromal PTSD is important because these individuals often suffer from stress symptoms that may be reduced in severity, but are still clinically meaningful and may complicate other conditions such as TBI.

Risk and Resilience

Only a small subset of individuals exposed to the same traumatic event will develop PTSD, suggesting that exposure to a traumatic event is necessary but not sufficient to cause the disorder. Over the last three decades, risk factors have been identified that have contributed to our knowledge of who develops PTSD and under what circumstances. An equally important question relates to resilience: How are some individuals able to cope and recover without suffering from PTSD symptomatology? Review of the literature suggests that the answers are complex; different factors appear to confer risk and protection in different populations.

Demographic and Psychosocial Factors

The demographic variables most frequently associated with PTSD vulnerability include socioeconomic, educational, and intellectual disadvantage, and gender (female > male) and race, although the effect sizes of these factors are generally small (Brewin, Andrews, & Valentine, 2000). African American, Hispanic, and Native American populations are at greater risk of developing PTSD (Schlenger et al., 1992), whereas being of Asian descent may be a protective factor (DiGrande et al., 2008; Friedman, Schnurr, Sengupta, Holmes, & Ashcraft, 2004).

Prior psychopathology and certain personality characteristics have also been linked to PTSD, although the effect sizes are again small (Brewin et al., 2000; Ozer, Best, Lipsey, & Weiss, 2003). Neuroticism, defined as emotional overresponsiveness in response to stress, has been linked to PTSD development (Casella & Motta, 1990; Cox, MacPherson, Enns, & McWilliams, 2004). By contrast, personality traits can also serve as protective factors. For example, individuals scoring high on "hardiness" (i.e., internal locus of control, commitment to one's existence and purpose, ability to view change as a challenge rather than a threat) are less likely to develop PTSD (King, King, Fairbank, Keane, & Adams, 1998; Zakin, Solomon, & Neria, 2003).

One of the most reliable factors associated with PTSD is perceived social support. In a sample of Vietnam veterans, Green, Grace, Lindy, Gleser, and Leonard (1990) found that support at homecoming was associated with decreased risk of PTSD. In addition, individuals who experience greater negative social reactions after a traumatic event show greater PTSD symptom severity (Andrews, Brewin, & Rose, 2003). However, the relationship between social support and PTSD is complex; there is evidence that trauma severity and stress symptomatology mediate whether an individual seeks or receives social support (King, Taft, King, Hammond, & Stone, 2006).

Trauma-Related Factors

Prior trauma exposure has been shown to be predictive of PTSD development (Brewin et al., 2000). Although the precise mechanism is presently unclear, it is possible that exposure to a previous trauma may sensitize the individual to a more significant stress response when reexposed. Furthermore, the impact of previous trauma may become more significant when prior exposure involves assaultive violence. A history of two or more traumatic events of assaultive violence in childhood, for example, has been shown to increase the risk of PTSD to an adulthood traumatic event by a factor of five (Breslau, Chilcoat, Kessler, & Davis, 1999). Clearly, these results may have implications for populations that are likely to be exposed to multiple traumatic events, such as military personnel (e.g., multiple combat tours), police and firemen, and first responders to disasters.

Across many studies and trauma populations, trauma severity emerges as a consistent predictor of PTSD. For example, extent of combat exposure was related to PTSD symptomatology in Vietnam veterans (Foy, Sipprelle, Rueger, & Carroll, 1984), as was severity of abuse among survivors of childhood sexual abuse (Rodriguez, Ryan, Vande Kemp, & Foy, 1997). Traumatic events that involve physical injury are related to greater risk for PTSD (Acierno, Resnick, Kilpatrick, Saunders, & Best, 1999; Koren, Norman, Cohen, Berman, & Klein, 2005) and having closer proximity to the event is associated with greater prevalence of PTSD (Schlenger et al., 2002). Furthermore, peritraumatic dissociation in response to a traumatic event may be an important risk factor for PTSD (Ozer et al., 2003). Symptoms of peritraumatic dissociation include depersonalization, derealization, out-of-body experiences, and altered time perception. In one study, individuals who developed PTSD at 6 months posttrauma reported higher levels of peritraumatic dissociation at the initial assessment (Shalev, Peri, Canetti, & Schreiber, 1996). Finally, in the aftermath of a traumatic event, experiencing additional stressors such as loss of employment, major illness, and divorce can drastically affect an individual's social and occupational functioning (Adams & Boscarino, 2006; Maes, Mylle, Delmeire, & Janca, 2001). Adams and colleagues (2006) found that individuals who experienced more negative life events after the September 11, 2001, attacks were more likely to develop PTSD 2 years later.

Increasing evidence suggests that suffering from an mTBI during the traumatic event is associated with greater risk for PTSD (Hoge et al., 2008; Schneiderman, Braver, & Kang, 2008), whereas more severe TBI, in the form of longer duration of posttraumatic amnesia, may serve as a protective factor (Bryant et al., 2009). Bryant et al. (2009) have underscored the importance of memory encoding and consolidation in the development of PTSD symptomatology. Posttraumatic amnesia may compromise memory for the traumatic event, resulting in fewer reexperiencing symptoms of the traumatic event. However, as discussed by Verfaellie, Amick, and Vasterling (Chapter 5, this volume), the relationship between degraded encoding of the trauma event and subsequent PTSD symptoms is likely to be complex, and these conclusions must be considered preliminary, as there are very few studies to date that have examined the effects of mild and severe TBI as risk factors for PTSD.

Genetic and Biological Factors

The mechanisms underlying genetic and biological risk factors are not fully understood. It is important to recognize that most studies have been unable to differentiate whether the impact of these variables is attributable merely to the likelihood of traumatic event exposure or, rather, to PTSD liability once exposed. Genetic studies of PTSD vulnerability illustrate this complexity, and have been one of the few literatures to examine this distinction. Twin studies have estimated the genetic heritability of exposure to trauma as falling between approximately 20 and 50% (Lyons et al., 1993; Stein, Jang, Taylor, Vernon, & Livesley, 2002). Furthermore, exposure to different types of trauma may be differentially mediated by genetic factors. The likelihood of exposure to traumatic events involving assaultive violence appears to be highly influenced by genetics, whereas event exposure involving nonassaultive trauma appears largely nongenetic (Stein et al., 2002). Once exposed to a traumatic event, the conditional risk of developing PTSD also appears to be significantly influenced by genetics. Both combat and civilian trauma twin studies estimate the genetic heritability of PTSD to be approximately 30–40% after adjusting for trauma exposure (Stein et al., 2002; True, Rice, Eisen, & Heath, 1993).

Biological risk factors for PTSD at the molecular and brain systems level have been examined and may be particularly relevant in trauma survivors who have incurred a TBI or other neural injury. A number of brain regions have been implicated in the pathogenesis of PTSD including the amygdala, the prefrontal cortex, and the hippocampus (see "Neural Mechanisms" section below). Although alterations in the morphology and function of these regions have been reliably reported, controversy has ensued about whether these differences represent a risk factor for or a consequence of PTSD. Smaller hippocampal volume, however, has emerged as a potential risk factor for predicting PTSD development. Gilbertson and colleagues (2002) examined this issue in pairs of combat-discordant monozygotic twins in which the combat-exposed index twin either did or did not develop PTSD. Results showed that combat veterans diagnosed with PTSD and their identical not-combat-exposed twin brothers had smaller hippocampi than combat veterans without PTSD and their brothers, suggesting that smaller volume confers pretrauma risk for PTSD (Gilbertson et al., 2002). Other neuroimaging evidence is not fully consistent with a "risk factor only" interpretation. Meta-analyses (Karl et al., 2006; Smith, 2005) have demonstrated that traumatized individuals without PTSD may also demonstrate some degree of reduced hippocampal volume, which suggests either trauma-induced atrophy or that hippocampal volume represents a risk factor for trauma exposure itself. To the degree that hippocampal volume differences exist, they may potentially represent both a predisposing factor and a neurotoxic product of trauma. In contrast to findings in the hippocampus, a study of combat-discordant twins has suggested that reduction in pregenual ACC (prefrontal cortex) may represent an acquired sign in PTSD, that is, trauma-induced reduction only seen in combat veterans with PTSD, as opposed to a preexisting vulnerability (Kasai, Yamasue, Gilbertson, Shenton, Rauch, & Pitman, 2008).

Several studies have examined levels of cortisol in patients with PTSD, which plays a critical role in the stress response by mobilizing the body's response to the stressor via the hypothalamus–pituitary–adrenal (HPA) axis. Results generally suggest that PTSD is associated with lower levels of cortisol (Delahanty, Raimonde, & Spoonster, 2000; Yehuda et al., 2000) and pretrauma glucocorticoid alterations may serve to increase the risk of developing PTSD once exposed to a traumatic event (Yehuda, 2009). However, other studies have found higher levels of cortisol in patients with PTSD, or no differences between trauma-exposed individuals and those who developed PTSD (Heim et al., 2000; Young & Breslau, 2004). The lack of uniformity indicates that the relationship between neuroendocrine function and PTSD is highly complex and subject to a number of individual difference variables.

Findings from psychophysiological research also play an important role in characterizing the psychobiology of PTSD. A consistent picture has emerged demonstrating greater peripheral (e.g., electrodermal, heart rate, and facial electromyogram) reactivity to stimuli that represent, or are related to, the traumatic events of individuals who develop, compared to those who do not develop PTSD (Orr, Metzger, & Pitman, 2002). Several studies have shown that increased heart rate in the aftermath of a traumatic event predicts the subsequent development of PTSD (Bryant, 2006). Although part of this effect may reflect diminished parasympathetic activity, the bulk is likely to reflect sympathetic overactivity, including the release of the emergency hormone epinephrine (adrenaline). Cerebrospinal norepinephrine levels are also elevated in chronic PTSD (Geracioti et al., 2001).

Finally, neurocognitive deficits (e.g., in memory, attention, executive function) are frequently reported in PTSD although it is not clear to what degree they represent pretrauma risk versus the consequence of trauma exposure and/or PTSD. Recent twin studies (Gilbertson et al., 2007; Gilbertson et al., 2006) and a prospective study (Marx, Doron-Lamarca, Proctor, & Vasterling, 2009) have suggested that a variety of pretrauma cognitive skills in attention, declarative verbal memory, executive function, and immediate visual recall may be associated with risk of developing PTSD upon exposure to trauma. These findings likely have particular relevance to TBI in which similar deficits may be observed and can lead to further complications in the differential diagnosis of PTSD and TBI. Further research will be required in order to better define these commonalities and elucidate to what degree cognitive deficits associated with TBI may impact the subsequent development of PTSD.

Neural Mechanisms of PTSD

In understanding both the clinical presentation of PTSD and its potential relationship to TBI, it is important to consider the underlying neural substrates of PTSD, including its neurobiology, neuroanatomical circuitry, and associated neurocognitive and information-processing correlates.

Neurobiology and Neuroanatomical Circuitry of PTSD

The experience of stress and anxiety serves the important function of preparing an individual to meet the demands and challenges of everyday life. The brain is evolutionarily hard-wired to dramatically mobilize the body's response to life-threatening situations to increase the chance for survival. However, in PTSD, such body reactions become persistent, maladaptive, unfounded, and interferes with one's ability to complete and maintain life goals.

The animal fear response is similar to the human stress response (LeDoux, 1996) and therefore can provide a viable model for understanding the manifestation of stress reactions after a traumatic event in humans. Analogous to animal models, learning theories of PTSD etiology and maintenance propose that the principles of conditioning play a major role in the development of PTSD symptomatology (Keane, Fairbank, Caddell, Zimering, & Bender, 1985). During Pavlovian fear conditioning, an organism learns that a conditioned stimulus (CS), such as a tone, is associated with a noxious unconditioned stimulus (UCS), such as a shock. After repeated pairings of the CS and the UCS, the CS begins to elicit the same fear response in the animal as the UCS. The neural fear circuitry mediating this response is involved in the release of stress hormones into the bloodstream, increased blood pressure and heart rate, and the expression of fear. The neural regions central to the fear response include the thalamus, amygdala, HPA axis, locus coeruleus, the bed nucleus of the stria terminalis (BNST), hippocampus, periaqueductal gray, and certain prefrontal cortex (PFC) regions. When an organism is confronted with a fearful stimulus, the sensory cortices (with the exception of olfaction) relay information to the thalamus, which has both direct and indirect connections (by way of sensory cortices) with the amygdala. In the face of threat, locus coeruleus and amygdalar projections to the HPA, BNST, and central gray matter result in a cascade of autonomic, neuroendocrine, and motor responses that prepare the body to respond, including freezing or flight, quicker reflexes, and pain suppression (Kim & Jung, 2006).

Importantly, the fear circuitry model represents a feedback loop, whereby particular brain regions down-regulate the fear response. Prefrontal cortical territories have been shown to suppress amygdala responses in the service of fear reduction (i.e., extinction; see below), whereas the hippocampus appears to play a critical role in processing relevant contextual information, for example, the ability to discern safe versus dangerous contexts (Corcoran & Maren, 2004; Milad & Quirk, 2002). The hippocampus has direct projections to the amygdala and is hypothesized to be involved in slowing down the release of stress hormones. With particular implications for chronic PTSD, studies have shown that prolonged stress can damage hippocampal cells (McEwen et al., 1992), reducing its effectiveness in regulating the amygdala response to fear.

Animal models have demonstrated that fear responses can be diminished through extinction learning. During extinction, the animal is presented with the CS without the UCS, which ultimately extinguishes the CS-mediated fear response. Extinction learning is mediated in part by a region within the PFC known as the ventromedial PFC (vmPFC), which may function to retain the extinction memory (Phelps, Delgado, Nearing, & LeDoux, 2004). Rodents who have lesions to the vmPFC show a perseverative fear response, unable to learn the new relationship between the CS and the UCS (Morgan, Romanski, & LeDoux, 1993). Extinction learning is likely to play an important role in exposure therapy, which has been shown to be an efficacious treatment for PTSD (Foa & Rauch, 2004).

Advances in elucidating the neural circuitry of PTSD have been made with the increasing popularity of neuroimaging techniques including functional and structural magnetic resonance imaging (MRI) and positron emission tomography (PET). These studies have highlighted the importance of similar neural regions identified in nonhuman animals as part of the putative neural circuitry underlying PTSD symptomatology, including the amygdala, hippocampus, and PFC (especially the vmPFC, including the anterior cingulate cortex [ACC]). In general, functional neuroimaging studies have shown that the amygdala is hyperresponsive in patients diagnosed with PTSD relative to trauma-exposed individuals, possibly reflecting hyperarousal and enhanced appraisal of threat (Rauch et al., 1996, 2000; Shin et al., 2005). A sizeable structural neuroimaging literature has revealed a relatively consistent pattern of volumetric reductions in both the hippocampus and the anterior cingulate cortex of adults diagnosed with chronic PTSD (Karl et al., 2006; Smith, 2005). Such findings would appear to be consistent with neural models of PTSD positing failures in these regions to provide adequate inhibitory control over the amygdala.

While amygdala activity is enhanced, activity in the vmPFC is reduced in PTSD (Bremner et al., 2005; Britton, Phan, Taylor, Fig, & Liberzon, 2005; Shin et al., 2005), although some studies have shown an increase in vmPFC activity in association with PTSD symptoms (Bryant et al., 2005; Morey, Petty, Cooper, LaBar, & McCarthy, 2008; Pannu Hayes, LaBar, Petty, McCarthy, & Morey, 2009). Interestingly, a recent functional MRI (fMRI) study showed that the vmPFC was reduced during extinction learning in patients with PTSD (Milad et al., 2009). Although greater research is warranted, it is possible that the function of the vmPFC will be more clearly elucidated within the context of extinction research, consistent with the nonhuman animal literature.

Prolonged PTSD may be associated with the inability to learn new, safe associations that would otherwise lead to an extinction response. Consistent with this notion, patients with PTSD continue to show a physiological fear response to the CS even after extinction learning (Orr et al., 2000), suggesting an impairment in extinction. Overall, structural and functional neuroimaging findings are broadly consistent with a model of PTSD that posits a reduced capacity of hippocampus and vmPFC to inhibit amygdala-based fear responses, likely reflecting a failure of these brain regions to effectively utilize cues in the environment to signal safety (hippocampus) and to adaptively maintain extinction of conditioned emotional responses (ACC) once traumatic experiences are no longer relevant. As summarized by Bigler and Maxwell (Chapter 2, this volume), there is overlap in the brain regions implicated in PTSD and mTBI, in particular, the hippocampus and prefrontal cortex.

Neurocognitive and Information-Processing Correlates of PTSD

By definition, PTSD is accompanied by memory and attentional disturbances including intrusive and repetitive memories, difficulty with retrieval of trauma memories, dissociative flashbacks, and difficulty with concentration. On neuropsychological tasks, patients with PTSD generally show mild deficits in sustained attention, working memory, initial acquisition of information, and inhibition of irrelevant information (Brandes et al., 2002; Leskin & White, 2007; Vasterling, Brailey, Constans, & Sutker, 1998). The nature of neuropsychological deficits is more closely related to inattention and interference during the encoding process than retention loss due to amnesia (Vasterling & Brailey, 2005) and may involve dysfunction of frontal–limbic circuits (Vasterling et al., 2002). PTSD is associated with greater disruptions in neural regions that subserve working memory and attention. A recent fMRI study found that reduced performance on a working memory task in individuals with PTSD symptoms was associated with deactivation in the dorsolateral prefrontal cortex (Morey et al., 2009), a region that has previously been implicated in active maintenance of task-relevant information in working memory (Dolcos & McCarthy, 2006). This study provides support for the theory that interference from distracters is a hallmark of the disorder.

The neuropsychological findings in PTSD, which typically employ neutral tasks without an emotional component, raise the important question of how emotional and cognitive systems interact to produce or maintain the disorder. Information-processing theories of PTSD have provided a framework for understanding cognitive alterations and attentional bias in PTSD in the presence of a threatening stimulus (Dalgleish, 2004). A typical task used to demonstrate threat bias is the emotional Stroop paradigm, in which individuals are asked to name the color of the ink that negative or trauma-related words are printed in. Longer response latencies during color naming indicate attentional preference toward threat stimuli in patients with PTSD (Constans, McCloskey, Vasterling, Brailey, & Mathews, 2004; Foa, Feske, Murdock, Kozak, & McCarthy, 1991). Event-related potential (ERP) studies have provided further support for information bias in PTSD. These studies typically employ modified oddball paradigms, in which infrequent salient target stimuli (e.g., emotional stimuli) are interspersed with frequent standard stimuli. During processing of infrequent stimuli, an enhanced P3 amplitude response was observed, which is thought to reflect heightened attention toward those stimuli (Attias, Bleich, Furman, & Zinger, 1996; Stanford, Vasterling, Mathias, Constans, & Houston, 2001). More recently, an fMRI study using a modified emotional oddball paradigm demonstrated that PTSD symptomatology was associated with greater activity in attentional circuitry for threat stimuli, accompanied by a reduction in activity for target, nonthreat stimuli in these regions (Pannu Hayes et al., 2009). Taken together, the behavioral, electrophysiological, and neuroimaging studies have demonstrated that threatening stimuli are given privileged attentional status, which may underlie hypervigilance symptoms in PTSD.

An intriguing question at the heart of controversy surrounding PTSD and of relevance to TBI is how traumatic memories are encoded, consolidated, and subsequently accessed at retrieval. As currently conceptualized, amnesia for traumatic event details may occur from repeated attempts at memory suppression and avoidance rather than from faulty encoding. However, some researchers have posited that inefficient encoding at the time of the traumatic event may underlie memory distortions seen in PTSD (Ehlers & Clark, 2000; Nadel & Jacobs, 1998). Direct evidence in support of these hypotheses in humans is lacking, as it is ethically and practically impossible to study the neurobiology of trauma memory while the trauma is occurring. Nevertheless, continued research in this area using animal models and encoding of trauma memory reminders as proxies are important given the broad implications this topic has for the recovered memory debate and eyewitness testimony (McNally, 2003).

The majority of memory and PTSD studies have examined retrieval mechanisms. PTSD is associated with difficulty in retrieval of detailed autobiographical memories, although the difficulty does not appear to be specific to traumatic memories (Kaspi, McNally, & Amir, 1995; McNally, Litz, Prassas, Shin, & Weathers, 1994). Rather, several studies have shown that patients with PTSD show an "overgeneral memory" during recollection of personal past events, including positive events (for a review, see Verfaellie & Vasterling, 2009). "Overgeneral memory" refers to the tendency to recall personal emotional memories with very few details and specific episodes and is thought to result from inadequate search of memory during retrieval, perhaps due to rumination, avoidance, and impairment in executive capacity (Williams et al., 2007). Interestingly, greater retrieval of specific memories is associated with successful psychosocial intervention for PTSD (Sutherland & Bryant, 2007).

Summary

A wealth of research in the last three decades has produced important discoveries regarding the nature of PTSD, risk and protective factors, and its neural substrates. Although controversies remain regarding several aspects of the disorder, there has been significant progress since the diagnosis became official in 1980. It has been demonstrated that trauma exposure is highly common, yet the development of PTSD is infrequent by comparison, suggesting that a host of individual and traumatic event variables influence development of the disorder. Whereas pretrauma variables such as demographic and personality characteristics appear to confer a modest risk of PTSD development, the most important variables to date appear to be related to features of the traumatic event itself, including severity of the trauma and the individual's response to the trauma, and posttrauma variables such as social support. However, greater understanding of premorbid neurobiological and cognitive risk factors, such as brain volume, HPA function in response to fear, and individual neurocognitive differences, hold promise in providing a comprehensive understanding of who develops PTSD in order to inform prevention and treatment efforts. Researchers have identified a working neurobiological model of PTSD that involves alterations in putative fear and cognitive circuits, primarily in the amygdala, hippocampus, and prefrontal cortex. Knowledge of the neuropsychological and biological factors associated with PTSD may help to uncover targeted treatments that act upon the functions of these regions.

In the next decade, we can expect a continuance of the surge in PTSD research that has generated a tremendous body of knowledge. Given the current geopolitical climate in which individuals are continually being exposed to combat and terrorism, research has focused more heavily on understanding PTSD and TBI comorbidity as well as the key features that distinguish the two disorders. In particular, PTSD and mTBI have been difficult to separate diagnostically and it is currently unknown whether the cognitive deficits observed in PTSD are different from the cognitive impairment associated with TBI. Greater research is needed with respect to differences in the neurobiology of PTSD and TBI, and treatment outcome of individuals who suffer from both PTSD symptoms and TBI. One intriguing question that needs to be addressed is whether individuals with comorbid PTSD and TBI benefit from the same interventions as individuals with PTSD only. Continued empirical work will help to answer these questions.

References

Acierno, R., Resnick, H., Kilpatrick, D., Saunders, B., & Best, C. (1999). Risk factors for rape, physical assault, and posttraumatic stress disorder in women: Examination of differential multivariate relationships. *Journal of Anxiety Disorders, 13*(6), 541–563.

Adams, R., & Boscarino, J. (2006). Predictors of PTSD and delayed PTSD after disaster: The impact of exposure and psychosocial resources. *The Journal of Nervous and Mental Disease, 194*(7), 485–493.

American Psychiatric Association. (2000). *Diagnostic and Statistical Manual of Mental Disorders.* (4th ed., text rev.). Washington DC. Author.

Andrews, B., Brewin, C., & Rose, S. (2003). Gender, social support, and PTSD in victims of violent crime. *Journal of Traumatic Stress, 16*(4), 421–427.

Asmundson, G., Frombach, I., McQuaid, J., Pedrelli, P., Lenox, R., & Stein, M. (2000). Dimensionality of posttraumatic stress symptoms: A confirmatory factor analysis of DSM-IV symptom clusters and other symptom models. *Behaviour Research and Therapy, 38*(2), 203–214.

Attias, J., Bleich, A., Furman, V., & Zinger, Y. (1996). Event-related potentials in post-traumatic stress disorder of combat origin. *Biological Psychiatry, 40*(5), 373–381.

Boscarino, J. (2008). A prospective study of PTSD and early-age heart disease mortality among Vietnam veterans: Implications for surveillance and prevention. *Psychosomatic Medicine, 70*(6), 668–676.

Brandes, D., Ben-Schachar, G., Gilboa, A., Bonne, O., Freedman, S., & Shalev, A. (2002). PTSD symptoms and cognitive performance in recent trauma survivors. *Psychiatry Research, 110*(3), 231–238.

Bremner, J. D., Vermetten, E., Schmahl, C., Vaccarino, V., Vythilingam, M., Afzal, N., et al. (2005). Positron emission tomographic imaging of neural correlates of a fear acquisition and extinction paradigm in women with childhood sexual-abuse-related post-traumatic stress disorder. *Psychological Medicine,* *35*(6), 791–806.

Breslau, N., Chilcoat, H., Kessler, R., & Davis, G. (1999). Previous exposure to trauma and PTSD effects of subsequent trauma: Results from the Detroit Area Survey of Trauma. *American Journal of Psychiatry, 156*(6), 902–907.

Breslau, N., Kessler, R., Chilcoat, H., Schultz, L., Davis, G., & Andreski, P. (1998). Trauma and posttraumatic stress disorder in the community: The 1996 Detroit Area Survey of Trauma. *Archives of General Psychiatry, 55*(7), 626–632.

Brewin, C., Andrews, B., & Valentine, J. (2000). Meta-analysis of risk factors for posttraumatic stress disorder in trauma-exposed adults. *Journal of Consulting and Clinical Psychology, 68*(5), 748–766.

Britton, J. C., Phan, K. L., Taylor, S. F., Fig, L. M., & Liberzon, I. (2005). Corticolimbic blood flow in posttraumatic stress disorder during script-driven imagery. *Biological Psychiatry, 57*(8), 832–840.

Bruns J. Jr., & Hauser, W. (2003). The epidemiology of traumatic brain injury: A review. *Epilepsia, 44*(Suppl.10), 2–10.

Bryant, R. (2006). Longitudinal psychophysiological studies of heart rate: Mediating effects and implications for treatment. *Annals of the New York Academy of Sciences, 1071,* 19–26.

Bryant, R., Creamer, M., O'Donnell, M., Silove, D., Clark, C., & McFarlane, A. (2009). Post-traumatic amnesia and the nature of post-traumatic stress disorder after mild traumatic brain injury. *Journal of the International Neuropsychological Society, 15*(6), 862–867.

Bryant, R. A., Felmingham, K. L., Kemp, A. H., Barton, M., Peduto, A. S., Rennie, C., et al. (2005). Neural networks of information processing in posttraumatic stress disorder: A functional magnetic resonance imaging study. *Biological Psychiatry, 58*(2), 111–118.

Casella, L., & Motta, R. (1990). Comparison of characteristics of Vietnam veterans with and without posttraumatic stress disorder. *Psychological Reports, 67*(2), 595–605.

Constans, J. I., McCloskey, M. S., Vasterling, J. J., Brailey, K., & Mathews, A. (2004). Suppression of attentional bias in PTSD. *Journal of Abnormal Psychology, 113*(2), 315–323.

Corcoran, K., & Maren, S. (2004). Factors regulating the effects of hippocampal inactivation on renewal of conditional fear after extinction. *Learning and Memory, 11*(5), 598–603.

Cox, B., MacPherson, P., Enns, M., & McWilliams, L. (2004). Neuroticism and self-criticism associated with posttraumatic stress disorder in a nationally representative sample. *Behaviour Research and Therapy, 42*(1), 105–114.

Dalgleish, T. (2004). Cognitive approaches to posttraumatic stress disorder: The evolution of multirepresentational theorizing. *Psychological Bulletin, 130*(2), 228–260.

Delahanty, D., Raimonde, A., & Spoonster, E. (2000). Initial posttraumatic urinary cortisol levels predict subsequent PTSD symptoms in motor vehicle accident victims. *Biological Psychiatry, 48*(9), 940–947.

DiGrande, L., Perrin, M., Thorpe, L., Thalji, L., Murphy, J., Wu, D., et al. (2008). Posttraumatic stress symptoms, PTSD, and risk factors among lower

Manhattan residents 2–3 years after the September 11, 2001 terrorist attacks. *Journal of Traumatic Stress, 21*(3), 264–273.

Dobie, D., Kivlahan, D., Maynard, C., Bush, K., Davis, T., & Bradley, K. (2004). Posttraumatic stress disorder in female veterans: association with self-reported health problems and functional impairment. *Archives of Internal Medicine, 164*(4), 394–400.

Dohrenwend, B., Turner, J., Turse, N., Adams, B., Koenen, K., & Marshall, R. (2006). The psychological risks of Vietnam for US veterans: A revisit with new data and methods. *Science, 313*(5789), 979.

Dolcos, F., & McCarthy, G. (2006). Brain systems mediating cognitive interference by emotional distraction. *Journal of Neuroscience, 26*(7), 2072–2079.

Ehlers, A., & Clark, D. M. (2000). A cognitive model of posttraumatic stress disorder. *Behaviour Research and Therapy, 38*(4), 319–345.

Foa, E. B., Feske, U., Murdock, T. B., Kozak, M. J., & McCarthy, P. (1991). Processing of threat-related information in rape victims. *Journal of Abnormal Psychology, 100*(2), 156–162.

Foa, E. B., & Rauch, S. (2004). Cognitive changes during prolonged exposure versus prolonged exposure plus cognitive restructuring in female assault survivors with posttraumatic stress disorder. *Journal of Consulting and Clinical Psychology, 72*(5), 879–884.

Foy, D., Sipprelle, R., Rueger, D., & Carroll, E. (1984). Etiology of posttraumatic stress disorder in Vietnam veterans: Analysis of premilitary, military, and combat exposure influences. *Journal of Consulting and Clinical Psychology, 52*(1), 79–87.

Friedman, M., Schnurr, P., Sengupta, A., Holmes, T., & Ashcraft, M. (2004). The Hawaii Vietnam Veterans Project: Is minority status a risk factor for posttraumatic stress disorder? *Journal of Nervous and Mental Disease, 192*(1), 42–50.

Geracioti T. Jr., Baker, D., Ekhator, N., West, S., Hill, K., Bruce, A., et al. (2001). CSF norepinephrine concentrations in posttraumatic stress disorder. *American Journal of Psychiatry, 158*(8), 1227–1230.

Gilbertson, M. W., Paulus, L. A., Williston, S. K., Gurvits, T. V., Lasko, N. B., Pitman, R. K., et al. (2006). Neurocognitive function in monozygotic twins discordant for combat exposure: Relationship to posttraumatic stress disorder. *Journal of Abnormal Psychology, 115*(3), 484–495.

Gilbertson, M. W., Shenton, M., Ciszewski, A., Kasai, K., Lasko, N., Orr, S., et al. (2002). Smaller hippocampal volume predicts pathologic vulnerability to psychological trauma. *Nature Neuroscience, 5*(11), 1242–1247.

Gilbertson, M. W., Williston, S., Paulus, L., Lasko, N., Gurvits, T., Shenton, M., et al. (2007). Configural cue performance in identical twins discordant for posttraumatic stress disorder: Theoretical implications for the role of hippocampal function. *Biological Psychiatry, 62*(5), 513–520.

Green, B., Grace, M., Lindy, J., Gleser, G., & Leonard, A. (1990). Risk factors for PTSD and other diagnoses in a general sample of Vietnam veterans. *American Journal of Psychiatry, 147*, 729–733.

Heim, C., Newport, D., Heit, S., Graham, Y., Wilcox, M., Bonsall, R., et al. (2000). Pituitary–adrenal and autonomic responses to stress in women after sexual and physical abuse in childhood. *Journal of the American Medical Association, 284*(5), 592–597.

Hoge, C. W., McGurk, D., Thomas, J., Cox, A., Engel, C., & Castro, C. (2008). Mild traumatic brain injury in US soldiers returning from Iraq. *New England Journal of Medicine, 358*, 453–463.

Hoge, C. W., Terhakopian, A., Castro, C., Messer, S., & Engel, C. (2007). Association of posttraumatic stress disorder with somatic symptoms, health care visits, and absenteeism among Iraq war veterans. *American Journal of Psychiatry, 164*(1), 150–153.

Hoge, C. W., Castro, C. A., Messer, S. C., McGurk, D., Cotting, D. I., & Koffman, R. L. (2004). Combat duty in Iraq and Afghanistan, mental health problems, and barriers to care. *New England Journal of Medicine, 351*(1), 13–22.

Karl, A., Schaefer, M., Malta, L., Dörfel, D., Rohleder, N., & Werner, A. (2006). A meta-analysis of structural brain abnormalities in PTSD. *Neuroscience and Biobehavioral Reviews, 30*(7), 1004–1031.

Kasai, K., Yamasue, H., Gilbertson, M. W., Shenton, M. E., Rauch, S. L., & Pitman, R. K. (2008). Evidence for acquired pregenual anterior cingulate gray matter loss from a twin study of combat-related posttraumatic stress disorder. *Biological Psychiatry, 63*, 550–556.

Kaspi, S. P., McNally, R. J., & Amir, N. (1995). Cognitive processing of emotional information in posttraumatic stress disorder. *Cognitive Therapy and Research, 19*(4), 433–444.

Keane, T., Fairbank, J., Caddell, J., Zimering, R., & Bender, M. (1985). A behavioral approach to assessing and treating post-traumatic stress disorder in Vietnam veterans. In C. R. Figley (Ed.), *Trauma and its wake: The study and treatment of post-traumatic stress disorder* (pp. 257–294). New York: Brunner/Mazel.

Kessler, R. C., Sonnega, A., Bromet, E., Hughes, M., & Nelson, C. B. (1995). Posttraumatic stress disorder in the National Comorbidity Survey. *Archives of General Psychiatry, 52*(12), 1048–1060.

Kim, J., & Jung, M. (2006). Neural circuits and mechanisms involved in Pavlovian fear conditioning: A critical review. *Neuroscience and Biobehavioral Reviews, 30*(2), 188–202.

King, D., Leskin, G., King, L., & Weathers, F. (1998). Confirmatory factor analysis of the Clinician-Administered PTSD Scale: Evidence for the dimensionality of posttraumatic stress disorder. *Psychological Assessment, 10*(2), 90–96.

King, D., Taft, C., King, L., Hammond, C., & Stone, E. (2006). Directionality of the association between social support and posttraumatic stress disorder: A longitudinal investigation. *Journal of Applied Social Psychology, 36*(12), 2980–2992.

King, L., King, D., Fairbank, J., Keane, T., & Adams, G. (1998). Resilience–recovery factors in post-traumatic stress disorder among female and male Vietnam veterans: Hardiness, postwar social support, and additional stressful life events. *Journal of Personality and Social Psychology, 74*(2), 420–434.

Koren, D., Norman, D., Cohen, A., Berman, J., & Klein, E. (2005). Increased PTSD risk with combat-related injury: A matched comparison study of injured and uninjured soldiers experiencing the same combat events. *American Journal of Psychiatry, 162*(2), 276–282.

Kulka, R., Schlenger, W., Fairbank, J., Hough, R., Jordan, B., Marmar, C., et al. (1990). *Trauma and the Vietnam War generation*: Brunner/Mazel.

LeDoux, J. E. (1996). *The emotional brain: The mysterious underpinnings of emotional life*. New York: Simon & Schuster.

Leskin, L., & White, P. (2007). Attentional networks reveal executive function deficits in posttraumatic stress disorder. *Neuropsychology, 21*(3), 275–284.

Lyons, M., Goldberg, J., Eisen, S., True, W., Tsuang, M., Meyer, J., et al. (1993). Do genes influence exposure to trauma?: A twin study of combat. *American Journal of Medical Genetics, 48*(1), 22–27.

Maes, M., Mylle, J., Delmeire, L., & Janca, A. (2001). Pre-and post-disaster negative life events in relation to the incidence and severity of post-traumatic stress disorder. *Psychiatry Research, 105*(1–2), 1–12.

Marx, B., Doron-Lamarca, S., Proctor, S., & Vasterling, J. (2009). The influence of pre-deployment neurocognitive functioning on post-deployment PTSD symptom outcomes among Iraq-deployed army soldiers. *Journal of the International Neuropsychological Society, 15*(06), 840–852.

McDonald, S., Beckham, J., Morey, R., Marx, C., Tupler, L., & Calhoun, P. (2008). Factorial invariance of posttraumatic stress disorder symptoms across three veteran samples. *Journal of Traumatic Stress, 21*(3), 309–317.

McEwen, B., Angulo, J., Cameron, H., Chao, H., Daniels, D., Gannon, M., et al. (1992). Paradoxical effects of adrenal steroids on the brain: Protection versus degeneration. *Biological Psychiatry, 31*(2), 177–199.

McNally, R. J. (2003). Progress and controversy in the study of posttraumatic stress disorder. *Annual Review of Psychology, 54*(1), 229–252.

McNally, R. J., Litz, B. T., Prassas, A., Shin, L. M., & Weathers, F. W. (1994). Emotional priming of autobiographical memory in post-traumatic stress disorder. *Cognition and Emotion, 8*(4), 351–367.

Milad, M. R., Pitman, R. K., Ellis, C. B., Gold, A. L., Shin, L. M., Lasko, N. B., et al. (2009). Neurobiological basis of failure to recall extinction memory in posttraumatic stress disorder. *Biological Psychiatry, 66*(12), 1075–1082.

Milad, M. R., & Quirk, G. (2002). Neurons in medial prefrontal cortex signal memory for fear extinction. *Nature, 420*(6911), 70–74.

Morey, R. A., Dolcos, F., Petty, C., Cooper, D., Hayes, J., LaBar, K., et al. (2009). The role of trauma-related distractors on neural systems for working memory and emotion processing in posttraumatic stress disorder. *Journal of Psychiatric Research, 43*(8), 809–817.

Morey, R. A., Petty, C. M., Cooper, D. A., LaBar, K. S., & McCarthy, G. (2008). Neural systems for executive and emotional processing are modulated by symptoms of posttraumatic stress disorder in Iraq War veterans. *Psychiatry Research: Neuroimaging, 162*(1), 59–72.

Morgan, M., Romanski, L., & LeDoux, J. (1993). Extinction of emotional learning: Contribution of medial prefrontal cortex. *Neuroscience Letters, 163*(1), 109–113.

Nadel, L., & Jacobs, W. J. (1998). Traumatic memory is special. *Current Directions in Psychological Science, 7*(5), 154–157.

Orr, S. P., Metzger, L., Lasko, N., Macklin, M., Peri, T., & Pitman, R. (2000). De novo conditioning in trauma-exposed individuals with and without posttraumatic stress disorder. *Journal of Abnormal Psychology, 109*(2), 290–298.

Orr, S. P., Metzger, L. J., & Pitman, R. K. (2002). Psychophysiology of posttraumatic stress disorder. *Psychiatric Clinics of North America, 25*(2), 271–293.

Ozer, E., Best, S., Lipsey, T., & Weiss, D. (2003). Predictors of posttraumatic stress disorder and symptoms in adults: A meta-analysis. *Psychological Bulletin, 129*(1), 52–73.

Pannu Hayes, J., LaBar, K., Petty, C., McCarthy, G., & Morey, R. (2009). Alterations in the neural circuitry for emotion and attention associated with posttraumatic stress symptomatology. *Psychiatry Research: Neuroimaging, 172*(1), 7–15.

Phelps, E., Delgado, M., Nearing, K., & LeDoux, J. (2004). Extinction learning in humans: Role of the amygdala and vmPFC. *Neuron, 43*, 897–905.

Rauch, S. L., van der Kolk, B. A., Fisler, R. E., Alpert, N. M., Orr, S. P., Savage, C. R., et al. (1996). A symptom provocation study of posttraumatic stress disorder using positron emission tomography and script-driven imagery. *Archives of General Psychiatry, 53*(5), 380–387.

Rauch, S. L., Whalen, P. J., Shin, L. M., McInerney, S. C., Macklin, M. L., Lasko, N. B., et al. (2000). Exaggerated amygdala response to masked facial stimuli in posttraumatic stress disorder: A functional MRI study. *Biological Psychiatry, 47*(9), 769–776.

Rodriguez, N., Ryan, S., Vande Kemp, H., & Foy, D. (1997). Posttraumatic stress disorder in adult female survivors of child sexual abuse: A comparison study. *Journal of Consulting and Clinical Psychology, 65*(1), 53–59.

Schlenger, W., Caddell, J., Ebert, L., Jordan, B., Rourke, K., Wilson, D., et al. (2002). Psychological reactions to terrorist attacks. *Journal of the American Medical Association, 288*(5), 581–588.

Schlenger, W., Kulka, R., Fairbank, J., Hough, R., Jordan, B., Marmar, C., et al. (1992). The prevalence of post-traumatic stress disorder in the Vietnam generation: A multimethod, multisource assessment of psychiatric disorder. *Journal of Traumatic Stress, 5*(3), 333–363.

Schneiderman, A., Braver, E., & Kang, H. (2008). Understanding sequelae of injury mechanisms and mild traumatic brain injury incurred during the conflicts in Iraq and Afghanistan: Persistent postconcussive symptoms and posttraumatic stress disorder. *American Journal of Epidemiology, 167*(12), 1446–1452.

Shalev, A. Y., Peri, T., Canetti, L., & Schreiber, S. (1996). Predictors of PTSD in injured trauma survivors: A prospective study. *American Journal of Psychiatry, 153*(2), 219–225.

Shin, L. M., McNally, R. J., Kosslyn, S. M., Thompson, W. L., Rauch, S. L., Alpert, N. M., et al. (1999). Regional cerebral blood flow during script-driven imagery in childhood sexual abuse-related PTSD: A PET investigation. *American Journal of Psychiatry, 156*(4), 575–584.

Shin, L. M., Wright, C. I., Cannistraro, P. A., Wedig, M. M., McMullin, K., Martis, B., et al. (2005). A functional magnetic resonance imaging study of amygdala and medial prefrontal cortex responses to overtly presented fearful faces in posttraumatic stress disorder. *Archives of General Psychiatry, 62*(3), 273–281.

Smith, M. (2005). Bilateral hippocampal volume reduction in adults with post-traumatic stress disorder: A meta-analysis of structural MRI studies. *Hippocampus, 15*(6), 798–807.

Stanford, M. S., Vasterling, J. J., Mathias, C. W., Constans, J. I., & Houston, R. J. (2001). Impact of threat relevance on P3 event-related potentials in combat-related post-traumatic stress disorder. *Psychiatry Research, 102*(2), 125–137.

Stein, M., Jang, K., Taylor, S., Vernon, P., & Livesley, W. (2002). Genetic and environmental influences on trauma exposure and posttraumatic stress disorder symptoms: A twin study. *American Journal of Psychiatry, 159*(10), 1675–1681.

Stein, M., & McAllister, T. (2009). Exploring the convergence of posttraumatic stress disorder and mild traumatic brain injury. *American Journal of Psychiatry, 166*(7), 768–776.

Stein, M., Walker, J., Hazen, A., & Forde, D. (1997). Full and partial posttraumatic stress disorder: Findings from a community survey. *American Journal of Psychiatry, 154*(8), 1114–1119.

Sutherland, K., & Bryant, R. (2007). Autobiographical memory in posttraumatic stress disorder before and after treatment. *Behaviour Research and Therapy, 45*(12), 2915–2923.

Tanielian, T., & Jaycox, L. (2008). *Invisible wounds of war: Psychological and cognitive injuries, their consequences, and services to assist recovery.* Santa Monica, CA: Rand Center for Military Health Policy.

True, W. R., Rice, J., Eisen, S. A., & Heath, A. C. (1993). A twin study of genetic and environmental contributions to liability for posttraumatic stress symptoms. *Archives of General Psychiatry, 50*(4), 257–265.

Vasterling, J. J., & Brailey, K. (2005). Neuropsychological findings in adults with PTSD. In J. Vasterling & C. R. Brewin (Eds.), *Neuropsychology of PTSD: Biological, Cognitive, and Clinical Perspectives* (pp. 178–207). New York: The Guilford Press.

Vasterling, J. J., Brailey, K., Constans, J., & Sutker, P. (1998). Attention and memory dysfunction in posttraumatic stress disorder. *Neuropsychology, 12*(1), 125–133.

Vasterling, J. J., Duke, L. M., Brailey, K., Constans, J. I., Allain, A. N. Jr., & Sutker, P. B. (2002). Attention, learning, and memory performances and intellectual resources in Vietnam veterans: PTSD and no disorder comparisons. *Neuropsychology, 16*(1), 5–14.

Verfaellie, M., & Vasterling, J. (2009). Memory in PTSD: A neurocognitive approach. In P. J. Shiromani, J. E. LeDoux, & T. Keane (Eds.), *Post-traumatic stress disorder: Basic science and clinical practice* (pp. 105–130). New York: Humana Press.

Williams, J., Barnhofer, T., Crane, C., Hermans, D., Raes, F., Watkins, E., et al. (2007). Autobiographical memory specificity and emotional disorder. *Psychological Bulletin, 133*(1), 122–148.

Yaffe, K., Vittinghoff, E., Lindquist, K., Barnes, D., Covinsky, K., Neylan, T., et al.

(2010). Posttraumatic stress disorder and risk of dementia among US veterans. *Archives of General Psychiatry, 67*(6), 608–613.

Yehuda, R., Bierer, L., Schmeidler, J., Aferiat, D., Breslau, I., & Dolan, S. (2000). Low cortisol and risk for PTSD in adult offspring of Holocaust survivors. *American Journal of Psychiatry, 157*(8), 1252–1259.

Yehuda, R. (2009). Status of glucocorticoid alterations in post traumatic stress disorder. *Annals of the New York Academy of Sciences, 1179*, 56–69.

Young, E., & Breslau, N. (2004). Cortisol and catecholamines in posttraumatic stress disorder: An epidemiologic community study. *Archives of General Psychiatry, 61*(4), 394–401.

Zakin, G., Solomon, Z., & Neria, Y. (2003). Hardiness, attachment style, and long term psychological distress among Israeli POWs and combat veterans. *Personality and Individual Differences, 34*(5), 819–829.

CHAPTER 5

Effects of Traumatic Brain Injury–Associated Neurocognitive Alterations on Posttraumatic Stress Disorder

Mieke Verfaellie, Melissa M. Amick, and Jennifer J. Vasterling

The high comorbidity of mild traumatic brain injury (mTBI) and posttraumatic stress disorder (PTSD) in those serving in Operation Enduring Freedom (OEF) and Operation Iraqi Freedom (OIF) (Hoge et al., 2008; Tanielian & Jaycox, 2008) has focused renewed attention on the nature of the relationship between the two disorders. In light of the high overlap in symptoms between mTBI and PTSD and their possible neural substrates (Vasterling, Verfaellie, & Sullivan, 2009), much of the current interest has focused on diagnostic questions, such as whether symptoms can best be understood as the result of physical or psychological trauma (Hoge, Goldberg, & Castro, 2009). Much less explored is the question as to how biomechanical injury to the brain may impact adjustment to psychological trauma.

This chapter examines the neurocognitive mechanisms by which mTBI may affect the development and course of PTSD. We make use of what is known about how sources of normal neurocognitive variance influence PTSD, on the assumption that the sequelae of mTBI represent another source of neurocognitive variance. To elucidate potential mechanisms of action, we draw on a cognitive model of PTSD (Ehlers & Clark, 2000) that postulates that PTSD is maintained by (1) an autobiographical memory disturbance, whereby memory cues trigger the traumatic memory in such a way that it is experienced as reliving of the trauma; and (2) excessive negative appraisals that lead to exaggerated estimates of harm and negative outcome. We consider possible neurocognitive mechanisms in light of how mTBI may (1) alter the creation and correction of the traumatic memory and (2) influence the appraisal of the event and its consequences.

Although the physical trauma that leads to TBI can be temporally distinct from the life-threatening trauma that results in PTSD (e.g., a veteran who sustains mTBI after deployment), more commonly the physical trauma occurs as part of the same discrete event (e.g., a motor vehicle accident in a civilian setting) or an ongoing series of events (e.g., blast explosion in the context of ongoing combat operations) that are perceived as life-threatening. Thus, mTBI may have the greatest potential to affect the expression of PTSD symptoms in the immediate aftermath of the injury, when cognitive alterations are most pronounced. Nonetheless, among at least a subset of mTBI victims, chronic neurocognitive abnormalities may also influence subsequent PTSD symptom expression. Regarding treatment, what little preliminary evidence we have suggests that evidence-based interventions for acute stress-related symptoms following psychological trauma can be applied successfully to patients with mTBI (Bryant, Moulds, Guthrie, & Nixon, 2003). However, as suggested by Bryant and Litz (Chapter 11, this volume), many questions remain regarding how the wide range of variance in mTBI-related cognitive deficits may moderate responses to various evidence-based PTSD interventions.

In keeping with the theme of this volume, we limit our discussion to mTBI. We first review the empirical evidence that suggests that mTBI may affect the development of PTSD. To set the stage for a consideration of cognitive mechanisms that may be responsible for the association between mTBI and PTSD, we next review neurocognitive alterations commonly observed in mTBI. Subsequent sections address ways in which these neurocognitive factors may influence the development and course of PTSD, and may have implications for treatment. Our considerations are restricted to the possible impact of mTBI in adulthood, as it is unknown how disruption of ongoing neurodevelopment in children or adolescents who sustain mTBI influences subsequent maturation (for discussion, see Yeates, 2010). Finally, although we acknowledge that other comorbidities, such as alcohol use or pain, may modulate the effects of mTBI on PTSD, consideration of these factors is beyond the scope of this chapter (see Najavits, Highley, Dolan, & Fee, Chapter 7, this volume; and Otis, Fortier, & Keane, Chapter 6, this volume, for discussion of comorbid substance abuse and pain, respectively).

The Impact of mTBI on PTSD

Systematic reviews of the literature suggest that mTBI increases risk of psychiatric disorders (Jorge, 2005; Kim et al., 2007). Further, compared to traumatic injury not associated with TBI, mTBI confers additional risk for common trauma-related psychopathologies such as PTSD and depression. For instance, studying Cambodian survivors of mass violence, Molica, Henderson, and Tor (2002) found that psychologically traumatic events involving brain injury were more strongly associated with depression and PTSD than psychologically traumatic events not involving brain injury. In a prospective study of traumatically injured patients admitted to the hospital for at least 24 hours, Bryant et al. (2010) reported that patients were at higher risk for subsequent development of PTSD and several other anxiety disorders if they had sustained mTBI. Similar findings hold in military veterans exposed to war-zone trauma, even when potential differences in combat exposure between veterans with and without TBI are taken into account. For instance, Chemtob and colleagues (1998) reported that patients who sustained TBI had higher levels of PTSD symptoms than their non-TBI counterparts, and Vasterling, Constans, and Hanna-Pladdy (2000) reported an increased severity of depression associated with TBI. Similar findings have been reported in OEF/OIF veterans (Hoge et al., 2008; Schneiderman, Braver, & Kang, 2008).

The association between mTBI and PTSD presents somewhat of a paradox, as the alterations in consciousness associated with TBI are thought to interfere with the formation of traumatic memories. According to one perspective (Sbordone & Liter, 1995), amnesia for the traumatic event might be incompatible with several core features of PTSD, including affective responses associated with the event, reexperiencing of trauma memories, and avoidance of trauma reminders. Consistent with this view, poorer memory for a traumatic event after mTBI is protective against select reexperiencing symptoms (Bryant, Creamer, O'Donnell, Silove, Clark, & McFarlane, 2009), and the likelihood of PTSD decreases as the severity of TBI increases (Glaesser, Neuner, Lutgehetmann, Schmidt, & Elbert, 2004). However, in patients with mTBI, amnesia for the event is not always complete, and some aspects of the trauma may be consciously accessible. Further, even when conscious retrieval fails completely, other mechanisms may be responsible for the development of symptoms: (1) affective and sensory–perceptual experiences associated with the trauma event may be encoded at an implicit, unconscious level, and subsequently impact on physiological, affective, and behavioral responses (Layton & Wardi-Zonna, 1995); (2) later reconstruction of memory from secondary sources such as family or observers may lead to the development of PTSD symptoms (Harvey & Bryant, 2001); and (3) the context of the trauma (e.g., sights and sounds upon regaining consciousness) and peritraumatic events (e.g., medical procedures) can be traumatic in their own right, and therefore lead to PTSD (McMillan, 1996).

In military combat and other contexts characterized by ongoing psychological stress, unique factors may further permit the coexistence of TBI and PTSD. Both war-zone stress exposures and domestic violence, for example, are rarely limited to a single discrete event, but more commonly involve a series of repeated or ongoing threatening events. Thus, even if a specific traumatic event is not remembered, it may be embedded in a larger context of psychological trauma. Moreover, less severe levels of mTBI, such as commonly reported in military personnel, may entail only momentary alteration of consciousness. As such, partial encoding of the trauma event may allow some aspects of the trauma to be accessed and reexperienced at a conscious level.

Recent findings in OEF and OIF veterans have further highlighted the association between mTBI and PTSD. Hoge and colleagues (2008) reported that of those service members who reported sustaining TBI with loss of consciousness, 44% met screening criteria for PTSD as compared to 27% of those who suffered TBI with altered consciousness and 16% of those with other injuries not including TBI. Similar findings have been reported by Schneiderman et al. (2008). On the one hand, given the considerable overlap in symptoms of mTBI and PTSD, it has been argued that the observed association may reflect inflated reporting of mTBI on the basis of psychiatric symptoms. On the other hand, such findings give added weight to the notion that mTBI may serve as a risk factor for PTSD. Consistent with the latter view, a recent analysis of data from a large sample of Vietnam-era veterans enrolled in the Vietnam Experience Study indicated that remote history of TBI increased the risk of current PTSD, on average 16 years after deployment (Vanderploeg, Belanger, & Curtiss, 2009).

Aside from its impact on the prevalence of PTSD, mTBI may also be associated with qualitative differences in the development of specific stress symptoms and the course of adjustment. Focusing specifically on acute stress disorder, Broomhall and colleagues (2009) found several differences in the nature of acute stress symptoms reported by patients with and without mTBI. Although some of these symptom differences were likely due to overlap in symptoms between mTBI and acute stress disorder, of note was a higher level of behavioral avoidance in patients with mTBI, a symptom that is not in itself associated with mTBI. In another study (Bryant & Harvey, 1999), patients with mTBI reported less fear and fewer intrusive memories than patients without TBI acutely posttrauma, but this difference was not apparent 6 months later. The lack of group differences at 6 months was attributable to the rate of intrusions increasing over the first 6 months in those with mTBI, but decreasing in those without mTBI.

There is inconclusive evidence as to whether posttraumatic stress symptoms in the context of mTBI may be more persistent. Harvey and Bryant (2000) followed individuals with mTBI due to motor vehicle accidents and found that of those who had acute stress disorder, 82% had a diagnosis of PTSD 6 months postinjury, and 80% still suffered from PTSD at 2-year follow-up. This outcome is comparable to that of survivors of motor vehicle accidents without TBI (Harvey & Bryant, 1999a). However, these findings are specific to acute stress disorder. Many individuals develop acute posttraumatic stress symptoms without meeting diagnostic criteria for acute stress disorder. Prospective studies of civilian trauma survivors without TBI show that more than half of individuals who show stress-related symptoms in the initial weeks after trauma exposure remit within 3 months (Blanchard et al., 1996; Riggs, Rothbaum, & Foa, 1995). It is unknown whether this trajectory is different for patients with mTBI.

Neurocognitive Alterations in mTBI

Insight into the neurocognitive effects of mTBI comes primarily from studies in a civilian context, including motor vehicle accidents and sports-related injury. As summarized by Bigler and Maxwell (Chapter 2, this volume), in civilian samples, the sequelae of mTBI are mostly transient and rapidly or gradually resolve in an overwhelming majority of patients (Caroll et al., 2004; Iverson, 2005), but in a minority of patients cognitive deficits and symptoms persist at 3 months postinjury (Pertab, James, & Bigler, 2009; Ponsford et al., 2000). In sports-related concussion, cognitive impairments typically resolve within 7–10 days (Belanger & Vanderploeg, 2005; McCrae et al., 2003), whereas in other clinical samples deficits on neuropsychological measures can persist for several months (Belanger, Curtiss, Demery, Lebowitz, & Vanderploeg, 2005). The temporal variability in the resolution of neurocognitive deficits may reflect individual differences in rate of recovery (McCrea et al., 2005), history of previous head injury (Belanger & Vanderploeg, 2005), and/or psychosocial factors including litigation (Belanger et al., 2005).

In the acute phase of mTBI, impairments in memory and executive function are most common. With regard to memory, deficient encoding of new information and delayed recall of this material frequently occur (Belanger et al., 2005; Belanger & Vanderploeg, 2005). Executive functions encompass a range of cognitive processes that are important for controlling or guiding behavior in a top–down manner. Specific executive control deficits that can follow mTBI include impaired ability to inhibit contextually inappropriate responses (McCrae et al., 2003), sustain and shift attention (Belanger et al., 2005; Belanger & Vanderploeg, 2005), manipulate information in working memory (Stuss, Stetham, & Poirier, 1989), and organize information into meaningful units (Bruce & Echemendia, 2003).

Despite a generally favorable recovery, considerable heterogeneity in outcome is observed across both neuropsychological measures and patients. Although not in the range of clinical impairment, patients with mTBI may continue to show reduced performance on measures of working memory and enhanced sensitivity to proactive interference years after injury (Vanderploeg, Curtiss, & Belanger, 2005). These residual deficits may reflect in part underlying deficits in speed of processing and a reduction in the amount of information that can be processed accurately (Crawford, Knight, & Alsop, 2007; Van Zomeren, Brouwer, & Deelman, 1984)—impairments that become apparent under conditions of high cognitive load or other sources of stress. Furthermore, symptoms of depression and anxiety disorders can follow a TBI (Bryant, O'Donnell, et al., 2010) and, as discussed by Iverson (Chapter 3, this volume), may exacerbate these cognitive impairments.

With respect to subject heterogeneity, Pertab et al. (2009) concluded from a reanalysis of meta-analytic studies that residual mild neuropsychological impairment may occur more reliably than previously acknowledged in a small subset of individuals. In this regard, it is of note that a history of multiple concussions is associated with worse long-term neuropsychological functioning, particularly in the domains of executive control (e.g., inhibition, set shifting, verbal fluency) and memory (Belanger, Spiegel, & Vanderploeg, 2010). Further, even in individuals who perform within normal limits on standard neuropsychological tests, deficits on more taxing executive control tasks may remain (Ellemberg, Leclerc, Couture, & Daigle, 2007; Pontifex, O'Connor, Broglio, & Hillman, 2009). For instance, in patients with chronic mTBI, residual impairments in inhibitory control have been documented on an experimental task in which responding to a central stimulus required inhibition of flanking stimuli (Pontifex et al., 2009). Impairments were observed even in the absence of deficient performance on standard clinical neuropsychological tests, and these became more pronounced with repetitive mTBI.

The constellation of cognitive deficits that may accompany mTBI suggests a disruption of functions mediated by the frontal and medial temporal regions of the brain. Evidence for such disruption comes from diffusion tensor imaging studies that measure the integrity of white matter tracts, which conduct neural impulses between brain regions. Several studies have demonstrated abnormalities in long white matter tracts that connect anterior and posterior regions of the brain in patients evaluated in the semiacute phase (Mayer et al., 2010; Messé et al., 2010), as well as more chronically in individuals with persistent symptoms (e.g., Huang et al., 2009; Lo, Shifteh, Gold, Bello, & Lipton, 2009). Such measures have also been linked to aspects of cognitive dysfunction (e.g., Kraus et al., 2007; Mayer et al., 2010). Studies using functional magnetic resonance imaging (fMRI) demonstrate that mTBI patients with normal structural imaging show alterations in neural activation relative to a control group. For instance, bilateral frontal and parietal lobe hypoactivation has been found on challenging tasks of working memory and spatial attention (Mayer et al., 2009; McAllister, Flashman, McDonald, & Saykin, 2006).

As shown by Bigler and Maxwell (Chapter 2, this volume), neuroimaging studies suggest that despite normal findings using the types of conventional MRI or computerized tomography (CT) commonly used in clinical settings, mTBI can alter brain microstructure and function in frontal and limbic regions. Given the significance of the limbic system to emotion, these regions are unsurprisingly also key in neural models of PTSD that postulate inadequate frontal lobe inhibition of the limbic system, and in particular a structure known as the amygdala, which is implicated in fear processing and learning (Rauch, Shin, & Phelps, 2006). In support of these models, a body of neuroimaging findings suggests that PTSD involves (1) exaggerated responsivity of the amygdala and (2) reduced activity in the frontal cortex (especially its medial, ventromedial, and orbital sections) and hippocampus (see Hayes & Gilbertson, Chapter 4, this volume). If mTBI affects the very same brain regions that account in part for the clinical presentation of PTSD, it stands to reason that mTBI may exacerbate symptoms associated with PTSD.

Cognitive Domains That May Influence the Development, Course, and Treatment of PTSD

Possibly the earliest evidence that sources of neurocognitive variance affect posttrauma psychological adjustment comes from studies examining the link between intellectual functioning and PTSD. Pitman, Orr, Lowenhagen, Macklin, and Altman (1991) reported that a lower score on the Arithmetic Reasoning subtest of the Armed Forces Qualification Test at enlistment predicted subsequent chronic PTSD, but their study remained inconclusive because it did not control for extent of combat exposure. Subsequent studies that adjusted for extent of stress exposure, however, have confirmed these findings (Macklin et al., 1998; Vasterling et al., 2002), although one study demonstrated that intellectual resources may be influential only at relatively lower levels of stress with less impact at higher stress levels (Thompson & Gottesman, 2008).

Regarding response to treatment, Rizvi, Vogt, and Resick (2009) found that lower general intelligence and education were associated with higher treatment dropout in a sample of 145 women being treated with a cognitive-behavioral therapy (CBT) for PTSD from sexual assault. Notably, however, general intelligence and education were not significantly associated with level-of-symptom reduction among treatment completers. These findings raise the possibility that cognitive deficits in patients with mTBI could potentially influence early treatment response (leading some patients to opt out early), but would not necessarily alter the eventual outcome of treatment for patients who became engaged for the full span of treatment.

Intellectual functioning is not a unitary construct, and as such, there are a number of possible mechanisms that may explain the observed association between intelligence and PTSD. Intellectual resources may broadly impact the ability to mobilize coping resources and problem-solving skills important for posttrauma adjustment, but may also have an impact through more specific neurocognitive processes that are potentially affected by mTBI independently of intellectual functioning. Possible candidates include (1) autobiographical memory; (2) executive control; and (3) verbal skills. We elaborate on each of these cognitive factors in turn, with special consideration of how they may be affected by mTBI.

Autobiographical Memory

Most cognitive theories of PTSD hold that autobiographical memory disturbance is a central element of the disorder, with enhanced involuntary recall of the trauma as well as decreased voluntary access to trauma memories (Brewin, 2007). Both in acute stress disorder (Harvey & Bryant, 1999b) and PTSD (Amir, Stafford, Freshman, & Foa, 1998), trauma memories have been described as being fragmented, disorganized, and lacking internal coherence. Such fragmentation is thought to result from disorganized initial encoding of the traumatic event, which leads to inconsistent consolidation and poorly regulated retrieval. Further, the failure to properly contextualize a memory by placing it in its appropriate spatial and temporal context may be responsible for the occurrence of involuntary intrusive memories, consisting of vivid, detailed images accompanied by a sense of reliving in the present. Evidence suggests that these characteristics of intrusions strongly predict PTSD severity (Michael, Ehlers, Halligan, & Clark, 2005) and that resolution of PTSD symptoms is associated with reduced frequency of intrusions (Hackmann, Ehlers, Speckens, & Clark, 2004) and establishment of a cohesive organization of the trauma memory (Foa, Molnar, & Cashman, 1995).

mTBI may exacerbate the development of PTSD by weakening the encoding and integration of a traumatic event into a temporally and conceptually organized autobiographical memory (Conway & Pleydell-Pearce, 2000). Disruption of consciousness during the mTBI is likely to interfere with the formation of a coherent memory of the trauma and altered mental status may have a blunting effect on memory abilities (Stuss et al., 1999). Even after consciousness returns to normal, however, difficulties with strategic learning and organization in the immediate aftermath of mTBI may continue to disrupt encoding of trauma-related information received from medical personnel or witnesses of the event. Thus, although degraded encoding of the trauma may be associated with protection against development of select reexperiencing symptoms (Bryant et al., 2009), reduced control over retrieval resulting from fragmented encoding could arguably be detrimental to recovery from psychological trauma.

Extending this line of reasoning, it is possible that accessibility to, and the coherence of, the trauma narrative would likewise be relevant to those PTSD interventions dependent on retrieval of the trauma memory. Evidence-based CBTs for PTSD typically include exposure-based components, which require retrieval of trauma memories so that new affective associations may be formed. Thus, even if an mTBI is fully resolved at the time of the intervention, it is plausible that acute neurocognitive impairment at the time of the trauma could influence the encoding of the trauma event, how associated emotions are processed, and therefore the degree to which trauma-related memories and affect can be retrieved in a controlled, verbally accessible manner during therapy (for fuller discussion of treating PTSD in the context of mTBI, see Bryant & Litz, Chapter 11, this volume).

In addition to the coherence of the trauma memory, more general aspects of autobiographical memory (extending to nontrauma memories) may also contribute to PTSD outcomes following trauma exposure. Specifically, trauma survivors with acute stress disorder (Harvey, Bryant, & Dang, 1998) or PTSD (McNally, Lasko, Macklin, & Pitman, 1995) tend to provide fewer specific details on autobiographical memory tasks, instead producing overgeneral memories, particularly in response to positive cues. Longitudinal studies have clarified that this tendency to produce overgeneral memories is a risk factor for the development of PTSD. For instance, Bryant, Sutherland, and Guthrie (2007) reported that a failure to retrieve specific memories in response to positive cues prior to trauma exposure in a group of firefighter trainees predicted symptom severity after trauma exposure.

To our knowledge, no studies have examined autobiographical memory in TBI samples limited to mTBI, although two studies have addressed autobiographical memory in samples with more severe TBI or in mixed severity groups. In the first study, more severe TBI was associated with significant difficulty in the retrieval of specific memories (Williams, Williams, & Ghadiali, 1998). Furthermore, the extent of overgeneral retrieval was related to impaired memory function on an immediate story recall task (Williams et al., 1998), suggesting a link between disruption of general memory formation and disturbance of autobiographical memory following TBI. In the second study, Bessel, Watkins, and Williams (2008) found that overgeneral memory was linked to depression in TBI. In that study, patients with mild and moderate–severe TBI showed reduced specificity of autobiographic memory retrieval following induction of depression-like ruminative self-focus. Moreover, baseline depression severity was inversely correlated with autobiographical memory retrieval. Thus, both general memory inefficiency and negative mood are associated with reduced ability to retrieve specific autobiographical memories in mTBI. One mechanism that may mediate these associations is reduced executive resources (Williams, 2006). Specifically, limited executive capacity may lead to a truncated search through the hierarchy of memory representations, resulting in the retrieval of memories at a general level of description rather than memories corresponding to specific events.

Executive Control

In addition to its role in guiding memory search, executive control may affect the development and course of PTSD through its impact on the control of memory retrieval, regulation of affective processing, and cognitive appraisal of the trauma and its sequelae. We discuss each of these possible mechanisms in turn.

Studies in normal cognition point to inefficient cognitive control as a vulnerability factor for reexperiencing symptoms. Specifically, the ability to inhibit interference from irrelevant emotionally neutral information in working memory has been linked to the presence of spontaneous intrusive memories (Verwoerd, Wessel, & de Jong, 2009) and experimentally induced undesirable intrusive memories (Wessel, Overwijk, Verwoerd, & de Vrieze, 2008). Likewise, in patients with PTSD, Vasterling, Brailey, Constans, and Sutker (1998) found that disinhibition and intrusion errors on emotionally neutral neuropsychological tasks were positively correlated with reexperiencing symptoms, suggesting that a more general deficit gating information contributes to difficulties with the control of emotional information. If extrapolated to mTBI, it is possible that TBI-related impairments in working memory and inhibitory control lead to difficulty suppressing intrusive information, thereby contributing to the development and maintenance of reexperiencing symptoms. Moreover, a reduction in executive resources may lead not only to an inability to control intrusive thoughts, but may additionally enhance precisely those thoughts that are intended to be controlled (Wegner, 1994).

The same executive impairments that potentially render mTBI patients more vulnerable to uncontrolled, intrusive memories may also compromise the controlled, voluntary retrieval of the trauma memory. This is so because controlled retrieval requires specification of appropriate retrieval cues and inhibition of inappropriate ones, as well as monitoring of the suitability of retrieved memories, all of which depend on the integrity of executive function. As discussed above, difficulty retrieving the trauma memory in a controlled manner may impede natural recovery from PTSD and hamper interventions with exposure components.

Executive control plays a similarly important role in affective regulation. Several studies have concluded that PTSD reflects an inability of dorsolateral prefrontal cortex to inhibit a hyperresponsive emotional system mediated by the limbic system (e.g., Bremner et al., 1999; Shin et al., 2005). Extending a framework on the normal interaction between cognition and emotion, Morey, Petty, Cooper, LaBar, and McCarthy (2008) examined how PTSD symptoms relate to the reciprocal relationship between executive functioning and processing of emotional information. They found that in a sample of OEF/OIF veterans recently returned from deployment, severity of PTSD symptoms was positively associated with activation in ventral frontal-limbic regions during processing of combat-related pictures and negatively associated with activation in dorsal-frontal regions during executive processing. Because these findings are correlational, they do not indicate whether alterations in brain function were caused by PTSD or were a precipitating factor. However, it stands to reason that reductions in executive control, as seen in mTBI, might exacerbate any imbalance between affective and executive processing in PTSD.

Aside from its effect on emotional experience, executive impairment may also impact the modulation of emotional expression. TBI-related difficulty monitoring and inhibiting behavioral expressions of anger, frustration, and other negative emotions may result in behaviors that are contextually inappropriate in non-life-threatening situations. It is possible that dysregulated emotional responses, such as irritability, anger, and aggression (Alderman, 2003; Johansson, Jamora, Ruff, & Pack, 2009), decrease feelings of control and lead to a negative self-perception. The emotional consequences of poor affect regulation, such as anger, shame, and guilt, have also been found to predict PTSD status (Andrews, Brewin, Rose, & Kirk, 2000; Marx et al., 2010). Emotional lability similarly may have deleterious effects on interpersonal relationships, reducing access to sources of social and economic support, thus further hindering recovery from psychological trauma. Dysfunctional emotional regulation could also interfere with relationships within a treatment context. For example, poor emotional control could potentially interfere with group treatment interventions, in which the focus of the group is vulnerable to inappropriate disruptions posed by individual group members.

Finally, executive dysfunction possibly adversely affects cognitive appraisal of the trauma and its consequences, a factor known to affect the development and maintenance of PTSD (Ehlers & Clark, 2000). More specifically, reduced cognitive flexibility in mTBI, due to compromised attentional switching and inhibitory processes, may interfere with the ability to reappraise stimuli in the environment as nonthreatening. This also has implications for the therapeutic context. Because cognitive therapy requires consideration of alternate appraisals of negative or distorted thoughts, with the goal of generating more realistic and constructive explanations (see Bryant & Litz, Chapter 11, this volume), cognitive flexibility may be particularly important for PTSD interventions with a cognitive component. Presumably, successful reappraisal would require both intact inhibition (of maladaptive thoughts) and cognitive flexibility (to reappraise thoughts), which may be particularly challenging for the subset of patients with mTBI who show lingering cognitive deficits. On the other hand, CBT offers a structured therapeutic context, which could arguably benefit patients with mild executive deficits. The success of CBT with patients with mTBI and acute stress disorder (Bryant et al., 2003) supports this perspective and argues for continued use of cognitive therapy with patients with mTBI and PTSD. The question remains, however, whether PTSD interventions with cognitive components would benefit from strategies that enhance the potential for efficient and adaptive reappraisal processes.

Verbal Skills

As described above, patients with mTBI may exhibit impairments in memory and executive functioning that affect both verbal and nonverbal information processing. Impairments in verbal processing may be particularly relevant to the development and course of PTSD. The association between impaired verbal memory and PTSD is well established (Brewin, Kleiner, Vasterling, & Field, 2006), and memory impairment appears to affect in particular the initial acquisition of verbal information into memory. Both prospective (Bustamante, Mellman, David, & Fins, 2001) and twin (Gilbertson et al., 2006) studies suggest that impaired verbal function, and especially verbal learning and memory, may be a risk factor for PTSD. Further, Bustamante and colleagues (2001) found that verbal learning and recall as well as verbal fluency measured in the first few weeks after trauma predicted the development of PTSD 6 weeks later.

There are a number of ways in which TBI-related deficits in verbal processing, including the ability to flexibly and effectively encode and manipulate verbal information, may impact on the development and maintenance of PTSD. Brewin (2005) has emphasized the relationship between verbal processing and the ability to suppress intrusive thoughts. In normal individuals, low verbal working memory has been associated with more intrusions of arbitrary (Brewin & Beaton, 2002) as well as personally relevant obsessive thoughts (Brewin & Smart, 2005). Further, in participants who watched a traumatic film, limiting spontaneous verbal processing by means of a concurrent verbal task enhanced the likelihood of intrusions, a finding that was interpreted as suggesting that intrusive memories are normally suppressed by verbal processes (Holmes, Brewin, & Hennessy, 2004). We highlighted above how deficiencies in cognitive control associated with mTBI may be a vulnerability factor for reexperiencing symptoms. Although not limited to the verbal domain, mTBI-related working memory impairments provide a possible mechanism by which top-down control of intrusive memories may be compromised.

The extent to which the trauma memory itself can be verbally accessed and processed also plays an important role in the course of PTSD. Brewin, Gregory, Lipton, and Burgess (2010) postulated that reexperiencing symptoms in PTSD occur when low-level sensory representations of the trauma are insufficiently integrated with corresponding contextual representations that allow an event to be placed in its appropriate spatial–temporal context. Sensory representations are triggered involuntarily by reinstatement of situational and affective cues, and it is by virtue of their association with contextual representations that they can be intentionally controlled and experienced as a memory from the past rather than relived in the present. Although contextual representations are not inherently verbal, they provide the basis for narrative memories, in that they allow information to be deliberately retrieved and manipulated and integrated into a person's individual history and knowledge base. Assimilation of trauma memories and their associated emotions into an ongoing life narrative may be critical for symptom resolution (Conway, 2005).

Contextual representations depend on functioning of the medial temporal lobe memory system, which may be compromised under conditions of extreme stress (Metcalfe & Jacobs, 1998). Because the hippocampus is uniquely vulnerable to the effects of brain injury (Lowenstein, Thomas, Smith, & McIntosh, 1992), even mTBI (and even more so repeated insult [Slemmer, Matser, De Zeeuw, & Weber, 2002]) may further exacerbate hippocampal dysfunction. Thus, mTBI may further interfere with the ability to establish contextual memory representations, leaving trauma memories largely dependent on sensory representations that are not verbally accessible. As discussed earlier in regard to autobiographical memory more generally, access to the trauma memory is key to successful implementation of exposure-based PTSD interventions. Given that these interventions rely specifically on the ability to form a verbal trauma narrative, verbal processing (both at the time of the trauma and subsequently during treatment) may be particularly important in the treatment context.

Conclusions

Although mTBI is associated with good short-term recovery, both acute neurocognitive deficits and subtle postacute deficits in a subgroup of patients potentially influence the development and course of PTSD. This possibility is borne out by empirical findings indicating that mTBI is associated with enhanced risk for PTSD. Little is currently known about the ways in which mTBI may affect how individuals cope with psychological trauma. It is apparent that a range of factors will need to be taken into account, including not only the neurocognitive sequelae of mTBI, but also its emotional and psychosocial consequences. Similarly, conditions that complicate recovery from mTBI, such as repeated head injury or alcohol abuse, will require consideration. In this chapter, we focused on the neurocognitive impairments associated with mTBI that may mediate vulnerability to PTSD, including impairments in autobiographical memory, executive function, and verbal processing. Given the lack of studies examining the effects of mTBI-related cognitive impairments upon the expression of PTSD, we drew on evidence regarding cognitive factors that have been postulated to mediate the variability in recovery from psychological trauma in the general population. Although theoretical considerations suggest multiple avenues by which mTBI-related neurocognitive impairment may influence the development, course, and recovery of PTSD, future empirical studies are clearly needed to evaluate these possibilities.

Treatment of course also potentially affects the course of PTSD, but limited data address whether PTSD treatments are as effective for patients with mTBI, and in particular for those with enduring deficits. What little evidence we have suggests that CBT is likely an effective treatment option for patients with comorbid mTBI and PTSD. Of less certainty is whether patients with mTBI would be more likely to terminate treatment prematurely, whether treatment response would be attenuated, and whether certain aspects of various CBT components could be enhanced via modifications that take into account cognitive deficits, or even via integrated treatments that address PTSD and mTBI sequelae concurrently, as described by Bryant and Litz (Chapter 11, this volume). Answers to these questions await carefully designed longitudinal studies and clinical trials that take into account the variability in outcome of mTBI and possible factors that may affect PTSD recovery.

References

Alderman, N. (2003). Contemporary approaches to the management of irritability and aggression following traumatic brain injury. *Neuropsychological Rehabilitation, 13*, 211–240.

Amir, N., Stafford, J., Freshman, M. S., & Foa, E. B. (1998). Relationship between trauma narratives and trauma pathology. *Journal of Traumatic Stress, 11*, 385–392.

Andrews, B., Brewin, C. R., Rose, S., & Kirk, M. (2000). Predicting PTSD symptoms in victims of violent crime: The role of shame, anger, and childhood abuse. *Journal of Abnormal Psychology, 109*, 69–73.

Belanger, H. G., Curtiss, G., Demery, J. A., Lebowitz, B. K., & Vanderploeg, R. D. (2005). Factors moderating neuropsychological outcomes following mild traumatic brain injury: A meta-analysis. *Journal of the International Neuropsychological Society, 11*, 215–227.

Belanger, H. G., Spiegel, E., & Vanderploeg, R. D. (2010). Neuropsychological performance following a history of multiple self-reported concussions: A meta-analysis. *Journal of the International Neuropsychological Society, 16*, 262–267.

Belanger, H. G., & Vanderploeg, R. D. (2005). The neuropsychological impact of sports-related concussion: A meta-analysis. *Journal of the International Neuropsychological Society, 11*, 345–357.

Bessel, A. L., Watkins, E. R., & Williams, W. H. (2008). Depressive rumination reduces specificity of autobiographical memory recall in acquired brain injury. *Journal of the International Neuropsychological Society, 14*, 63–70.

Blanchard, E. B., Hickling, E. J., Taylor, A. E., Loos, W. R., Forneris, C. A., & Jaccard, J. (1996). Who develops PTSD from motor vehicle accidents? *Behaviour Research and Therapy, 34*, 1–10.

Bremner, J. D., Staib, L. H., Kaloupek, D., Southwick, S. M., Soufer, R., & Charney, D. S. (1999). Neural correlates of exposure to traumatic pictures and sound in Vietnam combat veterans with and without posttraumatic stress disorder: A positron emission tomography study. *Biological Psychiatry, 55*, 612–620.

Brewin, C. R. (2005). Implications for psychological intervention. In J. J. Vasterling & C. R. Brewin (Eds.), *Neuropsychology of PTSD: Biological, cognitive and clinical perspectives* (pp. 271–291). New York: Guilford Press.

Brewin, C. R. (2007). Autobiographical memory for trauma: Update on four controversies. *Memory, 15*, 227–248.

Brewin, C. R., & Beaton, A. (2002). Thought suppression, intelligence, and working memory capacity. *Behaviour Research and Therapy, 40*, 923–930.

Brewin, C. R., Gregory, J. D., Lipton, M., & Burgess, N. (2010). Intrusive images in psychological disorders: Characteristics, neural mechanisms, and treatment implications. *Psychological Review, 117*, 210–217.

Brewin, C. R., Kleiner, J. S., Vasterling, J. J., & Field, A. P. (2006). Memory for emotionally neutral information in posttraumatic stress disorder: A meta-analytic investigation. *Journal of Abnormal Psychology, 116*, 448–463.

Brewin, C. R., & Smart, L. (2005). Working memory capacity and suppression of obsessional thoughts. *Journal of Behavior Therapy and Experimental Psychiatry, 36*, 61–68.

Broomhall, L. G. J., Clark, R., McFarlane, A. C., O'Donnell, M., Bryant, R. A., Creamer, M., et al. (2009). Early stage assessment and course of acute stress disorder after mild traumatic brain injury. *Journal of Nervous and Mental Disease, 197*, 178–181.

Bruce, J. M., & Echemendia, R. J. (2003). Delayed-onset deficits in verbal encoding strategies among patients with mild traumatic brain injury. *Neuropsychology, 17*, 622–629.

Bryant, R. A., Creamer, M., O'Donnell, M., Silove, D., Clark, C. R., & McFarlane, A. C. (2009). Posttraumatic amnesia and the nature of posttraumatic stress disorder after mild traumatic brain injury. *Journal of the International Neuropsychological Society, 15*, 862–867.

Bryant, R. A., & Harvey, A. G. (1999). The influence of traumatic brain injury on acute stress disorder and posttraumatic stress disorder following motor vehicle accidents. *Brain Injury, 13*, 15–22.

Bryant, R. A., Moulds, M., Guthrie, R., & Nixon, R. D. V. (2003). Treating acute stress disorder following mild traumatic brain injury. *American Journal of Psychiatry, 160*, 585–587.

Bryant, R. A., O'Donnell, M. L., Creamer, M., McFarlane, A. C., Clark, C. R., & Silove, D. (2010). The psychiatric sequelae of traumatic injury. *American Journal of Psychiatry, 167*, 312–320.

Bryant, R. A., Sutherland, K., & Guthrie, R. M. (2007). Impaired specific autobiographical memory as a risk factor for posttraumatic stress after trauma. *Journal of Abnormal Psychology, 116*, 837–841.

Bustamante, V., Mellman, T. A., David, D., & Fins, A. I. (2001). Cognitive functioning and the early development of PTSD. *Journal of Traumatic Stress, 14*, 791–797.

Caroll, L. J., Cassidy, J. D., Peloso, P. M., Borg, J., von Holst, H., Holm, L., et al. (2004). Prognosis for mild traumatic brain injury: Results of the WHO Collaborating Center Task Force on mild traumatic brain injury. *Journal of Rehabilitation Medicine* (Suppl. 43), 84–105.

Chemtob, C. M., Muraoka, M. Y., Wu-Holt, P., Fairbank, J. A., Hamada, R. S., & Keane, T. M. (1998). Head injury and combat-related posttraumatic stress disorder. *Journal of Nervous and Mental Disorders, 186*, 701–708.

Conway, M. A. (2005). Memory and the self. *Journal of Memory and Language, 53*, 594–628.

Conway, M. A., & Pleydell-Pearce, C. W. (2000). The construction of autobiographical memories in the self-memory system. *Psychological Review, 107*, 261–288.

Crawford, M. A., Knight, R. G., & Alsop, B. L. (2007). Speed of word retrieval in postconcussion syndrome. *Journal of the International Neuropsychological Society, 13*, 178–182.

Ehlers, A., & Clark, D. M. (2000). A cognitive model of posttraumatic stress disorder. *Behaviour Research and Therapy 38*, 319–345.

Ellemberg, D., Leclerc, S., Couture, S., & Daigle, C. (2007). Prolonged neuropsychological impairment following a first concussion in female university soccer athletes. *Clinical Journal of Sport Medicine 17*, 369–374.

Foa, E. B., Molnar, C., & Cashman, L. (1995). Change in rape narratives during exposure therapy for posttraumatic stress disorder. *Journal of Traumatic Stress, 8*, 675–690.

Gilbertson, M. W., Paulus, L. A., Williston, S. K., Gurvits, T. V., Lasko, N. B., Pitman, R., et al. (2006). Neurocognitive function in monozygotic twins discordant for combat exposure: Relationship to posttraumatic stress disorder. *Journal of Abnormal Psychology, 115*, 484–495.

Glaesser, J., Neuner, F., Lutgehetmann, R., Schmidt, R., & Elbert, T. (2004). Posttraumatic stress disorder in patients with traumatic brain injury. *BMC Psychiatry, 4*, 5–6.

Hackmann, A., Ehlers, A., Speckens, A., & Clark, D. M. (2004). Characteristics and content of intrusive memories in PTSD and their changes with treatment. *Journal of Traumatic Stress, 17*, 231–240.

Harvey, A. G., & Bryant, R. A. (1999a). The relationship between acute stress disorder and posttraumatic stress disorder: A 2-year prospective evaluation. *Journal of Consulting and Clinical Psychology, 67*, 985–988.

Harvey, A. G., & Bryant, R. A. (1999b). A qualitative investigation of the organization of traumatic memories. *British Journal of Clinical Psychology, 38*, 401–405.

Harvey, A. G., & Bryant, R. A. (2000). A two-year prospective evaluation of the relationship between acute stress disorder and posttraumatic stress disorder following mild traumatic brain injury. *American Journal of Psychiatry, 157*, 626–628.

Harvey, A. G., & Bryant, R. A. (2001). Reconstructing trauma memories: A prospective study of "amnesic" trauma survivors. *Journal of Traumatic Stress, 14*, 277–282.

Harvey, A. G., Bryant, R. A., & Dang, S. T. (1998). Autobiographical memory in acute stress disorder. *Journal of Consulting and Clinical Psychology, 66*, 500–506.

Hoge, C. W., Goldberg, H. M., & Castro, C. A. (2009). The care of war veterans with mild traumatic brain injury—Flawed perspectives. *New England Journal of Medicine, 360*, 1588–1591.

Hoge, C. W., McGurk, D., Thomas, J. L., Cox, A. L., Engel, C. C., & Castro, C. A. (2008). Mild traumatic brain injury in U.S. soldiers returning from Iraq. *New England Journal of Medicine, 358*, 453–463.

Holmes, E. A., Brewin, C. R., & Hennessy, R. G. (2004). Trauma films, information processing, and intrusive memory development. *Journal of Experimental Psychology: General, 133*, 3–22.

Huang, M. X., Theilmann, R., Robb, A., Angeles, A., Nichols, S., Drake, A., et al. (2009). Integrated imaging approach with MEG and DTI to detect mild traumatic brain injury in military and civilian patients. *Journal of Neurotrauma, 26*, 1213–1226.

Iverson, G. L. (2005). Outcome from mild traumatic brain injury. *Current Opinions in Psychiatry, 18*, 301–317.

Johansson, S. H., Jamora, C. W., Ruff, R. M., & Pack, N. M. (2008). A biopsychosocial perspective of aggression in the context of traumatic brain injury. *Brain Injury, 22,* 999–1006.

Jorge, R. E. (2005). Neuropsychiatric consequences of traumatic brain injury: A review of recent findings. *Current Opinion in Psychiatry, 18,* 289–299.

Kim, E., Lauerback, E. C., Reeve, A., Arciniegas, D. B., Coburn, K. L., Mendez, M. F., et al. (2007). Neuropsychiatric complications of traumatic brain injury: A critical review of the literature (a report by the ANPA Committee on Research). *Journal of Neuropsychiatry and Clinical Neuroscience, 19,* 106–127.

Kraus, M. F., Susmaras, T., Caughlin, B. P., Walker, C. J., Sweeney, J. A., & Little, D. M. (2007). White matter integrity and cognition in chronic traumatic brain injury: A diffusion tensor imaging study. *Brain 130,* 2508–2519.

Layton, B. S., & Wardi-Zonna, K. (1995). Posttraumatic stress disorder with neurogenic amnesia for the traumatic event. *Clinical Neuropsychologist, 9,* 2–10.

Lo, C., Shifteh, K., Gold, T., Bello, J. A., & Lipton, M. L. (2009). Diffusor tensor imaging abnormalities in patients with mild traumatic brain injury and neurocognitive impairment. *Journal of Computer Assisted Tomography, 33,* 293–297.

Lowenstein, D. H., Thomas, M. J., Smith, D. H., & McIntosh, T. K. (1992). Selective vulnerability of dentate hilar neurons following traumatic brain injury: A potenial mechanistic link between head trauma and disorders of the hippocampus. *Journal of Neuroscience, 12,* 4846–4853.

Macklin, M. L., Metzger, L. J., Litz, B. T., McNally, R. J., Lasko, N. B., Orr, S. P., et al. (1998). Lower precombat intelligence is a risk factor for posttraumatic stress disorder. *Journal of Consulting and Clinical Psychology, 66,* 323–326.

Marx, B. P., Foley, K. M., Feinstein, B. A., Wolf, E. J., Kaloupek, D. G., & Keane, T. M. (2010). Combat-related guilt mediates the relations between exposure to combat-related abusive violence and psychiatric diagnoses. *Depression and Anxiety, 27,* 287–293.

Mayer, A. R., Ling, J., Mannell, M. V., Gasparovic, C., Phillips, J. P., Doezema, D., et al. (2010). A prospective diffusion tensor imaging study in mild traumatic brain injury. *Neurology, 74,* 643–650.

Mayer, A. R., Mannell, M. V., Ling, J., Elgie, R., Gasparovic, C., Phillips, J. P., et al. (2009). Auditory orienting and inhibition of return in mild traumatic brain injury: A fMRI study. *Human Brain Mapping, 30,* 4152–4166.

McAllister, T. W., Flashman, L. A., McDonald, B. C., & Saykin, A. J. (2006). Mechanisms of working memory dysfunction after mild and moderate TBI: Evidence from functional MRI and neurogenetics. *Journal of Neurotrauma, 23,* 1450–1467.

McCrea, M., Barr, W. B., Guskiewicz, K., Randolph, C., Marshall, S. W., Cantu, R., et al. (2005). Standard regression-based methods for measuring recovery after sport-related concussion. *Journal of the International Neuropsychological Society, 11,* 58–69.

McCrae, M., Guskiewicz, K. M., Marshall, S. W., Barr, W., Randolph, C., Cantu, R. C., et al. (2003). Acute effects and recovery time following concussion in collegiate football players. *Journal of the American Medical Association, 290*, 2556–2563.

McMillan, T. M. (1996). Post-traumatic stress disorder following minor and severe closed head injury: 10 single cases. *Brain Injury, 10*, 749–758.

McNally, R. J., Lasko, N. B., Macklin, M. L., & Pitman, R. K. (1995). Autobiographical memory disturbance in combat-related posttraumatic stress disorder. *Behaviour, Research, and Therapy, 33*, 619–630.

Messé, A., Caplain, S., Paradot, G., Garrigue, D., Mineo, J. F., Soto Ares, G., et al. (2010). Diffusion tensor imaging and white matter lesions at the subacute stage in mild traumatic brain injury with persistent neurobehavioral impairment. *Human Brain Mapping, 32*, 999–1011.

Metcalfe, J., & Jacobs, W. J. (1998). Emotional memory: The effects of stress on "cool" and "hot" memory systems. In G. H. Bower (Ed.), *The psychology of learning and motivation* (Vol. 38, pp. 187–222). New York: Academic Press.

Michael, T., Ehlers, A., Halligan, S. L., & Clark, D. M. (2005). Unwanted memories of assault: What intrusion characteristics are associated with PTSD? *Behaviour Research and Therapy, 43*, 613–628.

Molica, R. F., Henderson, D. C., & Tor, S. (2002). Psychiatric effects of traumatic brain injury events in Cambodian survivors of mass violence. *British Journal of Psychiatry, 181*, 339–347.

Morey, R. A., Petty, C. M., Cooper, D. A., LaBar, K. S., & McCarthy, G. (2008). Neural systems for executive and emotional processing are modulated by symptoms of posttraumatic stress disorder in Iraq War veterans. *Psychiatry Research: Neuroimaging, 162*, 59–72.

Pertab, J. L., James, K. M., & Bigler, E. D. (2009). Limitations of mild traumatic brain injury meta-analyses. *Brain Injury, 23*, 498–508.

Pitman, R. K., Orr, S. P., Lowenhagen, M. J., Macklin, M. L., & Altman, B. (1991). Pre-Vietnam contents of PTSD veterans' service medical and personnel records. *Comprehensive Psychiatry, 32*, 1–7.

Ponsford, J., Willmott, C., Rothwell, A., Cameron, P., Kelly, A. M., Nelms, R., et al. (2000). Factors influencing outcome following mild traumatic brain injury in adults. *Journal of the International Neuropsychological Society, 6*, 568–579.

Pontifex, M. B., O'Connor, P. M., Broglio, S. P., & Hillman, C. H. (2009). The association between mild traumatic brain injury history and cognitive control. *Neuropsychologia, 47*, 3210–3216.

Rauch, S. L., Shin, L. M., & Phelps, E. A. (2006). Neurocircuitry models of posttraumatic stress disorder and extinction: Human neuroimaging research—Past, present, and future. *Biological Psychiatry, 60*, 376–382.

Riggs, D. S., Rothbaum, B. O., & Foa, E. B. (1995). A prospective examination of symptoms of posttraumatic stress disorder in victims of non-sexual assault. *Journal of Interpersonal Violence, 10*, 201–213.

Rizvi, S. L., Vogt, D. S., & Resick, P. A. (2009). Cognitive and affective predictors of treatment outcome in cognitive processing therapy and prolonged exposure for posttraumatic stress disorder. *Behaviour Research and Therapy, 47*, 737–743.

Sbordone, R. J., & Liter, J. C. (1995). Mild traumatic brain injury does not produce posttraumatic stress disorder. *Brain Injury, 9*, 405–412.

Schneiderman, A. I., Braver, E. R., & Kang, H. K. (2008). Understanding sequelae of injury mechanisms and mild traumatic brain injury incurred during the conflicts in Iraq and Afghanistan: Persistent postconcussive symptoms and posttraumatic stress disorder. *American Journal of Epidemiology, 167*, 1446–1452.

Shin, L. M., Wright, C. I., Cannistraro, P. A., Wedig, M. M., McMullin, K., Martis, B., et al. (2005). A functional magnetic resonance imaging study of amygdala and medial prefrontal cortex responses to overtly presented fearful faces in posttraumatic stress disorder. *Archives of General Psychiatry, 62*, 273–281.

Slemmer, J. E., Matser, E. J. T., De Zeeuw, C. I., & Weber, J. T. (2002). Repeated mild injury causes cumulative damage to hippocampal cells. *Brain, 125*, 2699–2709.

Stuss, D. T., Binns, M. A., Carruth, F. G., Levine, B., Brandys, C. E., Moulton, R. J., et al. (1999). The acute period of recovery from traumatic brain injury: Posttraumatic amnesia or posttraumatic confusional state? *Journal of Neurosurgery, 90*(4), 635–643.

Stuss, D. T., Stetham, L. L., & Poirier, C. A. (1989). Comparison of three tests of attention and rapid information processing across six age groups. *Clinical Neuropsychologist, 1*, 139–152.

Tanielian, T., & Jaycox, L. H. (2008). *Invisible wounds of war: Psychological and cognitive injuries, their consequences, and services to assist recovery.* Santa Monica, CA: RAND Corp.

Thompson, W., & Gottesman, I. (2008). Challenging the conclusion that lower preinduction cognitive ability increases risk for combat-related post-traumatic stress disorder in 2,375 combat-exposed, Vietnam War veterans. *Military Medicine, 173*, 576–582.

Vanderploeg, R. D., Belanger, H. G., & Curtiss, G. (2009). Mild traumatic brain injury and posttraumatic stress disorder and their associations with health symptoms. *Archives of Physical and Medical Rehabilitation, 90*, 1084–1093.

Vanderploeg, R. D., Curtiss, G., & Belanger, H. G. (2005). Long-term neuropsychological outcomes following mild traumatic brain injury. *Journal of the International Neuropsychological Society, 11*, 228–236.

Van Zomeren, A. H., Brouwer, W. H., & Deelman, B. G. (1984). Attentional deficits: The riddles of selectivity, speed and alertness. In N. Brooks (Ed.), *Closed head injury: Psychological, social and family consequences* (pp. 74–107). Oxford: Oxford University Press.

Vasterling, J. J., Brailey, K., Constans, J. I., & Sutker, P. B. (1998). Attention and memory dysfunction in posttraumatic stress disorder. *Neuropsychology, 12*, 125–133.

Vasterling, J. J., Constans, J. I., & Hanna-Pladdy, B. (2000). Head injury as a predictor of psychological outcome in combat veterans. *Journal of Traumatic Stress, 13*, 441–451.

Vasterling, J. J., Duke, L. M., Brailey, K., Constans, J. I., Allain, A. N., & Sutker,

P. B. (2002). Attention, learning, and memory performances and intellectual resources in Vietnam veterans: PTSD and no disorder comparisons. *Neuropsychology, 16*, 5–14.

Vasterling, J. J., Verfaellie, M., & Sullivan, K. D. (2009). Mild traumatic brain injury and posttraumatic stress disorder in returning veterans: Perspectives from cognitive neuroscience. *Clinical Psychology Review, 29*, 674–684.

Verwoerd, J., Wessel, I., & de Jong, P. J. (2009). Individual differences in experiencing intrusive memories: The role of the ability to resist proactive interference. *Journal of Behavior Therapy and Experimental Psychiatry, 40*, 189–201.

Wegner, D. M. (1994). Ironic processes of mental control. *Psychological Review, 101*, 34–52.

Wessel, I., Overwijk, S., Verwoerd, J., & de Vrieze, N. (2008). Pre-stressor cognitive control is related to intrusive cognition of a stressful film. *Behaviour Research and Therapy, 46*, 496–513.

Williams, J. M. G. (2006). Capture and rumination, functional avoidance, and executive control (CaR-Fa-X): Three process that underlie overgeneral memory. *Cognition and Emotion, 20*, 548–568.

Williams, W. H., Williams, J. M. G., & Ghadiali, E. J. (1998). Autobiographical memory in traumatic brain injury: Neuropsychological and mood predictors of recall. *Neuropsychological Rehabilitation, 8*, 43–60.

Yeates, K. O. (2010). Mild traumatic brain injury and postconcussive symptoms in children and adolescents. *Journal of the International Neuropsychological Society, 16*, 953–960.

PART III

COMMONLY ASSOCIATED CONDITIONS

CHAPTER 6

Chronic Pain

John D. Otis, Catherine B. Fortier, and Terence M. Keane

Although pain is typically a transient experience, for some people pain persists past the point where it is considered an adaptive reaction to an acute injury and results in emotional distress, increased disability, and prolonged use of health care system resources. Consistent with a biopsychosocial model of illness, individuals with chronic pain often report that pain interferes with their ability to engage in occupational, social, or recreational activities. Their limited ability to engage in these activities may contribute to increased isolation, negative mood (e.g., feelings of worthlessness and depression), and physical deconditioning, each of which in turn can exacerbate or contribute to the experience of pain. Pain that persists for longer than 3 months, that initially accompanies a disease process or bodily injury that may have resolved or healed, may be referred to as "chronic" pain (Merskey & Bogduk, 1994).

Pain is one of the most common complaints made to primary care providers and has significant implications for health care costs (Gureje, Von Korff, Simon, & Gater, 1998; Otis, Reid, & Kerns, 2005). In fact, the National Institute of Health identified chronic pain as the costliest medical problem in America, affecting nearly 100 million individuals (Byrne & Hochwarter, 2006). Pain is the second leading cause of medically related work absenteeism, resulting in more than 50 million lost workdays each year (Fox et al., 2000). Headaches are the most common type of pain, and it is estimated that industry loses $50 billion per year due to absenteeism and medical expenses caused by headaches. Chronic pain is a significant problem among U.S. veterans, with nearly 50% of veterans reporting that they experience pain on a regular basis (Kerns, Otis, Rosenberg, & Reid, 2003). High rates of pain have also been reported among Operation Enduring Freedom (OEF)/Operation Iraqi Freedom (OIF) returnees seeking care (Ruff, Ruff, & Wang, 2009). Current estimates are that the budgetary costs of providing disability compensation benefits and medical care to OEF/OIF veterans over the course of their lives will be from $350 to $700 billion dollars (Bilmes, 2007). Given the negative impact that pain can have on quality of life and its financial impact on both civilian and government health care systems, providing accurate assessment and effective treatment for patients with chronic pain is a priority.

Chronic pain is often related to naturally occurring degenerative changes in the body that develop gradually over time; however, some pain conditions may develop secondary to injury related to life events such as occupational injuries, motor vehicle accidents, or participation in military combat. With respect to the latter, whereas blast injuries caused by improvised explosive devices (IEDs) and suicide bombers can result in injuries that one can see (i.e., physical injuries), they can also cause injuries that may be less visually apparent (e.g., traumatic brain injury [TBI] and posttraumatic stress disorder [PTSD]) but equally debilitating. Injuries associated with current combat operations have led to a growing interest in the relationships among chronic pain, PTSD, and TBI, as clinical practice and research reveals that these disorders frequently co-occur and may interact in ways that complicate assessment and treatment. Pain, PTSD, and TBI are characterized by overlapping symptoms (e.g., headache, irritability, sleep disturbance, memory impairments), and in the absence of accurate assessment information or a diagnosis, symptoms may be inaccurately attributed to another condition. This type of error can negatively influence the treatment plan and expectations of recovery (Hoge et al., 2008). It is important that clinicians have a clear understanding of how these conditions may interact, and knowledge of what steps they can take to provide the most effective treatment.

The primary aim of this chapter is to provide a critical review and synthesis of the existing literature on the comorbidity among pain, PTSD, and TBI and its implication for clinical treatment. The chapter begins with a review of the epidemiological literature on the comorbidity among pain, PTSD, and TBI. The neurobiology, pathophysiology, and symptom presentation of each condition is outlined. Specific treatment strategies for managing pain when comorbid with PTSD or TBI are also presented. Finally, the chapter closes with a section on future directions for treatment as well as a call for continued research to further refine existing treatments for these comorbid conditions.

Epidemiology

Pain and PTSD

Many empirical studies have examined the extent to which PTSD is present in chronic pain samples. Asmundson, Norton, Allerdings, Norton, and Larson (1998) assessed the extent to which work-related injuries were associated with PTSD in a sample of 139 injured workers with chronic pain referred to a rehabilitation program and found that 34.7% reported PTSD symptoms. Studies suggest that rates of PTSD in patients with pain related to motor vehicle accidents (MVAs) range from 30 to 50% (Chibnall & Duckro, 1994; Hickling & Blanchard, 1992; Taylor & Koch, 1995). Further, 24 to 47% of patients with fibromyalgia attribute the onset of their symptoms to a physical injury caused during a MVA (Sherman, Turk, & Okifuji, 2000; Turk, Okifuji, Starz, & Sinclaire, 1996). More recently, Otis, Gregor, Hardway, Morrison, Scioli, and Sanderson (2010) found that in a sample of 149 veterans who completed self-report questionnaires as part of their participation in a pain management program, 49% met criteria for PTSD.

Research examining the prevalence of chronic pain in individuals with PTSD has reported slightly higher comorbidity rates. White and Faustman (1989) reviewed discharge summaries of 543 veterans treated for PTSD to assess the frequency and nature of medical problems. Their results indicated that 25% of the sample showed some type of musculoskeletal or pain problem. McFarlane, Atchison, Rafalowicz, and Papay (1994) reported that in a sample of patients with PTSD also reporting physical symptoms, pain was the most common physical complaint (45% reported back pain and 34% reported headaches). Amir et al. (1997) examined a sample of 29 patients with PTSD and found the prevalence of fibromyalgia syndrome to be 21%. Further, Beckham et al. (1997) noted that in a sample of 129 combat veterans with PSTD, 80% reported the presence of a chronic pain condition. In a more recent study, Shipherd et al. (2007) reported that of 85 veterans seeking treatment for PTSD, 66% had a chronic pain diagnosis at pretreatment.

The co-occurrence of chronic pain and PTSD may have implications in terms of an individual's experience of each condition. Some research suggests that patients with chronic pain related to PTSD experience more intense pain and affective distress (Geisser, Roth, Bachman, & Eckert, 1996; Toomey, Seville, Abashian, Finkel, & Mann, 1994), higher levels of life interference (Turk & Okifuji, 1996), and greater disability (Sherman et al., 2000) than pain patients without trauma or PTSD. For example, Sherman et al. (2000) found that in a sample of 93 treatment-seeking fibromyalgia patients, those who experienced PTSD-related symptoms reported significantly greater levels of pain, life interference, emotional distress, and inactivity than did patients who did not report PTSD-like symptoms. However, a close examination of these studies reveals a number of methodological weaknesses including the reliance on patient samples with specialized chronic pain conditions (e.g., fibromyalgia, chronic fatigue, or injury secondary to MVAs), and variability in the manner used to diagnose PTSD. Otis et al. (2010) recently examined the interaction between pain and PTSD in a sample of 149 veterans using psychometrically sound measures of pain, PTSD, and depression, and a more conservative analytical approach (multivariate analysis of covariance). The analyses indicated that after controlling for the effects of age, gender, pain duration, and depressive symptom severity, the presence of PTSD was significantly associated with the overall experience of chronic pain. In contrast with previous research, PTSD was not significantly associated with increased pain severity or disability; the largest proportion of the association between PTSD and the experience of pain was attributable to "pain-relevant affective distress," which was composed of items assessing anxiety, negative mood, and irritability. The results suggest that pain-relevant distress may be particularly affected by PTSD and that psychological interventions for patients with comorbid chronic pain and PTSD may require a greater emphasis on cognitive restructuring to address negative ways of thinking.

Several theoretical models attempt to explain the comorbidity between chronic pain and PTSD, and the manner in which these two conditions may interact with one another. For example, the mutual maintenance model (Sharp & Harvey, 2001) suggests that pain can serve as a reminder of a traumatic event and trigger PTSD symptoms (e.g., "Every time my back starts hurting I think about the day our humvee was hit by the IED"). Similarly, this model proposes that reexperiencing a traumatic event can trigger thoughts about pain and increase its perceived intensity. Other models, such as the shared vulnerability and triple vulnerability models suggest that there may be preexisting underlying vulnerabilities in some individuals, such as elevated "anxiety sensitivity," that places them at higher risk for developing chronic pain following an injury or PTSD after being involved in a traumatic event (Asmundson, Coons, Taylor, & Katz, 2002; Otis, Pincus, & Keane, 2006). To test these models, future studies may benefit from using path analysis techniques to examine the contribution of psychological vulnerabilities such as affective distress, catastrophizing, or anxiety sensitivity to pain outcome measures.

Pain and TBI

To examine the prevalence and interaction between pain and TBI, Uomoto and Esselman (1993) evaluated 104 patients seen in an outpatient rehabilitation facility. They reported that 89% of individuals with minor traumatic brain injury (mTBI) reported headache pain, whereas only 18% of individuals with severe TBI reported headache pain. Similar rates were found for neck, back, and other pain syndromes. The mTBI group also had a higher frequency of pain syndromes (in addition to headache). Nampiaparampil (2008) performed a meta-analysis involving 23 studies published between 1951 and 2008 assessing TBI and pain. The results indicated that among civilians, the prevalence of headache pain was greater among those with mTBI (75%) as compared to moderate-to-severe TBI (32.1%). The prevalence of headache pain among veterans with TBI was 35.9%. It was hypothesized that the fact that civilians reported more pain than veterans may have been due to the types of traumatic injuries experienced (combat/assault vs. sports trauma) or reduced willingness to report pain on the part of veterans.

A recent study performed by Ruff et al. (2009) examined the prevalence of headache in OEF/OIF veterans who reported mTBI caused by blast exposure during deployment. Among the 126 veterans who were evaluated, 80 had impairments on neurological examination that were best attributed to mTBI. Results indicated that veterans with impairments experienced more explosions and were more likely to have headache, features of migraine, more severe pain, and more frequent headaches. Theeler, Flynn, and Erickson (2010) examined the prevalence of headache in a sample of soldiers undergoing postdeployment evaluation after a 1-year tour in Iraq. All soldiers screening positive for a deployment-related concussion were given a 13-item headache questionnaire. A total of 1,033 (19.6%) out of 5,270 returnees met criteria for a deployment-related concussion. Among those with a concussion, 957 (97.8%) reported having headaches during the final 3 months of deployment. No veterans in the sample had moderate or severe TBI. In total, 58% of posttraumatic headaches were classified as migraine. In many cases, head trauma was temporally associated with either the onset of headaches or the worsening of preexisting headaches, implicating trauma as a precipitating or exacerbating factor. Overall, research supports the conclusion that headache is a common pain feature among individuals who experience a TBI. Although headache may be more prevalent in patients with mTBI, it is important to consider that some patients with moderate-to-severe TBI may have more difficulty reporting their symptoms due to memory or executive functioning deficits.

Pain, PTSD, and TBI

Only a few studies have reported on the coprevalence of pain, PTSD, and TBI. Although these injuries certainly occur in combination among civilians who have been involved in accidents, the available literature has primarily focused on veteran samples, as recent data obtained from OEF/OIF veterans receiving care at Level 1 and Level 2 polytrauma rehabilitation centers (PRC) have served to inform and heighten awareness of the level of comorbidity among these three conditions. A study by Sayer et al. (2009) found that in a sample of 188 combat-injured service members treated at a Level 1 PRC, 93% of veterans incurred a combat-related TBI, 81% endorsed a pain problem, and 52.6% received some type of mental health services. In a study of 50 OEF/OIF veterans treated at a Level 1 PRC, 80% of patients reportedly incurred a combat related TBI (penetrating = 58%, closed = 22%), 96% reported at least one pain problem, and 44% reported experiencing PTSD (Clark, Bair, Buckenmaier, Gironda, & Walker, 2007). Lew et al. (2007) found that in a sample of 62 patients evaluated at a Level 2 PRC, 97% reported three or more postconcussive symptoms (e.g., headache, dizziness, fatigue), 97% complained of chronic pain, and 71% met criteria for PTSD. Lew et al. (2009) performed a comprehensive review on the medical records of 340 OEF/OIF veterans seen at a Level 2 PRC. Analyses indicated a high prevalence of all three conditions in this population, with chronic pain, PTSD, and mTBI being present in 81.5%, 68.2%, and 66.8%, respectively. Only 12 of the veterans (3.5%) had no reported pain, PTSD, or mTBI. The frequency at which these three conditions were present in isolation (10.3%, 2.9%, and 5.3%, respectively) was significantly lower than the frequency at which they were present in combination with one another, with 42.1% of the sample being diagnosed with all three conditions simultaneously. The most common chronic pain symptoms were back pain (58%) and headache (55%). Taken together, the results of these studies demonstrate the high coprevalence rates among pain, PTSD, and mTBI. In the next section, we examine the pathophysiology associated with each of these conditions and explore the manner in which the overlapping symptom presentation can complicate assessment and treatment.

The Pathophysiology and Neurocognitive Outcomes of mTBI, PTSD, and Pain

Neuropathology and Neurocognition of mTBI

As described in detail in Bigler and Maxwell (Chapter 2, this volume), the primary neuropathology underlying mTBI is diffuse axonal injury (DAI) caused by shearing forces that result from sudden deceleration, as well as traumatic axonal injury (TAI), a progressive process evoked by the tensile forces of injury. Shearing and tensile forces primarily affect white matter spreading from the cortex to the midbrain. Axonal injury has been quantified in mTBI as well as more severe TBI (Kraus et al., 2007). Although more common in moderate-to-severe TBI, in some cases mTBI may also cause focal damage to the anterior and inferior surfaces of the frontal and temporal lobes (Bigler, 2007), where the brain may impact on bony protrusions of the skull, or focal injury may occur as a result of coup (site of impact with an object) and contrecoup (the side opposite to the impact) forces. Although less well documented, there is some evidence that the amygdala may be affected in some cases of TBI (e.g., Wilde et al., 2007).

The nature and course of postacute cognitive recovery from mTBI remains controversial (Belanger, Curtiss, Demery, Lebowitz, & Vanderploeg, 2005). The majority of cases show complete resolution of symptoms within the first 1 to 3 months postinjury (Iverson, 2005), but a minority of patients still complain of symptoms that limit their everyday activities months and even years postinjury (Alexander, 1995; Hartlage, Durant-Wilson, & Patch, 2001; Levin et al., 1987; Powell, Collin, & Sutton, 1996). Memory, complex attention, and executive function are the neurocognitive domains that remain most frequently impaired in the postacute phase following mTBI (Vanderploeg, Curtiss, & Belanger, 2005). As described by Iverson (Chapter 3, this volume), long-term neurocognitive impairments are likely a result of a complex interation of neurologic, somatic, and psychological factors. Even well-recovered mTBI patients may experience reduced mental efficiency under conditions of physical or psychological stress (Stuss et al., 1985).

Functional outcome and quality of life following TBI typically follows a spectrum of severity such that those with more severe injuries fare worse. However, the relationship between severity and outcome is an indirect one that appears to be mediated primarily by postacute neurocognitive variables and not by physical or behavioral difficulties (Novack, Bush, Meythaler, & Canupp, 2001). Specifically, memory and executive function are inversely related to long-term functional outcome (Rassovsky et al., 2006). Other psychological and health-related factors are also likely to influence outcome (Hoge et al., 2008; Lippa, Pastorek, Benge, & Thornton), but because these factors also affect neuropsychological functioning, it is difficult to ascertain whether they mediate outcome directly, or indirectly, through their impact on neurocognition.

Neuropathology and Neurocognition of PTSD

Evidence from the neuroimaging data and neurocircuitry literature suggests that PTSD may be mediated by an exaggerated amygdala response secondary to impaired inhibitory regulation by the prefrontal cortex (Shin, Rauch, & Pitman, 2006). For example, functional imaging studies have demonstrated hypoactivation of the medial prefrontal cortex during fear processing (Lanius, Bluhm, Lanius, & Pain, 2006), and structural imaging studies have shown smaller volume of medial prefrontal cortex structures (e.g., Woodward et al., 2006). The literature suggests diminished volume, neuronal integrity, and functional integrity of the hippocampus in PTSD (Shin et al., 2006), and hippocampal volumetric differences may covary with PTSD severity (Karl et al., 2006). For example, a recent functional imaging study demonstrated reduced hippocampal activity under conditions of high stress and arousal, and reduction in left hippocampal activity was associated with high PTSD arousal symptoms (Hayes et al., 2010).

The literature examining neurocognitive functioning in PTSD is in line with the neuroimaging findings generated by PTSD studies. There is a large body of literature showing impaired memory, monitoring, and cognitive disinhibition in PTSD (e.g., Leskin & White, 2007), and these impairments are associated with PTSD-related behavioral disturbances such as reexperiencing (Leskin & White, 2007). Verbal memory impairment in particular has been associated with PTSD (Brewin, Kleiner, Vasterling, & Field, 2007; Johnsen & Asbjornsen, 2008).

Neuropathology and Neurocognition of Pain

Pain is a frequent comorbidity of mTBI and a common problem in polytrauma cases, with headaches as the primary pain condition (Nicholson & Martelli, 2004). Interestingly, pain, particularly posttraumatic headache, is a more frequent complaint following mTBI than more severe head injuries (Couch & Bearss, 2001; Uomoto & Esselman, 1993).

Although a detailed literature exists regarding the brain network for pain (e.g., the "pain matrix"; Melzack, 1999), the primary neurologic substrates of pain involve forebrain areas such as the prefrontal cortex (particularly the anterior cingulate cortex), the amygdala (Neugebauer, Galhardo, Maione, & Mackey, 2009), and the white matter tracts connecting these regions (Lutz et al., 2008). As part of the reward–aversion circuitry, these structures most likely subsume the emotional, affective, and cognitive aspects of pain. These regions also play an essential role in higher order cognitive processes and executive functioning such as planning, decision making, reward expectancy, and goal-directed behaviors (Goldman-Rakic, 1996). As such, pain may be associated with neuropsychological deficits in attention and executive functioning (Hart, Wade, & Martelli, 2003), and, similarly to PTSD, pain may involve frequent thought (pain or memory-related) intrusions and heightened anxiety that compromise the resources available for cognitive tasks. This constellation of deficits typically leads to complaints of difficulty concentrating, forgetfulness, and inability to complete tasks (Iverson & McCracken, 1997).

Overlapping Neural Substrates

TBI, PTSD, and pain commonly co-occur in civilian and military populations. As evident in the brief reviews above, there is considerable convergence in the neural pathways among the three conditions. Specifically, pain, PTSD, and TBI all likely involve prefrontal cortical dysfunction, either directly (e.g., changes in the function and/or structure of the cortex itself) or via axonal connectivity. White matter abnormalities have been well documented in TBI (Kraus et al., 2007), and to a lesser degree in PTSD (Villarreal et al., 2002) and chronic pain (Lutz et al., 2008). It has been suggested that white matter changes to regions of the pain matrix may underlie the perception of both pain intensity and fatigue in pain syndromes (Lutz et al., 2008).

The compromise of the inhibitory control of the limbic system that can occur in each of the disorders independently may exacerbate frontal system dysfunction when these syndromes co-occur (e.g., monitoring, inhibition, planning, reward expectancy). These declines may be additive or possible even multiplicative. For example, even mild stress-related symptomatology and anxiety immediately following mTBI have been identified as important predictors of poor long-term outcome (Ponsford et al., 2000).

The amygdala is also compromised in pain and PTSD (perhaps via decreased inhibitory control from the prefrontal cortex) and, although less common, can be affected in mTBI as well. Hippocampal function may also be affected in all three syndromes. It is possible that the coexistence of afferents from the amygdala and the hippocampus may suggest an anatomical complement to the pervasive negative memory traces that may underlie traumatic reexperiencing as well as "pain memory" involved in neuropathic pain (Metz, Yau, Centeno, Apkarian, & Martina, 2009).

Overlapping Neurocognitive Impairment and Symptom Presentation

Accurate assessment and treatment of chronic pain, PTSD, and mTBI are complicated by their shared clinical features, including sleep problems, irritability, cognitive complaints (e.g., concentration difficulties), and performance deficits (e.g., memory, executive, and attentional impairment). In the acute phase of TBI, signs such as alteration of mental status (e.g., being dazed or confused) may overlap with dissociative symptoms of acute stress disorder. Postcombat, postconcussive symptoms (e.g., irritability, difficulty concentrating, sleep disturbance) are likely to overlap with symptoms of PTSD, pain, and other disorders, such as depression. However, even when this symptom overlap is accounted for, PTSD remains the strongest factor associated with neuropsychiatric symptoms (headaches, dizziness, memory problems, balance problems, ringing in the ears, irritability, and sleep problems) attributable to TBI (Schneiderman, Braver, & Kang, 2008).

Although researchers have looked to performance-based neuropsychological assessments to differentiate TBI, PTSD, and pain, there is also considerable overlap in this domain. TBI may alter/impair an individual's perception of his or her physiological state and produce a heightened emotional response, leading to the development and/or maintenance of PTSD (Williams et al., 2006) and pain syndromes. Emotional responses, particularly fear responses underlying PTSD, are generated by the same brain structures and systems that are often impacted by TBI (e.g., amygdala/limbic system) and that have been implicated in pain (e.g., "pain matrix"). However, the relationship is likely not linear. Consider that individuals with mTBI may experience reduced cognitive capacity and mental efficiency under conditions of stress (Stuss et al., 1985), which could be mediated by either PTSD, pain, or their combination. Thus, the psychological symptoms of each disorder (such as memory intrusions and heightened anxiety in PTSD; attentional impairment in pain) may exacerbate the neurocognitive features of TBI and vice versa. As suggested above, patients who have less severe brain injuries may in fact develop more pain symptoms, so the relationship is a complex one that may be mediated and moderated by multiple neurological and psychiatric constructs. The negative emotions and stress associated with pain potentially affect cognitive functioning independently of the effects of pain intensity (Hart et al., 2003). Furthermore, PTSD may mediate chronic pain symptoms, but TBI appears to have an independent correlation (above and beyond PTSD) with chronic pain even in mild cases of TBI (Hoge et al., 2008; Nampiaparampil, 2008).

Pain Management with Comorbid PTSD and/or mTBI

Dobscha et al. (2009) conducted a review of the literature from 1950 to 2008 addressing the assessment and management of pain in patients with polytrauma injuries including TBI and blast-related headache. A total of 94 studies met inclusion criteria. Their results indicated no studies examining the validity or reliability of measures of pain intensity or pain-related functioning in patients with blast-induced headache. Dobscha and colleagues also found no randomized controlled trials (RCTs) testing the efficacy of psychological pain treatment approaches for individuals with polytrauma. Further, while the Dobscha et al. review supported the association between TBI and headache, the authors found no RCTs that addressed treatment of blast-induced headache. The authors acknowledge that despite the high rate of reported comorbidity between TBI and pain, there is very little evidence-based guidance available in the literature to guide clinicians in assessing pain among patients with cognitive deficits due to TBI, treating pain related to polytrauma, and managing blast-related headache.

Since publication of the Dobscha et al. (2009) review, only a few studies have reported the results of treatments, or models for treatment, for individuals with comorbid pain, PTSD, and/or TBI. Ruff et al. (2009) examined the effectiveness of a sleep intervention program for veterans with blast-induced mTBI and headache. The sample included 126 veterans with blast-induced mTBI caused by an explosion during deployment in OEF/OIF. Of the 126 veterans included, 74 reported headaches and deficits in neurological functioning. Of those veterans, 71 had PTSD and 69 had poor sleep. Treatment included sleep hygiene counseling (9 weeks) and nightly oral prazosin. At posttreatment, 65 of 69 veterans reported restful sleep, headache pain decreased from 7.28 to 4.08 when rated on a 0 to 10 scale, headaches per month decreased from 12.4 to 4.77, and Montreal Cognitive Assessment Scores improved from 24.5 to 28.6. These gains were maintained at 6-month follow-up. The results suggest that addressing sleep is a good first step in treating posttraumatic headache.

Otis, Keane, Kerns, Monson, and Scioli (2009) described the development and pilot testing of an integrated treatment for veterans with comorbid chronic pain and PTSD. Using a multistep approach that included meetings with collaborators to decide on key elements of treatment, developing treatment manuals, and tailoring the manuals based on feedback from study therapists and participants, a 12-session integrated treatment for chronic pain and PTSD was created. The triple vulnerability model (Otis et al., 2006) served as a guide for determining some of the essential elements of treatment. The integrated treatment included components of cognitive processing therapy (CPT) for PTSD and cognitive-behavioral therapy (CBT) for chronic pain management. Core treatment elements of the integrated treatment included relaxation training, activity goal setting and weekly goal completion, cognitive restructuring (i.e., safety, trust, powerful others, self-esteem, and intimacy), pleasant activity scheduling and pacing, and relapse prevention. Additional elements included interoceptive exposure to address "anxiety sensitivity." A number of important themes emerged from the pilot testing of the treatment including the importance of establishing the trust of the participant, taking steps to reduce avoidance, and completing treatment goals.

Overall, participants who completed the integrated treatment program responded well to therapy and reported that they generally liked the format of treatment, and appreciated learning about the ways that chronic pain and PTSD share some common symptoms and the ways that the two disorders can interact with one another. Following the completion of the pilot study, we initiated an RCT to investigate the efficacy of the integrated treatment when compared to evidence-based treatments for chronic pain and PTSD. This study is still ongoing. Given the physical and psychological problems often faced by injured soldiers, if future well-controlled research studies find that the positive effects observed in participants receiving the integrated treatment are greater than the effects observed in participants who receive evidence-based treatments for either chronic pain or PTSD, then this line of research could have direct benefits for the improved care of individuals with comorbid pain and PTSD. Based on feedback received by OEF/OIF veterans and in an effort to develop a more expedient form of therapy, Otis and colleagues are currently investigating the efficacy of an intensive, 3-week treatment approach for veterans with comorbid chronic pain and PTSD. This study will also include participants with mTBI and will assess the relationships among participation in treatment, treatment outcome, and cognitive functioning across a variety of domains.

A Model of Care for Polytrauma Injuries

Walker, Clark, and Sanders (2010) described a model of integrated care for individuals with the clinical triad of symptoms of pain, PTSD, and mTBI (persistent postconcussive syndrome), which they term "postdeployment multisymptom disorder," or PMD. The integrated care model begins with an initial screening of all patients for symptoms of PMD and other comorbid conditions (e.g., sleep disturbance, substance abuse, and anxiety). Individuals who have at least two clusters of PMD symptoms along with evidence of significant life impairment and/or dissatisfaction are referred to the Center for Post-deployment Health and Education (CPHE). Treatment is based on established cognitive-behavioral models of brief intervention delivered in an interdisciplinary setting and targets clusters of thoughts, feelings, and behaviors that are interfering with reintegration into the community and satisfaction with life. The core components of the program include sleep hygiene training, stress management training, cognitive restructuring, substance misuse education, physical reactivation, and mood stabilization/medication management. The core is mandatory for all participants and addresses the most frequent clusters of behaviors that impede functioning. Focused component modules are delivered following core treatment and are based on participant needs. Modules include anger management, relaxation training, fear avoidance reduction, headache management, pain management, cognitive adaptation, and relationship enhancement. The integrative nature of this program, and the manner in which it can be tailored to the specific needs of the individual, are strengths of this model; however, controlled trials investigating the efficacy of this model of care are not yet available.

Summary and Conclusions

Research suggests that chronic pain, PTSD, and TBI are common problems among veterans who have experienced a blast-related injury. With respect to pain, there is a particularly high prevalence of headache reported in individuals who have experienced mTBI. One of the challenges in providing accurate assessment and treatment for individuals with chronic pain, PTSD, and mTBI is the high degree of shared symptom presentation. Studies examining the neuropathology and functional impairments associated with each of these conditions have helped to explain clinical observations that these conditions tend to interact with one another in a negative manner, causing exacerbation of symptoms and adding to the complexity of accurate assessment and treatment. Given the recognition of this problem, there are a number of issues that should gain attention from clinical researchers. First, pain is a subjective experience and continued research is needed on ways to reliably and accurately assess pain in individuals who have experienced a TBI. Although there are measures that have been validated and are commonly used when assessing pain in patients with impaired functioning or noncommunicative patients, such as the Wong–Baker Faces Scale (Wong & Baker, 1998), these measure have not been validated on a TBI population. Second, at present there is little available information available to guide clinicians on the appropriate course of treatment for individuals with comorbid chronic pain, PTSD, and mTBI. Walker et al. (2010) have a described a flexible model for providing care, but this model of care has yet to be fully tested. Although preliminary research supports the efficacy of an integrated treatment approach for comorbid pain and PTSD, continued research is needed to examine the efficacy of these treatments for individuals with TBI. It is likely that clinical materials used in pain management will need to be modified when working with individuals who have an mTBI. Modification may include simplification of forms, larger font size, less time between treatment sessions or more frequent sessions, added psychoeducation on how mTBI interacts with PTSD and pain symptoms, homework reminders, therapy "handouts" summarizing key points of each session to aid memory-impaired patients and reinforce concepts, repetition of key points in different modalities (verbal and visual), and simplification and repetition of cognitive restructuring tools when needed. Each modification should be based on the specific needs of the individual. Clinicians might also consider that although pain, PTSD, and mTBI appear to have high rates of comorbidity, there are other issues commonly associated with these conditions (e.g., substance abuse, sleep difficulties, lack of employment, marital/relationship issues) that are likely to have a significant impact on daily function. Clinicians and researchers who specialize in helping people who have experienced a traumatic injury will need to work together to gain a broader understanding of how the experience of injury has impacted the individual, to recognize the importance of treating the entire person—not just a particular disorder, and to prioritize the development of innovative and effective treatment approaches for this population.

References

Alexander, M. P. (1995). Mild traumatic brain injury: Pathophysiology, natural history, and clinical management. *Neurology, 45*, 1253–1260.

Amir, M., Kaplan, Z., Neumann, L., Sharabani, R., Shani, N., & Buskila, D. (1997). Posttraumatic stress disorder, tenderness and fibromyalgia. *Journal of Psychosomatic Research, 42*, 607–613.

Asmundson, G. J. G., Coons, M. J., Taylor, S., & Katz, J. (2002). PTSD and the experience of pain: Research and clinical implications of shared vulnerability and mutual maintenance models. *Canadian Journal of Psychiatry, 47*, 930–937.

Asmundson, G. J. G., Norton, G., Allerdings, M., Norton, P., & Larson, D. (1998). Post-traumatic stress disorder and work-related injury. *Journal of Anxiety Disorders, 12*, 57–69.

Beckham, J. C., Crawford, A. L., Feldman, M. E., Kirby, A. C., Hertzberg, M. A., Davidson, R. J. T., et al. (1997). Chronic post-traumatic stress disorder and chronic pain in Vietnam combat veterans. *Journal of Psychosomatic Research, 43*, 379–389.

Belanger, H. G., Curtiss, G., Demery, J. A., Lebowitz, B. K., & Vanderploeg, R. D. (2005). Factors moderating neuropsychological outcomes following mild traumatic brain injury: A meta-analysis. *Journal of the International Neuropsychological Society, 11*, 215–227.

Bigler, E. D. (2007). Anterior and middle cranial fossa in traumatic brain injury: Relevant neuroanatomy and neuropathology in the study of neuropsychological outcome. *Neuropsychology, 21*, 515–531.

Bilmes, L. (2007). *Soldiers returning from Iraq and Afghanistan: The long-term costs of providing veterans medical care and disability benefits* (RWP07-001; KSG Faculty Research Working Paper Series). Cambridge, MA: Harvard University.

Brewin, C. R., Kleiner, J. S., Vasterling, J. J., & Field, A. P. (2007). Memory for emotionally neutral information in posttraumatic stress disorder: A meta-analytic investigation. *Journal of Abnormal Psychology, 116*, 448–463.

Byrne, Z. S., & Hochwarter, W. A. (2006). I get by with a little help from my friends: The interaction of chronic pain and organizational support and performance. *Journal of Occupational Health Psychology, 11*, 215–227.

Chibnall, J. T., & Duckro, P. N. (1994). Post-traumatic stress disorder and motor vehicle accidents. *Headache, 34*, 357–361.

Clark, M. E., Bair, M. J., Buckenmaier, C. C., Gironda, R. J., & Walker, R. L. (2007). Pain and combat injuries in soldiers returning from Operations Enduring Freedom and Iraqi Freedom: Implications for research and practice. *Journal of Rehabilitation Reseach and Development, 44*(2), 179–194.

Couch, J. R., & Bearss, C. (2001). Chronic daily headache in the posttrauma syndrome: Relation to extent of head injury. *Headache, 41,* 559–564.

Dobscha, S. K., Clark, M. E., Morasco, B. J., Freeman, M., Campbell, R., & Helfand, M. (2009). Systematic review of the literature on pain in patients with polytrauma including traumatic brain injury. *Pain Medicine, 10,* 1200–1217.

Fox, C. D., Berger, D., Fine, P. G., Gebhard, G. F., Grabois, M., Kulich, R. J., et al. (2000). Pain assessment and treatment in the managed care environment: A position statement from the American Pain Society. Retrieved from *www. ampainsoc.org/advocacy/assess_treat_mce.htm.*

Geisser, M. E., Roth, R. S., Bachman, J. E., & Eckert, T. A. (1996). The relationship between symptoms of post-traumatic stress disorder and pain, affective disturbance and disability among patients with accident and non-accident related pain. *Pain, 66,* 207–214.

Goldman-Rakic, P. S. (1996). The prefrontal landscape: Implications of functional architecture for understanding human mentation and the central executive. *Philosophical Transactions of the Royal Society B: Biological Sciences, 351,* 1445–1453.

Gureje, O., Von Korff, M., Simon, G. E., & Gater, R. (1998). Persistent pain and well-being: A World Health Organization study in primary care. *Journal of the American Medical Association, 280,* 147–151.

Hart, R. P., Wade, J. B., & Martelli, M. F. (2003). Cognitive impairment in patients with chronic pain: The significance of stress. *Current Pain and Headache Reports, 7,* 116–126.

Hartlage, L. C., Durant-Wilson, D., & Patch, P. C. (2001). Persistent neurobehavioral problems following mild traumatic brain injury. *Archives of Clinical Neuropsychology, 16,* 561–570.

Hayes, J. P., Labar, K. S., McCarthy, G., Selgrade, E., Nasser, J., Dolcos, F., et al. (2010). Reduced hippocampal and amygdala activity predicts memory distortions for trauma reminders in combat-related PTSD. *Journal of Psychiatric Research.* (Online prepublication)

Hickling, E. J., & Blanchard, E. B. (1992). Post-traumatic stress disorder and motor vehicle accidents. *Journal of Anxiety Disorders, 6,* 285–291.

Hoge, C. W., McGurk, D., Thomas, J. L., Cox, A. L., Engel, C. C., & Castro, C. A. (2008). Mild traumatic brain injury in U.S. soldiers returning from Iraq. *New England Journal of Medicine, 358,* 453–463.

Iverson, G. L. (2005). Outcome from mild traumatic brain injury. *Current Opinion in Psychiatry, 18,* 301–317.

Iverson, G. L., & McCracken, L. M. (1997). "Postconcussive" symptoms in persons with chronic pain. *Brain Injury, 11,* 783–790.

Johnsen, G. E., & Asbjornsen, A. E. (2008). Consistent impaired verbal memory in PTSD: A meta-analysis. *Journal of Affective Disorders, 111,* 74–82.

Karl, A., Schaefer, M., Malta, L. S., Dorfel, D., Rohleder, N., & Werner, A. (2006). A meta-analysis of structural brain abnormalities in PTSD. *Neuroscience and Biobehavioral Reviews, 30,* 1004–1031.

Kerns, R. D., Otis, J. D., Rosenberg, R. A., & Reid, C. (2003). Veterans' reports of pain and associations with ratings of health, health-risk behaviors, affective distress, and use of healthcare system. *Journal of Rehabilitation Research and Development, 40,* 371–380.

Kraus, M. F., Susmaras, T., Caughlin, B. P., Walker, C. J., Sweeney, J. A., & Little, D. M. (2007). White matter integrity and cognition in chronic traumatic brain injury: A diffusion tensor imaging study. *Brain, 130,* 2508–2519.

Lanius, R. A., Bluhm, R., Lanius, U., & Pain, C. (2006). A review of neuroimaging studies in PTSD: Heterogeneity of response to symptom provocation. *Journal of Psychiatric Research, 40,* 709–729.

Leskin, L. P., & White, P. M. (2007). Attentional networks reveal executive function deficits in posttraumatic stress disorder. *Neuropsychology, 21,* 275–284.

Levin, H. S., Mattis, S., Ruff, R. M., Eisenberg, H. M., Marshall, L. F., Tabaddor, K., et al. (1987). Neurobehavioral outcome following minor head injury: A three-center study. *Journal of Neurosurgery, 66,* 234–243.

Lew, H. L., Otis, J. D., Tun, C., Kerns, R. D., Clark, M. E., & Cifu, D. X. (2009). Prevalence of chronic pain, posttraumatic stress disorder and persistent post-concussive symptoms in OEF/OIF veterans: The polytrauma clinical triad. *Journal of Rehabilitation, Research and Development, 46,* 697–702.

Lew, H. L., Poole J. H., Vanderploeg R. D., Goodrich G. L., Dekelboum, S., Guillory, S. B., et al. (2007). Program development and defining characteristics of returning military in a VA polytrauma network site. *Journal of Rehabilitation, Research and Development, 44,* 1027–1034.

Lippa, S. M., Pastorek, N. J., Benge, J. F., & Thornton, G. M. (2010). Postconcussive symptoms after blast and nonblast-related mild traumatic brain injuries in Afghanistan and Iraq war veterans. *Journal of the International Neuropsychological Society, 16,* 856–866.

Lutz, J., Jäger, L., de Quervain, D., Krauseneck, T., Padberg, F., Wichnalek, M., et al. (2008). White and gray matter abnormalities in the brain of patients with fibromyalgia: A diffusion-tensor and volumetric imaging study. *Arthritis and Rheumatism, 58,* 3960–3969.

McFarlane, A. C., Atchison, M., Rafalowicz, E., & Papay, P. (1994). Physical symptoms in posttraumatic stress disorder. *Journal of Psychosomatic Research, 42,* 607–617.

Melzack, R. (1999). Pain—An overview. *Acta Anaesthesiologica Scandinavica, 43,* 880–884.

Merskey, H., & Bogduk, N. (1994). *IASP Task Force on Taxonomy* (pp. 209–214). Seattle: IASP Press.

Metz, A. E., Yau, H. J., Centeno, M. V., Apkarian, A. V., & Martina, M. (2009). Morphological and functional reorganization of rat medial prefrontal cortex in neuropathic pain. *Proceedings of the National Academy of Sciences of the United States of America, 106,* 2423–2428.

Nampiaparampil, D. E. (2008). Prevalence of chronic pain after traumatic brain injury: A systematic review. *Journal of the American Medical Association, 300,* 711–719.

Neugebauer, V., Galhardo, V., Maione, S., & Mackey, S. C. (2009). Forebrain pain mechanisms. *Brain Research Reviews, 60,* 226–242.

Nicholson, K., & Martelli, M. F. (2004). The problem of pain. *Journal of Head Trauma Rehabilitation, 19,* 2–9.

Novack, T. A., Bush, B. A., Meythaler, J. M., & Canupp, K. (2001). Outcome after traumatic brain injury: Pathway analysis of contributions from premorbid, injury severity, and recovery variables. *Archives of Physical Medicine and Rehabilitation, 82,* 300–305.

Otis, J. D., Gregor, K., Hardway, C., Morrison, J., Scioli, E., & Sanderson, M. (2010). An examination of the co-morbidity between chronic pain and posttraumatic stress disorder on U.S. veterans. *Psychological Services, 7,* 126–135.

Otis, J. D., Keane, T., Kerns, R. D., Monson, C., & Scioli, E. (2009). The development of an integrated treatment for veterans with comorbid chronic pain and posttraumatic stress disorder. *Pain Medicine, 10,* 1300–1311.

Otis, J. D., Pincus, D. B., & Keane, T. M. (2006). Comorbid chronic pain and posttraumatic stress disorder across the lifespan: A review of theoretical models. In G. Young, A. Kane, & K. Nicholson (Eds.), *Causality: Psychological knowledge and evidence in court* (pp. 242–268). New York: Kluwer Academic/Plenum Press.

Otis, J. D., Reid, M. C., & Kerns, R.D. (2005). The management of chronic pain in the primary care setting. In L. C. James & R. A. Folen (Eds.), *Primary care clinical health psychology: A model for the next frontier* (pp. 41–59). Washington, D.C.: American Psychological Association Press.

Ponsford, J., Willmott, C., Rothwell, A., Cameron, P., Kelly, A. M., Nelms, R., et al. (2000). Factors influencing outcome following mild traumatic brain injury in adults. *Journal of the International Neuropsychological Society, 6,* 568–579.

Powell, T. J., Collin, C., & Sutton, K. (1996). A follow-up study of patients hospitalized after minor head injury. *Disability and Rehabilitation, 18,* 231–237.

Rassovsky, Y., Satz, P., Alfano, M. S., Light, R. K., Zaucha, K., McArthur, D. L., et al. (2006). Functional outcome in TBI I: Neuropsychological, emotional, and behavioral mediators. *Journal of Clinical and Experimental Neuropsychology, 28,* 567–580.

Ruff, R. L., Ruff, S. S., & Wang, X. (2009). Improving sleep: Initial headache treatment in OIF/OEF veterans with blast-induced mild traumatic brain injury. *Journal of Rehabilitation Research and Development, 46,* 1071–1084.

Sayer, N. A., Cifu, D. X., McNamee, S., Chiros, C. E., Sigford, B. J., Scott, S., et al. (2009). Rehabilitation needs of combat-injured service members admitted to the VA polytrauma rehabilitation centers: The role of PM&R in the care of wounded warriors. *Physical Medicine and Rehabilitation, 1,* 23–28.

Schneiderman, A. I., Braver, E. R., & Kang, H. K. (2008). Understanding sequelae of injury mechanisms and mild traumatic brain injury incurred during the conflicts in Iraq and Afghanistan: Persistent postconcussive symptoms and posttraumatic stress disorder. *American Journal of Epidemiology, 167,* 1446–1452.

Sharp, T. J., & Harvey, A. G. (2001). Chronic pain and posttraumatic stress disorder: Mutual maintenance? *Clinical Psychology Review, 21,* 857–877.

Sherman, J. J., Turk, D. C., & Okifuji, A. (2000). Prevalence and impact of posttraumatic stress disorder-like symptoms on patients with fibromyalgia syndrome. *Clinical Journal of Pain, 16,* 127–134.

Shin, L. M., Rauch, S. L., & Pitman, R. K. (2006). Amygdala, medial prefrontal cortex, and hippocampal function in PTSD. *Annals of the New York Academy of Sciences, 1071,* 67–79.

Shipherd, J. C., Keyes, M., Jovanic, T., Ready, D. J., Baltzell, D., Worley, V., et al. (2007). Veterans seeking treatment for posttraumatic stress disorder: What about comorbid chronic pain? *Journal of Rehabilitation Research and Development, 44,* 153–166.

Stuss, D. T., Ely, P., Hugenholtz, H., Richard, M. T., LaRochelle, S., Poirier, C. A., et al. (1985). Subtle neuropsychological deficits in patients with good recovery after closed head injury. *Neurosurgery, 17,* 41–47.

Taylor, S., & Koch, W. J. (1995). Anxiety disorders due to motor vehicle accidents: Nature and treatment. *Clinical Psychology Review, 15,* 721–738.

Theeler, B. J., Flynn, F. G., & Erickson, J. C. (2010). Research submissions: Headaches after concussion in US soldiers returning from Iraq or Afghanistan. *Headache: The Journal of Head and Face Pain, 50,* 1262–1272.

Toomey, T. C., Seville, J. L., Abashian, S. W., Finkel, A. G., & Mann, J. D. (1994, November). *Circumstances of chronic pain onset: Relationship to pain description, coping and psychological distress.* Poster presented at the American Pain Society meeting, Miami Beach, FL.

Turk, D. C., & Okifuji, A. (1996). Perception of traumatic onset, compensation status, and physical findings: Impact on pain severity, emotional distress, and disability in chronic pain patients. *Journal of Behavioral Medicine, 19,* 435–453.

Turk, D. C., Okifuji, A., Starz, T. W., & Sinclaire, J. D. (1996). Effects of type of symptom onset on psychological distress and disability in fibromyalgia syndrome patients. *Pain, 68,* 678–681.

Uomoto, J. M., & Esselman, P. C. (1993). Traumatic brain injury and chronic pain: Differential types and rates by head injury severity. *Archives of Physical Medicine and Rehabilitation, 74,* 61–64.

Vanderploeg, R. D., Curtiss, G., & Belanger, H. G. (2005). Long-term neuropsychological outcomes following mild traumatic brain injury. *Journal of the International Neuropsychological Society, 11,* 228–236.

Villarreal, G., Hamilton, D. A., Petropoulos, H., Driscoll, I., Rowland, L. M., Griego, J. A., et al. (2002). Reduced hippocampal volume and total white matter volume in posttraumatic stress disorder. *Biological Psychiatry, 52*(2), 119–125.

Walker, R. L., Clark, M. E., & Sanders, S. H. (2010). The post-deployment multisymptom disorder: An emerging syndrome in need of a new treatment paradigm. *Psychological Services, 7,* 136–147.

White, P., & Faustman, W. (1989). Coexisting physical conditions among inpatients with posttraumatic stress disorder. *Military Medicine, 154,* 66–71.

Wilde, E. A., Bigler, E. D., Hunter, J. V., Fearing, M. A., Scheibel, R. S., Newsome, M. R., et al. (2007). Hippocampus, amygdala, and basal ganglia morphometrics in children after moderate-to-severe traumatic brain injury. *Developmental Medicine and Child Neurology, 49,* 294–299.

Williams, L. M., Kemp, A. H., Felmingham, K., Barton, M., Olivieri, G., Peduto,

A., et al. (2006). Trauma modulates amygdala and medial prefrontal responses to consciously attended fear. *Neuroimage, 29*(2), 347–357.

Wong, D. L., & Baker, C. (1998). Pain in children: Comparison of assessment scales. *Pediatric Nursing, 14*, 9–17.

Woodward, S. H., Kaloupek, D. G., Streeter, C. C., Martinez, C., Schaer, M., & Eliez, S. (2006). Decreased anterior cingulate volume in combat-related PTSD. *Biological Psychiatry, 59*, 582–587.

CHAPTER 7

Substance Use Disorder

Lisa M. Najavits, Jennifer Highley, Sara L. Dolan,
and Frank A. Fee

Substance use disorder (SUD) is the second most common psychiatric disorder in the U.S. population, affecting 14.6% during their lives (Kessler et al., 2005). The term "substance dependence" refers to the most severe form of the disorder and "substance abuse" the less severe form (American Psychiatric Association, 2000). Among SUDs, alcohol is the most common (13.2% lifetime rate). Most people with SUD have one or more co-occurring diagnoses, including psychiatric conditions, cognitive impairment, and/or physical health problems (Corrigan & Deutschle, 2008; Graham & Cardon, 2008; Kessler et al., 1997; Najavits, 2004).

Two prominent disorders that co-occur with SUD are posttraumatic stress disorder (PTSD) and mild traumatic brain injury (mTBI) (Graham & Cardon, 2008; Najavits, 2004). These three disorders have important linkages over time, causal connections, and additional clinical implications when occurring together. The trimorbidity affects a wide range of populations, including military service members and veterans, the homeless, abused or neglected children, victims of domestic violence, and survivors of motor vehicle accidents.

We will review three key areas: background, assessment, and treatment. We focus primarily on how SUD impacts PTSD/mTBI. Much prior literature has addressed the SUD–PTSD connection per se (e.g., Ouimette & Brown, 2002). We focus on practical implications and clinically relevant information and emphasize the importance of a compassionate approach that recognizes that SUD is a medical disorder and not a moral failing, a character flaw, or a lack of will. Historically, treatment has been characterized by (1) judgmental attitudes toward SUD patients (Najavits et al., 1995); (2) a lack of SUD-specific treatments; and (3) a lack of understanding of how SUD relates to co-occurring psychiatric disorders. In contrast, enlightened approaches to SUD emphasize careful assessment, treatments that are relevant to SUD and its comorbidities, and training of providers to increase effective ways to interact with SUD patients. Many trimorbid patients can improve, with recovery possible (either partial or full) for each disorder alone and in combination.

The Interplay between TBI, SUD, and PTSD

Risk Factors

In contrast to other disorders that increase after TBI (including PTSD), SUD rates go down in a majority of patients (Graham & Cardon, 2008; Parry-Jones, Vaughan, & Miles Cox, 2006). For some, reduced consumption is motivated by recognition that the substance use may have been implicated in the incidence of TBI (e.g., a driving-drunk accident). We might call this "post-TBI growth" or a "teachable moment" in which there is recognition of what substances have wrought. For others, it may reflect a narrowing of social life that is common after TBI (Temkin, Corrigan, Dikmen, & Machamer, 2009) (i.e., less social drinking); decreased craving for substances (perhaps physically related to changes in brain function); confinement to a rehabilitation facility as a result of injury; or decreased functioning that simply results in less activities generally, including substance use. However, this reduction in substance use has been termed a "honeymoon period" because it may be followed by an increase in use in the longer term 2–3 years post-TBI (Ponsford, Whelan-Goodinson, & Bahar-Fuchs, 2007; Bjork & Grant, 2009).

　　　Yet for some patients, substance use increases after TBI (e.g., Halbauer et al., 2009; Graham & Cardon, 2008), and it is important to attend to this subset. Among drugs (aside from alcohol), people with a history of TBI most frequently use marijuana, followed by opiates, cocaine, and stimulants (Kreutzer, Wehman, Harris, Burns, & Young, 1991). According to Halbauer et al. (2009), TBI may instill "weakened self-control or somatic pains that lead to excessive use of a substance, followed by dependence" (p. 780). Also, substances may have more of an effect on some people due to deficiencies in brain function, a sort of sensitization to the impact of substances (Halbauer et al., 2009). Substance use may also reflect simply greater vulnerability due to a host of factors not necessarily specifically related to the TBI (e.g., poverty, homelessness, lack of social support). The presence of PTSD may also be a key determinant, as PTSD consistently shows elevated rates after TBI (Rogers & Read, 2007). Use of opiates to treat TBI and/or physical pain may also become addictive (Graham & Cardon, 2008).

The clinical picture is complex when considering order of onset of the different disorders. SUD typically precedes TBI, but follows PTSD; and PTSD typically follows TBI (Rogers & Read, 2007; Graham & Cardon, 2008; Ouimette & Brown, 2002). Each disorder has been shown to be a risk factor for the others, at least to some degree. For example, PTSD is consistently found to be a risk factor for SUD (Ouimette & Brown, 2002), a pattern that is often understood as self-medication (substances help people cope in the short term with PTSD symptoms such as nightmares and flashbacks). SUD is a risk factor for TBI (Rogers & Reade, 2007; Bjork & Grant, 2009): people who misuse substances are at heightened risk of accidents, falls, and fights that may incur brain injury. PTSD is often comorbid with TBI (Graham & Cardon, 2008), although causal relationships between PTSD and TBI may be complex (see Vasterling, Bryant, & Keane, Chapter 14, this volume).

Such patterns among the trimorbid conditions may have implications for treatment and prevention work. For example, according to Corrigan and Cole (2008), up to 66% of TBI patients have a prior history of alcohol use, and up to one-half were intoxicated at the time of their injuries. According to Olson-Madden et al. (2010), among veterans seeking outpatient substance abuse treatment, 55% screened positive for TBI that included loss of consciousness, and 37% of the injuries were reportedly sustained while the individual was using alcohol (24%), drugs (3%), or both (10%). Approximately 80% of the TBIs were classified as mTBI. Alcohol-related diagnoses were assigned to 40% of the sample; 37% had both drug- and alcohol-related diagnoses; and 20% had a drug misuse diagnosis, primarily cocaine and marijuana. Because of the strong relationship between SUD and TBI, it is important to educate patients in SUD treatment about their increased risk for TBI due to substances. Even if patients have already suffered a TBI, they are at heightened risk for later ones as well (Saunders et al., 2009), especially if they incur an additional TBI before they recover from the first one. Thus, for any individual, it is important to identify how the disorders arose over time, which may vary from patient to patient.

The trimorbidity can affect anyone. However, the typical pattern is young, male, and from a disadvantaged background (Corrigan, Lamb-Hart, & Rust, 1995), especially among certain populations, such as the military and the homeless. It is thus important to remember that "any statistical association between TBI and psychiatric diagnosis may simply be a product of the overlap in risk factors" (Rogers & Read, 2007, p. 1331).

More research is needed to better understand how sociodemographics play a role in the onset of the disorders. For example, poverty is a risk factor for all three disorders and may serve as a "third variable" to help explain their high co-occurrence. Clinically, such sociodemographics may be important for public health prevention efforts to target high-risk groups. Also, as Bjork and Grant (2009) have noted, research on the association between TBI and SUD is at a very early stage. For example, we need studies of patients with no SUD history prior to TBI to better address whether substance use increases post-TBI; also, preclinical animal studies are needed to explore the impact of experimentally induced TBI on self-administration of substances.

Relationships among Trimorbid Disorder Symptoms

Symptoms of any of the three disorders may be misinterpreted by clinicians and others who are unfamiliar with the trimorbidity. In relation to TBI, for example, deficits in attention and concentration characteristic of TBI may mimic PTSD, depression, or mild mental retardation. Deficits in immediate or delayed memory may be interpreted as treatment resistance or labeled with clinical pejoratives such as "noncompliant," "difficult to engage," or "poor historian." Blurting and other inappropriate speech can be mistaken as rudeness or personality disorder, and the altered states of consciousness common to patients with TBI are sometimes falsely attributed to dependence on opiates or other drugs. Similarly, clinicians who focus on PTSD or TBI may be unfamiliar with SUD. The memory deficits, disinhibition, denial, lack of insight, and shame that characterize chronic substance use often stymie clinicians, creating negative emotional responses to patients (Najavits et al., 1995). Likewise, clinicians unfamiliar with PTSD may misinterpret symptoms such as distrust, dissociation, and hypervigilance. Some symptoms may also be caused by any of the disorders, and thus it can be difficult to determine whether they arose from one or the other once the person has the trimorbidity. Impairment in social relationships, for example, is common to all three, and may take the form of isolation, anger problems, difficulty initiating and maintaining relationships, problems with authority, communication problems, and inappropriate social skills.

Neurocognitive impairments may also relate to each disorder alone and their combination. For example, SUD is associated with neuropsychological deficits, during intoxication, acute withdrawal (3-5 days after the last use), and postacute withdrawal (1–6 weeks after last use) (Scheurich, 2005). Although these deficits recover with increasing length of sobriety, some patients continue to experience deficits even years later (Parsons, 1996). Whether neurocognitive deficits result from the direct effects of the substance on the brain, TBIs incurred while intoxicated or from some other cause (e.g., psychiatric comorbidities such as PTSD) can have a confounding effect on assessment and diagnosis of each of the disorders.

Patients with SUD display deficits in a variety of neuropsychological functions, including attention, processing speed, learning and memory, visuospatial functions, executive functions (e.g., monitoring, goal-directed behavior, planning, organization), cognitive efficiency (see, e.g., Ratti, Bo, Giardini, & Soragna, 2002), in addition to exhibiting neurologically based impulsivity and emotional dysregulation (Verdejo-Garcia, Recknor, Bechara, & Perez-Garcia, 2007). For example, approximately 33–75% of alcoholics entering treatment display mild-to-moderate neuropsychological deficits, and in particular executive dysfunction (Meek, Clark, & Solana, 1989; Morgenstern & Bates, 1999). The presence of cognitive deficits can influence an assessment (e.g., a patient with memory dysfunction who cannot recall information that would be useful to a diagnostic evaluation).

It is also important to consider the overlapping neurocognitive problems present in the comorbidity of PTSD/SUD. The neuropsychological impairments found in PTSD are also found, at least to some extent, in persons with SUD. Studies have found deficits in certain aspects of learning and memory, attention, and executive functioning among both patients with PTSD (Leskin & White, 2007; Vasterling et al., 2002) and patients with SUD (Verdejo-Garcia et al., 2005); however, not all aspects of these broad domains are affected by either PTSD or SUD (Gilbertson, Gurvits, Lasko, Orr, & Pitman, 2001; Verdejo-Garcia et al., 2005). Moreover, SUD cognitive deficits are quite variable, depending on the specific substance, extent of use, and recency of use (Copersino et al., 2009).

Little research has examined the concurrent and potentially overlapping neuropsychological deficits in SUD, PTSD, and TBI. As described elsewhere in this volume, neuropsychological impairment often resolves among patients with mTBI; however, there is evidence that a subset of patients with mTBI may continue to exhibit deficits such as decreased attention, slowed processing speed, learning and memory problems, executive dysfunction, and emotional dysregulation, which may also be observed in PTSD and some SUDs (Corrigan & Cole, 2008). The extent to which substance use retards recovery from mTBI remains unknown.

Assessment

Barriers to Assessment

Known difficulties in the assessment of trimorbid PTSD, mTBI, and SUD may in part reflect obstacles inherent in the systems of care in which patients present for treatment (Taylor, Kreutzer, Demm, & Meade, 2003).

Typically, SUD providers may have little formal training in neuropsychological assessment or specialized PTSD assessment. In a similar way, not all PTSD specialists and neuropsychologists have had specialized training in assessing or treating SUD. Additionally, the importance of assessment of TBI has only recently received widespread attention, and the techniques necessary to do so have yet to be mainstreamed into the core curricula of many health care advanced degree programs. Compounding the problem, some states have separate funding streams for the treatment of psychiatric illness, medical illness, and SUD, preventing treatment facilities from being reimbursed for providing treatment for these three commonly comorbid disorders concurrently. As a result, clinicians who learn at these facilities as residents, interns, or externs may not be trained to look for all three disorders.

Lack of expertise in the proper assessment of co-occurring SUD, TBI, and psychiatric disorders including PTSD can contribute to "revolving door" utilization of substance abuse detoxification, rehabilitation, and long-term residential treatment facilities as well as inpatient psychiatric units. Misdiagnosis can result in improper treatment, and can contribute to loss of productivity, medico-legal liability, redundant treatment, and patient demise.

There are also obstacles to assessment that may be difficult for clinicians to acknowledge because they relate to emotional reactions to this population (e.g., bias against SUD patients within the medical community) (Dackis & O'Brien, 2005). A typical example is the patient who presents to an emergency department staggering, smelling of alcohol, and unable to give a coherent history, only to be written off as intoxicated and allowed to "sleep it off" until he is discharged from the emergency department, any TBI or psychiatric illness he may suffer having gone untreated. Indeed, it has been reported that "for each person who dies from a TBI, five are hospitalized and 27 are sent home from the ER" (Kraus & McArthur, 1996, p. 439).

It is also notable that substance use and/or substance withdrawal can mimic nearly every psychiatric illness, and thus it is essential that the clinician be aware of the effects of the various substances on their patients (Modesto-Lowe & Kranzler, 1999). Stimulants such as cocaine and methamphetamine can mask the symptoms of depression by their stimulant effects; mimic mania by producing pressured speech, delusions of grandeur, and psychomotor agitation; and induce psychosis in the form of paranoia and auditory, visual, or tactile hallucinations during substance intoxication. In withdrawal from stimulants, patients may look as though they are severely depressed and may feign symptoms of psychosis (suicidal or homicidal ideation) to gain access to inpatient psychiatric units so that they can rest after several weeks on a so-called "run." Benzodiazepine and alcohol intoxication and dependence can both cause and masquerade as major depression. Withdrawal from both alcohol and benzodiazepine dependence can produce anxiety, suicidality, and psychosis in the form of delirium tremens, whereas opiate intoxication produces psychomotor retardation and stupor and mimics depression or catatonia (American Psychiatric Association, 2000).

Similarly, PTSD has been called "the great pretender" as it too can masquerade as other psychiatric illnesses, especially if the patient is being diagnosed in an emergency or urgent-care facility, where the clinician is only privy to a "snapshot" of the patient. PTSD sufferers may present emergently with acute anxiety, with pressured speech that is nearly uninterruptible, and may be misdiagnosed with bipolar I affective disorder and admitted. Because PTSD is often comorbid with depression (American Psychiatric Association, 2000), a patient who presents for treatment while depressed may be admitted for treatment of major depressive disorder. In each case, the patient will not usually be assessed for a history of trauma, and may be treated with an antipsychotic, a mood stabilizer, and an antidepressant, respectively, only the last of which will have much efficacy in treating the patient's symptoms. Compounding the confusion, the patient may have been informed of these (false) diagnoses in the past, and when asked about prior diagnoses, may report being bipolar, or having schizophrenia or major depression. Indeed, if clinicians overrely on patient report or even medical records, they may misdiagnosis patients with PTSD. In some cases, clinicians may feel pressed to provide certain diagnostic categories because of systems limitations. For example, if a patient with PTSD presents emergently for care as a result of suicidality, the clinician may emphasize non-PTSD diagnoses because most health insurance companies will not reimburse an inpatient stay for PTSD.

Moreover, depending on the context of care, TBI may go undiagnosed and untreated, and its symptoms can be mistaken for other disorders. Even in mTBI, impulsivity, which is common to both SUD and mTBI (Hibbard, Uysal, Kepler, Bogdany, & Silver, 1998; Corrigan & Deutschle, 2008), can be interpreted as mania, personality disorder, or impulse control disorder. Finally, the altered states of consciousness that accompanied the mTBI at the time of injury can be (falsely) attributed to dependence on opiates or other central nervous system (CNS) depressants.

Conducting the Assessment

As other chapters in this book focus on assessment of PTSD and TBI, we elaborate here on assessment of SUD. Per Table 7.1, there are numerous assessment measures for SUD, including those used for screening, diagnosis, identification of levels of substance use, verification of substance

TABLE 7.1. Areas of SUD Assessment

1. Screening for SUD

Key question: Might the patient have an SUD?

Examples of measures: for alcohol—Michigan Alcohol Screening Test (Seltzer, 1971); for drugs—DAST (Skinner, 1982).

Notes: Brief, requires little or no training, some available online or in community programs (e.g., National Alcohol Screening Day).

2. Diagnosis of SUD

Key question: Does the patient truly have an SUD?

Examples of measures: Structured Clinical Interview for DSM-IV (Spitzer, Williams, & Gibbon, 1997), Mini-International Neuropsychiatric Interview (Sheehan, Lecrubier, Harnett Sheehan, Amorim, Janavs, Weiller, et al., 1998).

Notes: Alcohol and drug use disorders have separate diagnostic criteria. Training in both the measure and diagnostic criteria are required (usually DSM-IV, but may be ICD-9 or other system). Interrater reliability usually needs to be established. Most measures are interview-based, but some self-report computerized versions also exist.

3. Level of substance use

Key question: What, how much, and how often is the patient using?

Examples of measures: Addiction Severity Index (McLellan, Kushner, Metzger, Peters, Smith, Grissom, et al., 1992), Timeline Follow-Back (Sobell & Sobell, 1992), Brief Addiction Monitor (McKay, Drapkin, Goodwin, & DePhillipis, 2010).

Notes: For clinical practice, the clinician often simply asks three questions at each session: What type of substances have you used in the past week? How much of each (e.g., number of drinks)? How often for each? More formal measures are typically used for detailed assessment and/or research. A related area is measures of *cravings* to use substances (see Abrams, 2000, for a review).

4. Verification of substance use

Key question: Is the patient telling the truth about use?

Examples of measures: Biological measures include urinalysis testing (home kit or laboratory), breath alcohol testing, and blood or hair analysis; collateral informant measures involve corroboration by family members or others (Maisto, Sobell, & Sobell, 1982).

Notes: Accuracy of biological measures depend in part on how long ago the patient used (e.g., alcohol may be detected only within a few hours, whereas marijuana may be days later). Random testing and chain-of-custody procedures enhance accuracy. Collateral informant measures require the patient's written consent.

5. Negative consequences of substance use

Key question: How is the substance use affecting the patient's life?

Examples of measures: Inventory of Drug Use Consequences (Tonigan & Miller, 2002), Addiction Severity Index (McLellan et al., 1992).

Notes: Typical areas of assessment include impact of substance on legal, psychiatric, social, vocational, medical, and family functioning.

(cont.)

TABLE 7.1. *(cont.)*

6. Motivation for substance abuse treatment

Key question: How motivated is the patient to engage in substance abuse treatment?

Examples of measures: Stages of Change Readiness and Treatment Eagerness Scale (Miller & Tonigan, 1994), University of Rhode Island Change Assessment Scale.

Notes: The widely used *stages of change* model evaluates the patient's readiness in terms of stages (e.g., precontemplation, action, maintenance).

7. Acute detoxification issues

Key question: Does the patient have any immediate medical issues related to addiction that need attention?

Examples of measures: CIWA

Notes: A patient who has had heavy abuse of alcohol or prescription medication usually needs medical evaluation and treatment prior to stopping. Referral to a detoxification program can be used, or to an outpatient physician or psychiatrist who can evaluate the patient's needs.

8. Cognition / belief measures

Key question: How does the patient view the addiction?

Examples of measures: Beliefs About Substance Use (Wright, 1992), Cocaine Expectancy Questionnaire (Jaffe & Kilbey, 1994).

Notes: These are used to evaluate patients' reasons for using substances, and their expectations about their ability to stop using.

Note. Adapted with permission from Najavits (2004). Copyright 2004 by The Guilford Press.

use, negative consequences of use, motivation for substance abuse treatment, acute detoxification issues, and cognitions/beliefs (Najavits, 2004). Depending on the setting, goal, and clinician background, any, all, or some combination of these may be used during a patient's treatment episode. However, such assessment tools, although validated for SUD populations, may need to be validated in patients with co-occurring TBI and PTSD, as their psychometric properties have not been assessed for this trimorbidity. Rogers and Read (2007) report that only one study employed a psychiatric outcome measure developed specifically for the TBI population and warn that measures designed for use with the general community may not be appropriate for this specific patient population.

It is also helpful to obtain a substance use history, including factors that contribute to substance onset, course, treatment response (including detoxifications and use of 12-step groups), and remission/abstinence periods. Ask when and how the patient first used a substance and whether the patient has been able to complete any substance abuse programs. In some cases, exacerbation of PTSD symptoms or cognitive impairment (or both) may render patients incapable of tolerating substance abuse treatment programs. Such information should be incorporated into the assessment to help guide treatment planning. For example, patients who self-medicate symptoms of PTSD with substances may have difficulty coping with a substance abuse treatment setting as their PTSD symptoms may emerge when they are no longer using drugs and alcohol. Thus, for treatment planning, it is beneficial to assess how they manage their PTSD symptoms.

It is also important to determine whether the patient has a substance-induced psychiatric disorder, or psychiatric disorders other than PTSD that underlie the substance use (Galanter & Kleber, 2008). Assessing for psychiatric symptoms during periods of "clean time" (no substance use) can help clarify these issues. For some patients, their only period without using substances may have occurred while in a controlled environment or context, such as prison, an inpatient hospital setting, military training, or during pregnancy. However, even under these conditions, patients may still have used substances, so it is important not to assume but instead to ask.

Finally, substance intoxication and withdrawal can negatively affect the assessment process. The accuracy of a patient's reporting may already be affected by the trimorbidity, but if a patient arrives intoxicated or in withdrawal, the cognitive difficulties associated with these conditions may complicate a diagnosis. If patients are intoxicated, they may be impulsive and difficult to understand due to slurred speech; consciousness may be altered to the point that assessment may not be possible (e.g., if they are passed out). Withdrawal symptoms can also include anxiety, agitation, and impulsivity if their substance is alcohol or opiates. If the substance is cocaine or another stimulant, withdrawal symptoms of excessive sleepiness and depressive-like symptoms may affect the willingness and ability of the patient to participate in an interview. If the patient has a history of recent substance use, ask the patient to abstain from substances the day of the interview and schedule the evaluation in the morning to minimize the possibility of substance withdrawal during the interview. Explain to the patient why this is essential (e.g., to help provide the most accurate assessment, which can impact the treatment plan).

Despite these complicating factors, it is unclear to what degree recent substance intoxication and withdrawal distort the actual diagnosis of PTSD and/or TBI. These syndromes may remain robust such that diagnostic accuracy may still be quite high even if particular symptoms are dampened or increased due to substance use or withdrawal (Najavits, 2004). In general, the goal is for the patient to be sober during the assessment (e.g., last use the day before) and to assess for psychiatric conditions and TBI as the patient may not be able to achieve sustained abstinence without treatment of co-occurring PTSD/TBI (Najavits, 2004).

Other Assessment Considerations

Najavits (2004) described various issues in relation to comorbid PTSD/SUD that also have relevance when TBI is present. In addition to those discussed in previous sections, these include avoiding unwarranted concerns about "labeling" patients; confusing the harm of substances with trauma per se; assuming that SUD is related to the amount of use, context of use (e.g., using alone), or type of substance (e.g., drugs rather than alcohol); and waiting too long to assess psychiatric conditions. We also recommend giving patients clear feedback about their assessment results and creating a kind yet direct style of questioning during the assessment.

Contextual issues may also impact assessment results (Najavits, 2004). For example, the legal implications of assessment may affect the patient's ability to retain custody of children or forensic charges being held against them. Similarly, institutional policies may affect a patient's self-report. For example, a patient with SUD who reports high levels of psychiatric disturbance (e.g., depression, suicidality) may be refused entry into SUD treatment until stabilized, and thus may minimize such symptoms. Likewise, a patient with PTSD who receives disability benefits for the disorder may hesitate to report decreased symptoms for fear of losing the benefits. Finally, the social context may affect the assessment (e.g., adolescents may fear restriction from friends or normal activities if they report substance use honestly). Although all of these factors may affect symptom validity, it is notable that self-reports, urine toxicology screens, and collateral reports tend to be convergent (Hoffman & Ninonuevo, 1994) unless there are major consequences related to reporting (e.g., potential loss of a job, home, treatment, or child) (Weiss et al., 1998).

Treatment

The literature on treatment of the trimorbidity is virtually nonexistent. Moreover, even the separate literatures are lacking in attention to comorbidities (Graham & Cardon, 2008). For example, according to a meta-analysis of rigorous randomized controlled trials of PTSD psychosocial treatments, 62% of the studies excluded patients with SUD (Bradley, Greene, Russ, Dutra, & Westen, 2005). Studies that include SUD typically just include substance abuse but not substance dependence and have other rule-outs (e.g., suicidal ideation, current domestic violence, homelessness, cognitive impairment) that result in limited generalizability to trimorbid populations. Similarly, SUD outcome studies, although not typically excluding for PTSD, do not generally report rates of co-occurring PTSD and sometimes exclude patients with cognitive impairment. The TBI outcome literature has not generally addressed either PTSD or SUD and is limited in terms of examining more chronic presentations. Nonetheless, as described below, some recommendations regarding treatment of the trimorbidty are now possible.

Culture of Care

Each disorder, PTSD, SUD, and TBI, has different care cultures and historical roots. PTSD is firmly situated in the mental health field. SUD treatment has historically had separate funding streams, oversight and research agencies, credentialing, and provider training. Thus, SUD treatment holds different assumptions (e.g., much more focus on peer support, open disclosure of treaters' own recovery, far more reliance on group over individual counseling, and different workforce training). The TBI field has focused primarily on cognitive and physical rehabilitation and is typically less well integrated with mental health or SUD treatment environments. It will be a major public health challenge to help providers in each system get "up to speed" on assessment, treatment, and sensitivity to each of the comorbidities as well as associated life problems beyond diagnoses.

There may also be notable disparities in terms of the quality of care given in relation to each of the three disorders, depending on which system of care they enter. For example, the homeless may receive substandard treatment in emergency departments because of their "homeless" appearance or other prejudices. As a result, TBIs sustained after the onset of homelessness may also go undetected and untreated. If a homeless patient presents to an emergency room staggering, incoherent, smelling of alcohol, and unable to give any history, he or she may be diagnosed as intoxicated and observed until discharge rather than evaluated for TBI. Specialty care settings for PTSD, SUD, and TBI also may have rigid criteria that leave gaps in care. For example, PTSD programs may require the patient to be abstinent or at least motivated to give up substances prior to starting PTSD treatment. SUD programs may require that the patient not be suicidal or have notable mental health problems. TBI programs may, similarly, have any number of such "closed door" policies. Clinician attitudes may also present barriers to treatment of the trimorbidity. In studies addressing clinician attitudes, comorbid PTSD/SUD patients were perceived as more difficult to treat than those with either disorder alone (Najavits, Norman, Kosten, & Kivlahan, 2010; Najavits, 2002a).

Safety Risks

Each disorder is a risk factor for suicidality and other harm to self and/or others. For example, individuals with TBI have a three- to fourfold increase in successful suicides, an increase in suicide attempts (18%), and an increase in suicidal ideation (21–22%) (Halbauer et al., 2009). Moreover, each disorder frequently co-occurs with depression (Whelan-Goodinson, Ponsford, Johnston, & Grant, 2009), chronic pain (Nampiaparampil, 2008), and other disorders that in and of themselves confer additional risk for harm to self and others. It is thus crucial to provide staff training to identify how each disorder can contribute to such harm, and to incorporate risk reduction into assessment and treatment.

Patient, Clinician, and Family Expectations

It is helpful to convey that prognoses for each disorder are positive in many cases. Patients can improve in each disorder, and it is likely that recovery in one may potentially also help recovery in the others. Indeed, it is often a surprise to clinicians who are not familiar with TBI that mTBI symptoms generally improve and/or resolve within 6 months postinjury (Carlson et al., 2010). However, if further insult to the CNS occurs, as is often the case among those in the military, homeless persons, and persons dependent on substances, further decrements in functioning may take place. For example, further injury in the context of street violence, explosions, and penetrating injuries may exacerbate the effects of mTBI. Similarly, chronic substance abuse, which even in the absence of TBI can cause cognitive impairment, may also retard recovery from TBI. Thus, patients need clear instruction and aid to prevent them from using substances, which can interfere with both TBI and PTSD recovery (Kelly, Johnson, Knoller, Drubach, & Winslow, 1997; Parry-Jones et al., 2006; Ouimette & Brown, 2002; Najavits, 2009).

Clinicians who are unfamiliar with PTSD and/or SUD may also not be aware that these disorders too generally have positive prognoses if patients are given evidence-based care for them, and if the patient attends treatment regularly (Bradley et al., 2005; Carroll & Onken, 2005). If the clinician believes there is no hope for recovery, he or she may "give up." However, in some patients, chronicity may reflect the patient never having received adequate assessment, and as a result, may not yet have received evidence-based treatment for all current comorbid psychiatric disorders. Families too can enhance patient outcomes by learning that outcomes can be positive for all three disorders, especially if, as a result of this knowledge, family members provide additional support to reinforce treatment goals.

Application of Single-Disorder Interventions to the Trimorbidity

It is unclear whether treatment models that work with each disorder will work with the trimorbidity. There are no treatment outcomes studies as yet for the trimorbidity, and few even for the comorbidity of TBI with PTSD or SUD. One of the most interesting is a study of TBI/SUD by Corrigan, Bogner, Lamb-Hart, Heinemann, and Moore (2005) who conducted a randomized controlled trial (RCT) on 195 TBI patients that compared motivational interviewing (MI), one of the standard evidence-based treatments in the SUD field, to financial incentives, barrier reduction (helping reduce logistical barriers to treatment), and an attention condition. Barrier reduction and financial incentives significantly and consistently outperformed the control on study outcomes (e.g., treatment attendance, retention in treatment, and amount of time to sign an individualized service plan), whereas MI did not.

According to Graham and Cardon (2008, p. 156), "The National Institutes of Health made a recommendation for the inclusion of substance-abuse evaluation and treatment in rehabilitation programs for TBI in 1999. However, little work has been done to determine if interventions that are effective in the general population are effective for persons with TBI." Graham and Cardon note that "traditional methods of substance-abuse treatment are often ineffective due to the cognitive, behavioral, physical, and emotional deficits that occur after brain injury" (p. 156).

Thus far, no psychosocial model for the trimorbidity has been evaluated. For PTSD–SUD comorbidity, Seeking Safety is the most empirically studied model thus far (Najavits et al., 2008). Seeking Safety is a present-focused coping skills approach that can be used with virtually any patient and conducted in group or individual format (Najavits, 2009). In contrast, for PTSD or SUD alone (single diagnosis models), there are numerous models. Single-diagnosis SUD models, for example, include Relapse Prevention, CBT for Substance Abuse, Contingency Management, and MI (Carroll & Onken, 2005). These are generally viewed as first-stage models that can typically be used with any patient and conducted in group or individual format. Single-diagnosis PTSD models include Prolonged Exposure, Eye Movement Desensitization and Reprocessing, and Cognitive Processing Therapy, for example (Institute of Medicine, 2007). These are generally viewed as second-stage models that require careful assessment of readiness (due to their emotional intensity) and are typically done in individual format. Readiness for such stage-2 models is particularly important for patients with significant vulnerability factors, such as substance dependence (the more severe form of SUD), homelessness, domestic violence, danger of violence to self or others, and treatment instability (e.g., Ruzek, Polusny, & Abueg, 1998). Clearly, more research is needed to determine which models will have relevance, safety, and efficacy for the trimorbidity. Moreover, given the general lack of significant differences between single-diagnosis SUD treatments when compared to each other (Imel, Wampold, Miller, & Fleming, 2008) and single-diagnosis PTSD treatments when compared to each other (Benish, Imel, & Wampold, 2007; Powers, Halpern, Ferenschak, Gillihan, & Foe, 2010), identifying which treatments are most feasible and least costly for a broad range of providers, settings, and patients will be key.

A helpful summary is provide by Graham and Cardon (2008). They state:

> (1) Community-based treatment for substance abuse for individuals with TBI is required. Inpatient or residential treatment for persons with TBI is seldom available or affordable. (2) Motivational interviewing techniques are not sufficient when used in isolation. Skills-based interventions show more promise for improved outcomes. (3) Inclusion of financial incentives and, to a lesser extent, barrier reduction helps to retain participants in treatment for at least the first month. (4) Peer-based support is generally well received by persons with TBI and their families, and has shown to benefit participants in a variety of ways (knowledge, a sense of empowerment, and coping capabilities). (5) Treatment has been shown to be effective using both individual counseling and group psychotherapy modalities in outpatient community settings. (pp. 158–159)

It is also useful to consider additional treatment options that may be helpful for the trimorbidity. For example, collaborative care, case management models, and recovery-oriented care principles may be particularly helpful, given the often long-term course of the trimorbidity, the need for multidisciplinary care, and the need for such diverse areas of care (e.g., psychosocial, medical, cognitive rehabilitative, employment-related) (Corrigan et al., 1995; Kreutzer & Harris, 1990). People with histories of brain injury have greater utilization of health care resources including hospital stays, admissions, and ER visits (Graham & Cardon, 2008). Future treatment-related research will need to include RCTs with larger sample sizes and longer follow-up periods to verify such conclusions.

Neurocognitive Predictors of Treatment Response

It will be important to identify which types of interventions impact which types of symptoms, as well as which patient and provider characteristics best predict good and poor outcomes. For example, a meta-analysis (Rohling, Faust, Beverly, & Demakis, 2009) of cognitive rehabilitation for brain injury provided evidence for efficacy of attention training with patients with TBI, but also noted that patient characteristics moderated treatment response. One important characteristic for TBI might be severity of injury. Indeed, the literature we have covered on comorbidity treatment studies (e.g., TBI/

SUD) does not specifically address outcomes based on level of TBI injury, and thus conclusions regarding mTBI await future research.

Neuropsychological deficits may constitute a class of predictors of particular relevance to the trimorbidity. There appears to be a positive relationship between neurocognitive abilities and success in treatment among patients with SUD (Allsop, Saunders, & Phillips, 2000; Morgenstern & Bates, 1999), with an effect size range from $d = 0.4$ to 0.5 between neuropsychological test performance measured at the beginning of treatment and treatment outcome, as defined by both completion of treatment and post-treatment substance use. If sufficiently severe, deficits in attention, learning, and memory can make it nearly impossible for a patient with SUD to acquire the information that is taught in treatment (Sanchez-Craig, 1982). Deficits in executive functions can impede the ability to integrate new behaviors (e.g., new skills taught in treatment) into a behavioral repertoire that to date had focused on negative coping such as drinking or using drugs. Executive dysfunction could also impair the ability to use what is taught in treatment in the real world (Morgenstern & Bates, 1999), as it would be difficult for a person with deficits in problem solving and abstract reasoning to apply the skills taught in treatment to novel situations. More specifically, deficits in abstract thinking may relate to a lack of generalizability of relapse prevention skills outside of treatment. Impairment in cognitive flexibility and verbal fluency may reduce the patient's ability to produce behavioral alternatives to substance use. Response inhibition problems may make it more likely that patients display prepotent responses (i.e., substance use) to environmental stimuli such as stress or high-risk situations. In fact, evidence bears out that neuropsychological deficits in substance abusers negatively relate to attainment of treatment objectives (Teichner, Horner, & Harvey, 2001). Further, the impulsivity and disinhibition that substance users exhibit may be misinterpreted by the provider as the patient being oppositional or resistant to treatment, resulting in termination from the treatment program. Although the deficits described in this paragraph stem from the SUD literature, they are also relevant to cognitive impairments associated with PTSD/mTBI in some patients, which may be exacerbated in the context of SUD.

Other Treatment Considerations

Treatment of each of the disorders generally focuses on symptom change. It is, however, also important to address the broader issue of identity in relation to each disorder (Najavits, 2002b). In TBI, it has been said that patients frequently describe a discrepancy between preinjury "self" and postinjury "self" (Halbauer et al., 2009). Learning to "tell a new story" occurs in PTSD (e.g., survivor rather than victim), in substance abuse (a clean-and-sober recovery-focused identity), and TBI (facing losses of some cognitive capacities). There may be a profound need to mourn the loss of memory and skills; loss of power and control; loss of independence; loss of the anticipated future (dreams, career); relationship problems (including the possible loss of some relationships); spiritual confusion and crisis; and potential isolation related to these issues. Patients may also have to face the reality that they have various behavioral, personality, social, and cognitive changes from the trimorbidity, and may need help adjusting to these.

There are various subpopulations with notable rates of PTSD, SUD, and/or TBI, such as military/veterans, abused children and adolescents, victims of domestic violence, and motor vehicle and other accident survivors. In addition to focusing on general principles, it will be important to develop sensitivity to how the needs of these subpopulations may differ. For example, in some settings, many patients with the trimorbidity may never have received medical or psychosocial attention. The injuries they suffered as children, as well as their neuropsychological sequelae, may have gone unreported and untreated. Abusive parents may have attempted to conceal their children's injuries; the impoverished circumstances in which some patients were raised may have resulted in limited access to affordable medical care; still others may have come from cultures in which receiving treatment for a mental disorder of any type would be considered a weakness.

Outcomes may correspondingly vary according to circumstances of the patient. There are also entire systems in which the rates of these disorders are especially high (criminal justice, military, VA), and thus a system-based approach may be important to develop as well. Finally, clinicians too may have their own histories of one or more of the three disorders, and thus clinician awareness of how their own history may impact treatment is also needed.

Summary and Future Directions

Understanding of the trimorbidity of PTSD/SUD/TBI is in its infancy. Yet drawing on existing research and clinical insight from the comorbidity field for pairs of these disorders indicates some overarching principles that can be helpful. We have reviewed various aspects related to background on the disorders, assessment, and treatment. It is hoped that patients will come to receive a level of care that is sensitive and respectful of the ways in which these disorders interact, and that clinicians and programs will receive the supports they need to provide the best quality care for what is a challenging set of problems.

References

Allsop, S., Saunders, B., & Phillips, M. (2000). The process of relapse in severely dependent male problem drinkers. *Addiction, 95,* 95–106.

American Psychiatric Association. (2000). *Diagnostic and statistical manual of mental disorders* (4th ed., text rev.). Washington, DC: Author.

Benish, S., Imel, Z., & Wampold, B. (2007). The relative efficacy of bona fide psychotherapies for treating post-traumatic stress disorder: a meta-analysis of direct comparisons. *Clinical Psychology Review, 28,* 746–758.

Bjork, J. M., & Grant, S. J. (2009). Does traumatic brain injury increase risk for substance abuse? *Journal of Neurotrauma, 26*(7), 1077–1082.

Bradley, R., Greene, J., Russ, E., Dutra, L., & Westen, D. (2005). A multidimensional meta-analysis of psychotherapy for PTSD. *American Journal of Psychiatry, 162,* 214–227.

Carlson, K. F., Nelson, D., Orazem, R. J., Nugent, S., Cifu, D. X., & Sayer, N. A. (2010). Psychiatric diagnoses among Iraq and Afghanistan war veterans screened for deployment-related traumatic brain injury. *Journal of Traumatic Stress, 23,* 17–24.

Carroll, K. M., & Onken, L. S. (2005). Behavioral therapies for drug abuse. *American Journal of Psychiatry, 162*(8), 1452–1460.

Copersino, M. L., Fals-Stewart, W., Fitzmaurice, G., Schretlen, D. J., Solokoff, J., & Weiss, R. D. (2009). Rapid cognitive screening of patients with substance use disorders. *Experimental and Clinical Psychopharmacology, 17,* 337–344.

Corrigan, J. D., Bogner, J., Lamb-Hart, G., Heinemann, A. W., & Moore, D. (2005). Increasing substance abuse treatment compliance for persons with traumatic brain injury. *Psychology of Addictive Behaviors, 19,* 131–139.

Corrigan, J. D., & Cole, T. B. (2008). Substance use disorders and clinical management of traumatic brain injury and posttraumatic stress disorder. *Journal of the American Medical Association, 300,* 720–721.

Corrigan, J. D., & Deutschle, J. J. Jr. (2008). The presence and impact of traumatic brain injury among clients in treatment for co-occurring mental illness and substance abuse. *Brain Injury, 22,* 223–231.

Corrigan, J. D., Lamb-Hart, G. L., & Rust, E. (1995). A programme of intervention for substance abuse following traumatic brain injury. *Brain Injury, 9,* 221–236.

Dackis, C., & O'Brien, C. (2005). Neurobiology of addiction: Treatment and public policy ramifications. *Nature Neuroscience, 8,* 1431–1436.

Galanter, M. & Kleber, H. D. (2008). *Textbook of substance abuse treatment* (4th ed., pp. 62–63) Arlington, VA: American Psychiatric Publishing.

Gilbertson, M. W., Gurvits, T. V., Lasko, N. B., Orr, S. P., & Pitman, R. K. (2001). Multivariate assessment of explicit memory function in combat veterans with posttraumatic stress disorder. *Journal of Traumatic Stress, 14,* 413–432.

Graham, D. P., & Cardon, A. L. (2008). An update on substance use and treatment following traumatic brain injury. *Annals of the New York Academy of Science, 1141,* 148–162.

Halbauer, J. D., Ashford, J. W., Zeitzer, J. M., Adamson, M. M., Lew, H. L., & Yesavage, J. A. (2009). Neuropsychiatric diagnosis and management of chronic sequelae of war-related mild to moderate traumatic brain injury. *Journal of Rehabilitation Research and Development, 46,* 757–796.

Hibbard, M., Uysal, S., Kepler, K., Bogdany, J., & Silver, J. M. (1998). Axis I psychopathology in individuals with TBI. *Journal of Head Trauma Rehabilitation, 13,* 24–39.

Hoffmann, N. G., & Ninonuevo, F. G. (1994). Concurrent validation of substance abusers self-reports against collateral information: Percentage agreement vs. Kappa vs. Yule's Y. *Alcoholism: Clinical and Experimental Research, 18,* 231–237.

Imel, Z., Wampold, B., Miller, S., & Fleming, R. (2008). Distinctions without a difference: Direct comparisons of psychotherapies for alcohol use disorders. *Psychology of Addictive Behavior, 22,* 533–543.

Institute of Medicine. (2007). *Treatment of PTSD: An assessment of the evidence.* Washington, DC: National Academies Press.

Iverson, G. L. (2005). Outcome in mild traumatic brain injury. *Current Opinion in Psychiatry, 18,* 301–317.

Jaffe, A. J., & Kilbey, M. M. (1994). The Cocaine Expectancy Questionnaire (CEQ): Construction and predictive validity. *Psychological Assessment, 6,* 18–26.

Kelly, M. P, Johnson, C. T., Knoller, N., Drubach, D. A., & Winslow, M. M. (1997). Substance abuse, traumatic brain injury, and neuropsychological outcome. *Brain Injury, 11,* 391–402.

Kessler, R. C., Berglund, P., Demler, O., Jin, R., Merikangas, K. R., & Walters, E. E. (2005). Lifetime prevalence and age-of-onset distributions of DSM-IV disorders in the National Comorbidity Survey replication. *Archives of General Psychiatry, 62,* 593–602.

Kessler, R. C., Crum, R. C., Warner, L. A., Nelson, C. B., Schulenberg, J., & Anthony, J. C. (1997). Lifetime co-occurence of DSM-III-R alcohol abuse and dependence with other psychiatric disorders in the National Comorbidity Survey. *Archives of General Psychiatry, 54,* 313–321.

Kraus, J., & McArthur, D. (1996). Epidemiologic aspects of brain injury. *Neurologic Clinics, 14,* 435–450.

Kreutzer, J. S., & Harris, J. (1990). Model systems of treatment for alcohol abuse following traumatic brain injury. *Brain Injury, 4,* 1–5.

Kreutzer, J. S., Wehman, P. H., Harris, J. A., Burns, C. T., & Young, H. F. (1991). Substance abuse and crime patterns among persons with traumatic brain injury referred for supported employment. *Brain Injury, 5,* 177–187.

Leskin, L. P., & White, P. M. (2007). Attentional networks reveal executive function deficits in posttraumatic stress disorder. *Neuropsychology, 21,* 275–284.

Maisto, S. A., Sobell, L. C., & Sobell, M. B. (1982). Corroboration of drug abuser's self-reports through the use of multiple data sources. *American Journal of Drug and Alcohol Buse, 83*(9), 301–308.

McKay, J., Drapkin, M., Goodman, J., & DePhillipis, D. (2010). *Brief Addiction Monitor. Unpublished measure, University of Pennsylvania.*

McLellan, A. T., Kushner, H., Metzger, D., Peters, R., Smith, I., Grissom, G., et al.

(1992). The fifth edition of the Addiction Severity Index. *Journal of Substance Abuse Treaetment, 9*, 199–213.

Meek, P. S., Clark, H. W., & Solana, V. L. (1989). Neurocognitive impairment: The unrecognized component of dual diagnosis in substance abuse treatment. *Journal of Psychoactive Drugs, 21*, 153–161.

Miller, W. R., & Tonigan, J. S. (1994). *Assessing drinkers' motivation for change: The Stages of Change Readiness and Treatment Eagerness Scale (SOCRATES).* Unpublished manuscript, Center on Alcoholism, Substance Abuse, and Addictions, University of New Mexico, Albuquerque, NM.

Modesto-Lowe, V., & Kranzler, H. R. (1999). Diagnosis and treatment of alcohol-dependent patients with comorbid psychiatric disorders. *Alcohol Research and Health, 23*, 144–149.

Morgenstern, J. B., & Bates, M. E. (1999). Effects of executive function impairment on change processes and substance use outcomes in 12-step treatment. *Journal of Studies on Alcohol, 60*, 846–855.

Najavits, L. M. (2002a). Clinicians' views on treating posttraumatic stress disorder and substance use disorder. *Journal on Substance Abuse Treatment, 22*, 79–85.

Najavits, L. M. (2002b). *Seeking Safety: A treatment manual for PTSD and substance abuse.* New York: Guilford Press.

Najavits, L. M. (2004). Assessment of trauma, PTSD, and substance use disorder: A practical guide. In J. P. Wilson & T. M. Keane (Eds.), *Assessment of psychological trauma and PTSD* (pp. 466–491). New York: Guilford Press.

Najavits, L. M. (2009). Psychotherapies for trauma and substance abuse in women: Review and policy implications. *Trauma, Violence, and Abuse: A Review Journal, 10*, 290–298.

Najavits, L. M., Griffin, M. L., Luborsky, L., Frank, A., Weiss, R. D., Liese, B. S., et al. (1995). Therapists' emotional reactions to substance abusers: A new questionnaire and initial findings. *Psychotherapy, 32*, 669–677.

Najavits, L. M., Norman, S. B., Kivlahan, D., & Kosten, T. R. (2010). Improving PTSD/substance abuse treatment in the VA: A survey of providers. *American Journal on Addictions, 19*(3), 257–263.

Najavits, L. M., Ryngala, D., Back, S. E., Bolton, E., Mueser, K. T., & Brady, K. T. (2008). Treatment for PTSD and comorbid disorders: A review of the literature. In E. B. Foa, T. M. Keane, M. J. Friedman, & J. Cohen (Eds.), *Effective treatments for PTSD: Practice guidelines from the International Society for Traumatic Stress Studies* (2nd ed., pp. 508–535). New York: Guilford Press.

Nampiaparampil, D. E. (2008). Prevalence of chronic pain after traumatic brain injury: A systematic review. *Journal of the American Medical Association, 300*, 711–719.

Olson-Madden, J. H., Brenner, L., Harwood, J. E., Emrick, C. D., Corrigan, J. D., & Thompson, C. (2010). Traumatic brain injury and psychiatric diagnoses in veterans seeking outpatient substance abuse treatment. *Journal of Head Trauma Rehabilitation, 25*, 470–479.

Ouimette, P., & Brown, P. J. (2002). *Trauma and substance abuse: Causes, consequences, and treatment of comorbid disorders.* Washington, DC: American Psychological Association Press.

Parsons, O. A. (1996). *Alcohol abuse and alcoholism*. In R. L. Adams & O. A. Parsons (Eds.), *Neuropsychology for clinical practice: Etiology, assessment, and treatment of common neurological disorders* (pp. 175–201). Washington, DC: American Psychological Association.

Parry-Jones, B. L., Vaughan, F. L., & Miles Cox, W. (2006). Traumatic brain injury and substance misuse: A systematic review of prevalence and outcomes research (1994–2004). *Neuropsychologial Rehabilitation, 16*, 537–560.

Ponsford, J., Whelan-Goodinson, R., & Bahar-Fuchs, A. (2007). Alcohol and drug use following traumatic brain injury: A prospective study. *Brain Injury, 21*(13–14), 1385–1392.

Powers, M. B., Halpern, J. M., Ferenschak, M. P., Gillihan, S. J., & Foa, E. B. (2010). A meta-analytic review of prolonged exposure for posttraumatic stress disorder. *Clinical Psychology Review, 30*(6), 635–641.

Ratti, M. T., Bo, P., Giardini, A., & Soragna, U. (2002). Chronic alcoholism and the frontal lobe: Which executive functions are impaired? *Acta Neurologica Scandinaviae, 105*, 276–281.

Rogers, J., & Read, C. (2007). Psychiatric comorbidity following traumatic brain injury. *Brain Injury, 21*, 1321–1333.

Rohling, M. L., Faust, M. E., Beverly, B., & Demakis, G. (2009). Effectiveness of cognitive rehabilitation following acquired brain injury: A meta-analytic re-examination of Cicerone et al.'s (2000, 2005) systematic reviews. *Neuropsychology, 23*, 20–39.

Ruzek, J. I., Polusny, M. A., & Abueg, F. R. (1998). Assessment and treatment of concurrent posttraumatic stress disorder and substance abuse. In V. M. Follette, J. I. Ruzek, & F. R. Abueg (Eds.), *Cognitive-behavioral therapies for trauma* (pp. 226–255). New York: Guilford Press.

Sanchez-Craig, M. W., K. (1982). Teaching coping skills to alcoholics in a coeducational halfway house: Assessment programme. *British Journal of Addiction, 15*, 35–50.

Saunders, L. L., Selassie, A. W., Hill, E. G., Nicholas, J. S., Horner, M. D., Corrigan, J. D., et al. (2009). A population-based study of repetitive traumatic brain injury among persons with traumatic brain injury. *Brain Injury, 23*, 866–872.

Scheurich, A. (2005). Neuropsychological functioning and alcohol dependence. *Current Opinion in Psychiatry, 18*, 319–323.

Seltzer, M. L. (1971). The Michigan Alcohol Screening Test: The quest for a new diagnostic instrument. *American Journal of Psychiatry, 127*, 1653–1658.

Sheehan, D., Lecrubier, Y., Harnett Sheehan, K., Amorim, P., Janavs, J., Weiller, E., et al. (1998). The Mini-International Neuropsychiatric Interview (M.I.N.I.): The development and validation of a structured diagnostic psychiatric interview for DSM-IV and ICD-10. *Journal of Clinical Psychiatry, 59*, 22–33.

Skinner, H. A. (1982). Drug Abuse Screening Test. *Addictive Behavior, 7*, 363–371.

Sobell, L. C., & Sobell, M. B. (1992). Timeline Follow-back: A technique for assessing self-reported alcohol consumption. In R. Litten & J. Allen (Eds.), *Measuring alcohol consumption* (pp. 41–72). New York: Humana Press.

Sobell, L. C., & Sobell, M. B. (1995). *Alcohol timeline followback users' manual*.

[Computer software; instructional training video.] Toronto, Canada: Addiction Research Foundation.

Spitzer, R. L., Williams, J. B. W., & Gibbon, M. (1997). *Structured Clinical Interview for DSM-IV—Patient Version*. New York: Biometrics Research Institute.

Taylor, L., Kreutzer, J., Demm, S., & Meade, M. (2003). Traumatic brain injury and substance abuse: A review and analysis of the literature. *Neuropsychological Rehabilitation, 13*, 165–188.

Teichner, G., Horner, M. D., & Harvey, R. T. (2001). Neuropsychological predictors of the attainment of treatment objectives in substance abuse patients. *International Journal of Neuroscience, 106*, 253–263.

Temkin, N. R., Corrigan, J. D., Dikmen, S. S., & Machamer, J. (2009). Social functioning after traumatic brain injury. *Journal of Head Trauma Rehabilitation, 24*, 460–467.

Tonigan, J. S., & Miller, W. R. (2002). The Inventory of Drug Use Consequences (InDUC): Test–retest stability and sensitivity to detect change. *Psychology of Addictive Behaviors, 16*, 165–168.

Vasterling, J. J., Duke, L. M., Brailey, K., Constans, J. I., Allain, A. N. Jr., & Sutker, P. B. (2002). Attention, learning, and memory processes and intellectual resources in Vietnam veterans: PTSD and no disorder comparisons. *Neuropsychology, 16*, 5–14.

Verdejo-Garcia, A., Lopez-Torrecillas, F., Aguilar de Arcos, F., & Perez-Garcia, M. (2005). Differential effects of MDMA, cocaine, and cannabis use severity on distinctive components on the executive functions of polysubstance abusers: A multiple regression analysis. *Addictive Behaviors, 30*, 89–101.

Verdejo-Garcia, A., Recknor, E. C., Bechara, A., & Perez-Garcia, M. (2007). Negative-emotion driven impulsivity predicts substance dependence problems. *Drug and Alcohol Dependence, 91*, 213–219.

Weiss, R. D., Najavits, L. M., Greenfield, S. F., Soto, J. A., Shaw, S. R., & Wyner, D. (1998). Reliability of substance use self-reports in dually diagnosed outpatients. *American Journal of Psychiatry, 155*, 127–128.

Whelan-Goodinson, R., Ponsford, J., Johnston, L., & Grant, F. (2009). Psychiatric disorders following traumatic brain injury: Their nature and frequency. *Journal of Head Trauma Rehabilitation, 24*, 324–332.

Wright, F. D. (1992). *Beliefs about substance use*. Philadelphia, PA: Unpublished scale, Center for Cognitive Therapy, University of Pennsylvania.

PART IV

CLINICAL MANAGEMENT

CHAPTER 8

Assessment

Erin W. Ulloa, Brian P. Marx, Rodney D. Vanderploeg,
and Jennifer J. Vasterling

The wars in Iraq and Afghanistan have brought increased attention to comorbid presentations of posttraumatic stress disorder (PTSD) and mild traumatic brain injury (mTBI) among military personnel and veterans. However, PTSD and mTBI also co occur in civilian survivors of physical trauma (e.g., motor vehicle accidents, assault). Assessing the singular presence of either one of these disorders can be challenging due to retrospective reporting biases and difficulties linking symptoms to specific precipitating events. Cases in which both conditions are diagnostic possibilities present an even greater challenge as a result of symptom overlap. Although determination of whether a person currently meets diagnostic criteria for PTSD or whether an mTBI occurred is typically possible, the attribution of current symptoms to PTSD or mTBI is far more complicated. Knowledge of the natural course of symptoms and typical trajectory of recovery for each condition can facilitate this process in most cases.

This chapter provides information pertinent to assessment of patients reporting risk factors for, and symptoms associated with, both PTSD and mTBI. Specifically, we present diagnostic criteria and descriptions of commonly used assessment methods for PTSD and mTBIand discuss the challenges associated with assessing comorbid PTSD and mTBI. We also discuss the assessment of functional impairment, as this is an important indicator of both disorder severity and recovery for both disorders. Given the vast number of available assessment tools, we focus on general methods used to assess both disorders rather than on specific tools. Assessment of symptom validity in contexts involving potential secondary gain is discussed by Elhai, Sweet, Guidotti Breting, and Kaloupek (Chapter 9, this volume) and will not be covered here.

Assessment of PTSD

Evaluation of the Traumatic Event

As detailed by Pannu-Hayes and Gilbertson (Chapter 4, this volume), the DSM-IV-TR characterizes PTSD as a syndrome that is the result of exposure to an event involving a serious threat of injury, death, or the physical integrity of oneself or others. This event also must prompt the individual to respond with extreme fear, helplessness, or horror (American Psychiatric Association, 2000). According to the specifications of DSM-IV-TR, the diagnosis of PTSD cannot be rendered until at least 1 month has passed since the traumatic event occurred (American Psychiatric Association, 2000). In actuality, however, Criterion A is usually assessed many months or years after it has occurred.

Similar to retrospective reports of mTBI injury events, retrospective reporting of psychologically traumatic events that may have happened in the distant past leaves the assessment of Criterion A vulnerable to a number of potential biases and errors (e.g., Rubin, Bernsten, & Bohni, 2008; Weathers & Keane, 2007). Of particular relevance to comorbid PTSD and TBI, reports and recall of Criterion A events can be subject to memory deficits (Candel & Merckelbach, 2004), social desirability concerns (e.g., Krinsley, Gallagher, Weathers, Kutter, & Kaloupek, 2003; Rosen & Lilienfeld, 2008), psychiatric symptom severity (e.g., King et al., 2000; Porter & Peace, 2007; Wilson et al., 2008), and other preexisting individual differences (e.g., Adler, Wright, Bliese, Eckford, & Hoge, 2008), as well as current attitudes and goals, such as secondary gain (Candel & Merckelbach, 2004; Rubin et al., 2008). Additionally, the temporal stability of self-reported trauma exposure may vary. Despite these potential threats to the reliability and validity of self-reported trauma exposure, in a reanalysis of National Vietnam Veterans Readjustment Study data, Dohrenwend et al. (2006) found relatively high correlations between veterans' self-report of war-zone stressor exposure and objective indices of war-zone stress.

Similar to the process of assessing mTBI history, because all sources of information relevant to the psychological trauma are fallible, it is always advisable to use multiple sources of information (e.g., military, medical, or occupational records; police or forensic reports; collateral reports from family, friends, or witnesses) to document the history of the exposure to a psychologically traumatic event of sufficient magnitude to meet the

DSM-IV stressor criterion. Obtaining a more detailed narrative of the psychological trauma exposure from the survivor typically constitutes another essential element of an in-depth PTSD evaluation, as the narrative often provides useful information for both assessment and treatment purposes and can avoid biased responding resulting from leading questions. Instead of using an unstructured approach to obtain detailed information about the exposure from the survivor, an assessor may wish to use a semistructured interview, such as the Evaluation of Lifetime Stressors (Krinsley, Gallagher, Weathers, Kutter, & Kaloupek, 2003), as these are reliable and valid assessment instruments.

There are also a variety of reliable and valid self-report measures that can be used to obtain information about the psychological trauma exposure. Some of these self-report measures, such as the Trauma History Questionnaire (Green, 1996) and the Brief Trauma Questionnaire (Schnurr, Vielhauer, Weathers, & Findler, 1999), are checklists that screen for the occurrence of potentially traumatic experiences without detailing event characteristics or Criterion A2, whereas other self-report measures, such as the Traumatic Life Events Questionnaire (Kubany, Leisen, Kaplan, & Kelly, 2000) and the Life Stressor Checklist–Revised (Wolfe, Kimerling, Brown, Chrestman, & Levin, 1996), do assess Criterion A2. Still other self-report measures, such as the Combat Exposure Scale (Keane et al., 1989) and the War Zone Stress Index (King, King, Gudanowski, & Vreven, 1995), assess the intensity, frequency, and duration of exposure to events that involve threat of danger, loss of life, or severe physical injury. Regardless of which self-report measure is chosen, it is best practice to use them as a means of screening for possible trauma exposure and identifying an index event for symptom inquiry. Once the event(s) have been identified via self-report, then a more detailed assessment of these specific events is needed to adequately assess Criterion A (i.e., the trauma event).

Assessment of PTSD Symptoms

A number of psychometrically sound self-report and interview measures have been developed to assess the presence and severity of the 17 cardinal symptoms of PTSD. Self-report scales of PTSD symptom severity include the PTSD Checklist (Weathers, Litz, Herman, Huska, & Keane, 1993) and the Posttraumatic Stress Diagnostic Scale (Foa, Cashman, Jaycox, & Perry, 1997). Other self-report measures, such as the Mississippi Scale for Combat-Related PTSD (Keane, Caddell, & Taylor, 1988) may assess trauma-relevant symptoms but do not correspond specifically to the diagnostic criteria. Interview measures include the Clinician-Administered PTSD Scale (CAPS; Blake, Weathers, Nagy, & Kaloupek, 1995) and the PTSD Symptom Scale-Interview (Foa, Riggs, Dancu, & Rothbaum, 1993).

Table 8.1 provides information regarding the diagnostic utility of the measures. In general, paper-and-pencil self-report measures are typically better conceptualized as screening instruments that may aid in providing additional information about symptom severity (McDonald & Calhoun, 2010). However, for PTSD clinical diagnosis, it is also important to include a structured interview, which is generally considered to be the "gold standard."

Abbreviated self-report instruments used to assess PTSD symptom severity may be particularly helpful in screening for the possible presence of PTSD in primary care and other nonspecialty health care settings. Such instruments are useful in the context of mass trauma and have important implications for providing services that may ultimately prevent the development of PTSD following trauma exposure. In his review of PTSD screening measures, Brewin (2005) noted that screening with a few items referring to core PTSD symptoms may be effective in screening for PTSD and that measures with fewer items, simpler response scales, and simpler methods of scoring do as well as or better than other measures in screening for PTSD. Since Brewin's review, additional research has explored the extent to which successful screening for PTSD can occur using even shorter screening instruments (Bliese et al., 2008; Kimerling et al., 2006). As with longer symptom-based PTSD self-report measures, however, abbreviated screening measures would not be considered sufficient to make or confirm a diagnosis. For additional information about PTSD screening and assessment measures and discussion of best assessment practices, clinicians and researchers can refer to Kaloupek et al. (2010) or the National Center for PTSD website (*www.ptsd.va.gov/professional/pages/assessments/assessment.asp*).

Assessment of mTBI

TBI Classification

As detailed by Bigler and Maxwell (Chapter 2, this volume), although there are several available definitions of mTBI, all require that an individual must experience an external force to the head that leads to an alteration in mental state such as loss of consciousness (LOC), posttraumatic amnesia (PTA), or transient confusion or disorientation (Carroll, Cassidy, Holm, Kraus, & Coronado, 2004; Ruff et al., 2009). Whereas most mTBI definitions stipulate that the person must experience a LOC of less than 30 minutes, PTA no longer than 24 hours, or a period of confusion/disorientation of any duration following the head injury, there is some variability across definitions with respect to these time frames (Carroll et al., 2004). Some definitions also incorporate the Glasgow Coma Scale (GCS), which classifies the

TABLE 8.1. Measures Commonly Used to Assess PTSD Symptoms

Name	Description	Strengths	Weaknesses
Structured Clinical Interview for DSM-IV (SCID; First et al., 1996)	Assessment of all PTSD DSM-IV symptoms	Multiple versions available; excellent psychometrics	Yields only present–absent ratings for symptoms and diagnosis
Clinician-Administered PTSD Scale (CAPS; Blake et al., 1995)	30-item interview assesses PTSD DSM-IV symptoms; frequency and intensity of each symptom rated	Excellent psychometrics; widely used; available in multiple languages	Lengthy; requires training
PTSD Symptom Scale–Interview (PSS-I; Foa et al., 1993)	17-item interview assessing severity of each PTSD symptom	Excellent psychometrics; brief and easy to administer; yields PTSD diagnosis and symptom severity scores	One question per symptom; relies on a single rationally derived scoring rule
Structured Interview for PTSD (SIP; Davidson, Malik, & Travers, 1997)	Interview assessing DSM-IV PTSD symptoms and trauma-related guilt	Excellent reliability; brief and easy to administer; includes follow-up prompts for ratings	Relies on a single rationally derived scoring rule
Detailed Assessment of Posttraumatic Stress (DAPS; Briere, 2001)	104-item self-report measure of all PTSD symptoms, trauma exposure, and functional impairment	Has response bias scale; assessment of peritraumatic response and other associated features	Longer than most self-report measures
Impact of Event Scale—Revised (IES-R; Weis & Marmar, 1997)	22-item self-report measure that assesses PTSD symptoms	Consistent and reliable measure of trauma-related symptoms	Does not directly correspond with criteria listed in DSM-IV
Mississippi Scale for Combat-Related PTSD (Keane et al., 1988)	35-item self-report measure of combat-related PTSD symptoms	Excellent psychometrics; civilian version available	Probable PTSD diagnosis validated in some but not all populations
PTSD Checklist (PCL; Weathers et al., 1993)	17-item self-report measure of how much participant was bothered by each PTSD symptom over past month	Excellent psychometrics; military, civilian, and specific stressor versions available	Identified cutoff scores not standardized; psychometrics cannot be generalized across all versions
Posttraumatic Stress Diagnostic Scale (PDS; Foa et al., 1997)	49-item self-report instrument assessing PTSD DSM-IV criteria	Yields both a continuous index of symptom severity and a PTSD diagnosis; excellent psychometrics	Relies on a single diagnostic scoring rule

initial injury severity based on degree of eye opening and motor and verbal response. However, GCS ratings will only be available for patients seen by emergency medical personnel or a physician during the acute postinjury period (Ruff & Jurica, 1999).

Focal neurological deficits (e.g., posttraumatic seizures, obvious gait/balance problems, changes in sense of smell) or evidence of injury on conventional clinical neuroimaging (e.g., CT) may be found in some cases of mTBI; however, they are relatively uncommon (Borg et al., 2004; Ruff et al., 2009). When neurological deficits or positive findings on conventional neuroimaging studies are present in injuries that would otherwise be categorized as mTBI, functional and neuropsychological outcomes are generally similar to individuals with at least moderately severe TBI (Goldstein, Levin, Goldman, Clark, & Kenehan-Altonen, 2001; Kashluba, Hanks, Casey, & Millis, 2008). This had led some experts to apply the term "complicated mTBI" to such cases (Levin et al., 1987).

Obtaining a TBI History

Regardless of which definition of mTBI is used, we recommend obtaining medical record documentation (e.g., GCS) and witness reports whenever possible to determine the severity of LOC, PTA, and other symptoms experienced shortly after injury (see Ponsford, Chapter 10, this volume, for a discussion of emergency department assessment and management). Because of the mild nature of the injury and relatively minor transient symptoms, individuals may not seek immediate medical attention. In the absence of hospital records, diagnosis is dependent upon patient self-report facilitated by an in-depth clinical interview (Corrigan & Bogner, 2007). Guidelines offered jointly by the Department of Veterans Affairs (VA) and the Department of Defense (DoD) suggest that questions focus on injury characteristics (e.g., evidence of direct or indirect blow to head, location of impact), the circumstances surrounding the injury (e.g., cause of injury, injury/death of others), and the patient's mental state at the time of the injury (e.g., LOC, PTA) and shortly thereafter (e.g., early signs of confusion) (Management of Concussion/mTBI Workgroup, 2009). In all cases, best practice is to document the history of head injury using multiple sources of information, as all sources of information can be fallible.

There are several caveats to consider when conducting an mTBI interview. First, interviews may vary in the degree to which questions are structured. To reduce clinician influence on patient response, we recommend first asking patients to provide a spontaneous description of the potential head injury event and immediate symptoms or problems, rather than asking them to respond to a series of closed-ended questions. Such closed-ended questions may instead be used as prompts, with discordance in spontaneous and cued recall reconciled by the clinician through further questioning.

To determine injury severity, it is also important to clarify distinctions between LOC and PTA. Spontaneous reports of gaps in memory or being unable to function cognitively at the scene of the injury (e.g., feeling dazed, confused, or incoherent) may provide evidence of physiological disruption of brain functioning. However, without a witness report, it may be challenging to attribute an inability to remember aspects of the injury to LOC or PTA. Patients may assume that gaps in memory reflect loss of consciousness when in reality the patient may have been walking and talking but unable to process information and form new memories (i.e., PTA; Arciniegas, Anderson, Topkoff, & McAllister, 2005). Thus, accurate estimates of LOC or PTA duration may be difficult for patients to provide, particularly as time since the injury increases (et. al., 1989).

PTA implies, therefore, that consciousness has been altered at least to the extent that encoding of new information is affected. Further, alteration of consciousness (e.g., confusion, disorientation), even without PTA or full loss of consciousness, constitutes a critical component of most mTBI classification systems. For the purposes of mTBI diagnosis, reports of feeling dazed, confused, and/or disoriented must reflect physiological disruption of brain functioning rather than a psychological response (e.g., fear, horror, dissociation) to a stressor. Although clinical interviewing techniques can be used to separate an individual's alteration in consciousness from his or her psychological responses during exposure to a stressor, it still can be difficult to tease apart these reactions under certain circumstances, such as when the psychological symptoms are more salient to the patient than the alteration in consciousness or when the patient cannot articulate such subtle distinctions in his or her responses. Under these conditions, it may be unwise to assume that an initial report of altered consciousness indicates mTBI because it might be the patient's way of describing an emotional reaction; conversely, to assume that the patient's report of an emotional response does not also encompass an injury-induced alteration of consciousness may also be inaccurate. One recently published structured interview for collecting information on the lifetime history of TBI using self- or proxy reports is called the Ohio State University TBI Identification Method. Prior studies have demonstrated acceptable levels of interrater and test–retest reliability and validity of this instrument (Corrigan & Bogner, 2007; Bogner & Corrigan, 2009).

In part because of difficulties in establishing alteration or loss of consciousness at the time of the injury, recent efforts have searched for potential "objective" markers of mTBI (Bazarian, 2010), such as tympanic membrane perforation found during neuro-otologic examinations for blast-related mTBI and tissue texture analysis, blood or cerebral spinal fluid markers, visual tracking tasks, and neuroimaging techniques for non-blast-related mTBI (Belanger, Vanderploeg, Curtiss, & Warden, 2007; Holli et. al., 2010; Maruta, Suh, Niogi, Múkherjec, & Ghajar, 2010). As summarized by Bigler and Maxwell (Chapter 2, this volume), studies using positron emission tomography (PET), functional magnetic resonance imaging (fMRI), magnetization transfer imaging (MTI), and magnetic resonance spectroscopy (MRS) have found that such methods may be sufficiently sensitive to identify individuals who have suffered mTBI. However, additional prospective research with larger samples and rigorous experimental methods are needed before these techniques can be used in routine clinical practice to detect mTBI (for reviews, see Belanger et al., 2007; Bigler, 2008).

Assessment of Postconcussion Syndrome

Postconcussion syndrome (PCS) refers to a set of symptoms that can arise after mTBI, often consisting of physical/somatic (e.g., headache, dizziness, photophobia, fatigue), cognitive (e.g., impaired memory, decreased concentration), and emotional (e.g., depression, irritability) symptoms (Hall, Hall, & Chapman, 2005). The *Diagnostic and Statistical Manual of Mental Disorders, Fourth Edition, Text Revision* (DSM-IV-TR; American Psychiatric Association, 2000) and the *International Classification of Diseases–10* (ICD-10; World Health Organization, 1994) include PCS as a diagnosis in their classification systems. Symptoms common to the disorder across both classification systems include headaches, irritability, fatigue, dizziness, and sleep disturbance (American Psychiatric Association, 1994; World Health Organization, 1994). In addition, DSM PCS diagnostic criteria require a minimum duration of 3 months (vs. 1 month in ICD-10), discrimination from preexisting symptoms, exclusion of other disorders, evidence of cognitive deficit based on formal testing, and interference with social functioning. Direct comparison of DSM-IV and ICD-10 PCS criteria found that any diagnostic discrepancies within specific patients were primarily attributable to DSM-IV's requirement for evidence of deficit on formal neuropsychological testing and clinical significance (Boake et al., 2004).

Although mTBI victims may experience some PCS symptoms in the immediate aftermath of a head trauma (Alexander, 1995), the overwhelming majority of mildly brain-injured people recover within hours to days after the injury (Carroll et al., 2004; Ponsford et al., 2000). A minority of people report PCS symptoms several months or more postinjury (Alexander, 1995; Vanderploeg, Curtiss, Luis, & Salazar, 2007). Some research suggests that this persistent PCS may be the result of structural damage in one or more neuroanatomical regions, such as the upper brainstem, base of the frontal lobe, hypothalamic–pituitary axis, medial temporal lobe, fornix, or corpus callosum (Bigler, 2008). In such instances, however, emotional and other contextual factors may also play a role in slowing recovery. For example, depression (Lange, Iverson, & Rose, 2010), chronic pain (Iverson & McCracken, 1997), traumatic injuries not affecting the brain

(Meares et al., 2008), and compensation claims (Cassidy, Carroll, Côté, Holm, & Nygren, 2004; Paniak, Reynolds, Toller-Lobe, Melnyk, Nagy, & Schmidt, 2002) have all been associated with persistent PCS. In most cases, PCS symptoms that begin weeks or months after mTBI (i.e., delayed onset) or symptoms that progressively worsen over time or are grossly disproportionate to the injury or objective examination findings may be more likely related to other co-occurring conditions than to the mTBI, although slowly developing TBI-related complications such as subdural hematoma should be ruled out (Arciniegas et al., 2005). In sum, persistent PCS is likely determined by organic, psychological, and environmental influences (see Iverson, Chapter 3, this volume) and they all should be considered in a thorough evaluation.

PCS can be assessed using a number of available self-report inventories that contain questions about the frequency or intensity of associated symptoms and behaviors (see Table 8.2). Although these measures can be useful for screening for PCS and monitoring changes in PCS symptoms, they cannot be used to diagnose the initial brain injury because they do not necessarily indicate that an mTBI occurred. Similarly, the lack of current symptoms does not address whether an injury occurred but is now resolved. Other potential limitations of these instruments include the lack of validity indicators and potential for biased or inaccurate responding (Iverson, Brooks, Ashton, & Lange, 2010; Lange et al., 2010).

Neuropsychological Assessment of mTBI Recovery

Although self-report measures can be useful for quantifying somatic and behavioral postconcussive complaints, neuropsychological testing may provide objective, performance-based indicators of neurocognitive recovery from mTBI. During the acute recovery period, mTBI has been associated with working memory abnormalities (McAllister, Flashman, McDonald, & Saykin, 2006) and deficits in information-processing speed (Barrow, Collins, & Britt, 2006; Barrow, Hough, et al., 2006), executive functioning, delayed memory, and verbal fluency (Alexander, 1995; Belanger, Curtiss, Demery, Lebowitz, & Vanderploeg, 2005). Meta-analyses of the neuropsychological deficits associated with mTBI have revealed that performance deficits on clinical neuropsychological tasks typically dissipate within 3 months of the injury (Belanger et al., 2005; Frencham, Fox, & Mayberry, 2005), although recent reanalysis of some of these data has suggested that a subset of individuals with mTBI may experience more enduring measurable neuropsychological impairments (Pertab, James, & Bigler, 2009). In particular, there is some evidence that mTBI can be associated with persistent yet subtle deficits in long-term and working memory, attention, and executive function (Bohnen, Jolles, & Twijnstra, 1992; Ruff &

TABLE 8.2. Measures Commonly Used to Assess Postconcussive Symptoms

Name	Description	Strengths	Weaknesses
Neurobehavioral Functioning Inventory (NFI; Kreutzer, Marwitz, Seel, & Serio, 1996)	70-item measure of symptom frequency	Widely used; versions for patient and family; six independent subscales	License and fees required; lengthy
Postconcussive Syndrome Symptom Scale (PSSS; Gunstad & Suhr, 2002)	97 items correspond to DSM-IV-TR criteria for PCS	Contains distracter items to minimize response set; evidence for reliability; no license or fees; maps to diagnostic criteria	Limited research base; lengthy
Neurobehavioral Symptom Inventory (NSI; Cicerone & Kalmar, 1995; Caplan et al., 2010)	22 items assess symptom severity	Widely used; no license or fees; excellent reliability	Symptoms highly confounded with PTSD in OIF veteran sample; assesses severity only
British Columbia Postconcussion Symptom Inventory (BC-PSI; Iverson & Lange, 2003)	16 items assess frequency and intensity of ICD-10 PCS criteria	Brief; widely used; maps to diagnostic criteria	Divergent validity not supported
Rivermead Post-Concussion Symptoms Questionnaire (PCSQ; King, Crawford, Wenden, Moss, & Wade, 1995)	16 items; preinjury symptoms compared with current symptoms	Brief; has companion measure of functional status	Conflicting data on factor structure; ratings based on perception of prior functioning may be biased
Postconcussion Syndrome Checklist (PCSC; Gouvier, Cubic, Jones, Brantley, & Cutlip, 1992)	9 items assess symptom frequency, intensity, and duration	Brief	Minimal evidence of psychometrics; needs more research

Jurica, 1999; Vanderploeg, Curtiss, & Belanger, 2005). Nonetheless, standardized clinical neuropsychological tests may not be optimally sensitive to subtle deficits or sufficiently specific to use as the basis of a diagnosis. Thus, their use is best construed as ancillary measures of recovery.

Additional Considerations in the Assessment of Comorbid PTSD and mTBI

Prevalence rates for comorbid PTSD and mTBI have ranged from 10 to 40%, depending upon the sample being examined (see Carlson et al., 2010, for a review). The potential presence of both PTSD and mTBI suggests a more complicated clinical presentation, with numerous targets for assessment and treatment. In such cases, an assessment must include a thorough evaluation of both PTSD and mTBI.

One important consideration when conducting an assessment of these comorbid conditions is that there is considerable symptom overlap between PCS and PTSD (Brenner, Vanderploeg, & Terrio, 2009; Stein & McAllister, 2009). In particular, anxiety, hyperarousal (e.g., sleep and concentration problems, irritability, sensitivity to noise), anhedonia, and posttraumatic amnesia (i.e., psychogenic vs. TBI-induced posttraumatic amnesia) symptoms overlap with postconcussive symptoms. Such symptom overlap may make it challenging for the examiner to render a correct diagnosis, particularly in situations in which a singular event is the source for both potential PTSD and mTBI. Although evidence-based guidance for assessment of the co-occurrence of these two conditions is limited (Carlson et al., 2010), we recommend careful questioning of symptom frequency, severity, onset, and course to link each reported symptom to TBI and/or psychologically traumatic events. In fact, when both PTSD and mTBI are possible diagnostic outcomes, it may be advisable to employ structured diagnostic interviews for both conditions to ensure that information about all aspects of the symptom presentation is obtained. It is also essential to assess for exposure to other psychological trauma and brain injuries and determine the extent to which these events might serve as potential anchors for symptom onset. Regardless of which tests and assessment methods are used, however, it will be difficult to attribute many of the current symptoms specifically to either PTSD or mTBI if both conditions are present and have similar onset and course.

The possible additional presence of other common comorbidities, such as depression, chronic pain, alcohol use, and drug use further complicates both the clinical presentation and the diagnosis. Regarding diagnosis, conditions comorbid to PTSD and mTBI also often share common symptoms (Dunn, Julian, Formolo, Green, & Chicoine, 2011; Iverson, 2006; Keane,

Brief, Pratt, & Miller, 2007; Lange et al., 2010). Given the frequent complexities of mTBI/PTSD cases, the importance of a multidisciplinary team approach to assessment and treatment of individuals with comorbid PTSD and mTBI has been consistently espoused, particularly in active-duty military and veteran settings (Sayer et al., 2009). Integrated evaluation of medical, psychological, vocational, and cognitive needs holds benefits for both patients and providers and represents a high standard of care.

Another consideration in the assessment of comorbid PTSD and mTBI is the role that various contextual factors may play in the information gathering during an assessment. For example, cultural differences in reporting style (Osterman & de Jong, 2007) or stigma associated with having a mental disorder (e.g., Hoge et al., 2004) may increase the likelihood that a patient will report physical problems rather than psychological ones. Patients may also be more willing to seek and accept care for problems associated with a physical injury, such as mTBI, rather than a mental health condition, such as PTSD (Brenner et al., 2009). Being aware of such contextual influences may help prevent the misattribution of symptoms.

Another consideration is that despite a variety of methods to assess PCS, PTSD, and mTBI all of the current methods have inherent limitations. Self-report scales and interview-based methods are vulnerable to response biases and memory failures (Frueh, Elhai, & Hamners, 2003; Iverson et al., 2010; Lange et al., 2010). More sophisticated assessment methods (e.g., psychophysiological and neuropsychological assessments, neuroimaging) are not always available due to their expense, requirement for advanced training, or lack of appropriate clinical norms relative to PTSD and mTBI to allow for valid interpretation of testing results. Reliance on a single assessment methodology or instrument may lead to an inaccurate diagnosis. As a result, it has become standard practice to employ multiple methods and measures to better inform diagnostic decisions (Belanger, Scott, Scholten, Curtiss, & Vanderploeg, 2005; Weathers, Keane, & Foa, 2009). Such multimethod assessment takes advantage of each method's relative strengths, overcoming the psychometric limitations of any single instrument and maximizing correct diagnostic decisions. However, as each patient's needs are different and determine the evaluation procedures to be used accordingly, each of these components may not always be used in every assessment case.

Finally, although there has been considerable debate on the question of whether it is possible for an individual to develop PTSD after sustaining an mTBI (Bryant, 2001), the most recent evidence suggests that PTSD can indeed develop after mTBI (e.g., Bryant & Harvey, 1998; Harvey & Bryant, 2000; Hoge et al., 2008). Two studies of returning veterans have even found that mTBI may increase PTSD prevalence (Hoge, McGurk, Thomas, Cox, Engel, & Castro, 2008; Schneiderman, Braver, & Kang,

2008). These findings suggest that clinicians should not be dissuaded from assessing for PTSD when it is a possible diagnostic outcome among those with an mTBI.

Assessment of Functional Impairment in PTSD and mTBI

For both PTSD and mTBI, the assessment of functional impairment is as important as diagnosis, particularly for the purposes of treatment planning and outcome monitoring. "Functional impairment" generally refers to the negative impact of one's symptoms on everyday functioning and is an important component of quality of life. This multidimensional construct includes functioning abilities in several important domains, such as physical, psychological, social, occupational, recreational, and cognitive. Although it is commonly assumed that symptoms and functioning are strongly related, such that amelioration of symptoms leads to improvements in functioning and vice versa, this is not uniformly the case.

According to DSM-IV-TR criteria, before a diagnosis of PTSD or PCS can be made, symptoms must be deemed to cause clinically significant distress or disruption to social or occupational functioning (American Psychiatric Association, 2000). Similar to the assessment of psychiatric symptoms and diagnoses, the assessment of functional impairment can be accomplished in a number of ways, such as via clinical interviews, self report instruments, and performance-based measures that assess functioning more broadly or within specific domains. As with symptom reports, information obtained via patient self-report or clinician rating should be supplemented with data from friends, family members, coworkers, supervisors, or teachers to provide a complete picture of current and premorbid functional status. Although these corroborating reports are also subjective, when combined with other data they may strengthen the conclusions that can be made and are less likely to be colored by the influence of postconcussive and trauma symptoms. It is beyond the scope of this chapter to review all available measures; however, references for assessment of functional impairment in individuals with PTSD (Holowka & Marx, in press) and mTBI (Temkin, Corrigan, Dikmen, & Machamer, 2009; Management of Concussion/mTBI Workgroup, 2009) can be found elsewhere.

One commonly used measure of functioning is the Medical Outcome Study (MOS) Short-form Health Survey–36 (SF-36; Ware, Snow, Kosinski, & Gandek, 1993), a self-report measure of functional health and well-being that has seen wide use in both PTSD (e.g., Power et al., 2002; Schnurr et al., 2003) and mTBI research (Maio et al., 2006; Stulemeijer et al., 2006), and is generally considered sensitive to change in these populations. Benefits of this measure include its strong psychometric qualities, long history of use in illness populations, ease of administration, and normative references. Another commonly used measure is the World Health Organization Disability Assessment Schedule–II (WHODAS-II; World Health Organization, 2000). The WHODAS-II is similar to the SF-36 in length, organization, and content; however, it can also be completed in interview format or via proxy. As a relatively new measure, the WHODAS-II has not been used extensively with individuals with PTSD or mTBI; however, emerging evidence suggests that it is likely to be a valid measure of impairment in mental health and TBI populations (Garin et al., 2010). A notable asset of the WHODAS-II is its relationship with the International Classification of Functioning, Disability, and Health (World Health Organization, 2001), an internationally recognized system of classifying the consequences of physical and mental health conditions.

Historically, patients with mTBI have been assessed for functional impairment in rehabilitation settings using a variety of other measures, such as the Glasgow Outcome Scale (Jennett & Bond, 1975), the Disability Rating Scale (Rappaport et al., 1982), and the Functional Independence Measure (Hamilton, Granger, Sherwin, Zielezny, & Tashman, 1987). However, these instruments have been criticized for ceiling effects even for moderate and severe TBI (Hall, Bushnick, Lakisic-Kazazic, Wright, & Cantagallo, 2001), rendering them insufficiently sensitive to deficits experienced by patients with mTBI. The Rivermead Head Injury Follow-Up Questionnaire (RHFUQ; Crawford, Wenden, & Wade, 1996) and the Functional Status Examination (FSE; Dikmen, Machamer, Miller, Doctor, & Temkin, 2001), both self-report measures of functioning, were developed and validated using samples with mild–moderate head injuries, which may make them more appropriate for use in mTBI; however, the RHFUQ and FSE also have limitations and require additional psychometric development with mTBI samples before their use can be supported.

In terms of functional measures applied to PTSD but not mTBI, the Global Assessment of Functioning (GAF; American Psychiatric Association, 2000) is commonly used as a measure of functioning in PTSD clinical and compensation settings. The GAF is a single-item clinician rating designed to assess both social/occupational functioning and symptom severity. However, the application of the GAF to PTSD has been criticized on the basis of inadequate psychometric properties in veteran PTSD samples (Söderberg, Tungström, & Armelius, 2005), a possible skew toward impairment (McNally, 2007), and its emphasis on symptoms of mood disorders and schizophrenia (Institute of Medicine, 2007). In a recent report on VA PTSD compensation and pension practices, the Institute of Medicine (2007) also noted that although the social and functional domains of the score provide some information, better measures of these domains exist, recommending that the VA identify and implement a suitable replacement for the GAF.

A growing body of evidence suggests that among individuals with comorbid physical and psychiatric conditions psychological consequences play a greater role in sustaining impairment than physical consequences (Laffaye, Kennedy, & Stein, 2003; Zatzick et al., 2002). Although only a handful of studies have examined the comparative impact of PTSD and mTBI on functioning, the results of these studies are consistent with this conclusion (Bryant et al., 2010; Pietrzak, Johnson, Goldstein, Malley, & Southwick, 2009). When assessing functional impairment among individuals with potential symptoms of PTSD and PCS, it is unlikely that the clinician will be able to determine conclusively whether the observed impairments are attributable to PTSD, to lingering effects of mTBI, or to common comorbidities of these two conditions (e.g., depression, alcohol misuse, chronic pain, sleep disturbance). Ultimately, the primary goal is to understand the impact of symptoms on daily functioning and to use this information to develop targeted interventions that will reduce symptoms and improve functioning across domains.

Conclusions

Our review of the literature on the assessment of comorbid mTBI and PTSD reveals that similar considerations may arise in the assessment of both disorders. For example, in addition to assessing symptoms, it is important to thoroughly assess events that may have precipitated the symptoms. It is also key to use a multimethod approach when assessing each disorder, as it is not prudent to rely on the results of a single instrument. Relatedly, there are response biases and errors that may similarly influence the reliability and validity of exposure and symptom reports. Both PTSD and mTBI may also lead to functional impairments and, as such, it is important to assess for such impairments across domains of functioning. Finally, the overlap in symptom presentation itself between PCS and PTSD may result in difficulties for the examiner in terms of determining the possible presence of one or both disorders.

Our review also indicates that there are some considerations that are unique to each disorder. For example, as already mentioned, there is currently only one available validated interview for assessing TBI, but it may be vulnerable to response bias as a result of "leading questions." Work by one of the authors of this chapter (R. Vanderploeg) is currently underway to develop a structured, reliable, and valid TBI interview that minimizes the potential for response bias. Another unique aspect of mTBI is that, similar to prior findings showing that a minority (ranging between 7 and

32%, depending on the sample) of individuals exposed to traumatic stress do not develop chronic PTSD (see Keane, Marx, Sloan, & Deprince, 2011, for a review), the overwhelming majority of those with such injuries recover from PCS symptoms shortly afterward. Specifically, it has been previously reported that only 10–20% of those who suffer an mTBI report continued problems (see Vasterling, Verfaellie, & Sullivan, 2009); further, persistent PCS is likely the result of a constellation of biological, psychological, and contextual factors, which may vary among individuals. Such individuals have been referred to as the "miserable minority" (Ruff, 2005). Unlike delayed-onset PTSD, which has now been shown to occur with some frequency and is usually an exacerbation of preexisting subsyndromal symptoms, depending upon the population (e.g., Andrews, Brewin, Philpott, & Stewart, 2007), delayed-onset PCS occurs rarely. When it is seen, it is thought to be the result of other neurological or psychiatric conditions, secondary gain motivations, adverse medication effects, medicolegal stressors, or a combination of these factors (Arciniegas et al., 2005). An issue that is of particular relevance to the assessment of PTSD is that, unlike mTBI, there are no available objective markers of the disorder. Previous research that has attempted to demonstrate that psychophysiological challenge tasks can be used to discriminate individuals with PTSD from those without the disorder have yielded mixed results (e.g., Blanchard, Hickling, & Taylor, 1991; Keane et al., 1998; Orr, Pitman, Lashko, & Herz, 1993). Thus, examiners must rely on self-report and interview methods to determine the presence of PTSD.

In terms of the methods and measures that are currently available to assess PTSD and mTBI, more work is needed to determine their generalizability across treatment settings, individual differences, and cultural contexts. It is also important to develop evidence-based methods for integrating the information collected using multiple methods or measures for the purpose of enhancing clinical decision making. Continued work to refine evidence-based PTSD and mTBI assessment practices will increase our understanding of the etiology and phenomenology of comorbid PTSD and mTBI. This additional work will also further help clinicians plan and implement more effective comorbid PTSD and mTBI treatment programs.

References

Adler, A. B., Wright, K. M., Bliese, P. D., Eckford, R., & Hoge, C. W. (2008). A2 diagnostic criterion for combat-related posttraumatic stress disorder. *Journal of Traumatic Stress, 21*, 301–308.

Alexander, M. P. (1995). Mild traumatic brain injury: Pathophysiology, natural history, and clinical management. *Neurology, 45*, 1253–1260.

American Psychiatric Association. (2000). *Diagnostic and statistical manual of mental disorders* (4th ed., text rev.). Washington, DC: Author.

Andrews, B., Brewin, C. R., Philpott, R., & Stewart, L. (2007). Delayed-onset posttraumatic stress disorder: A systematic review of the evidence. *American Journal of Psychiatry, 164,* 1319–1326.

Arciniegas, D. B., Anderson, C. A., Topkoff, J., & McAllister, T. W. (2005). Mild traumatic brain injury: A neuropsychiatric approach to diagnosis, evaluation, and treatment. *Neuropsychiatric Disease and Treatment, 1,* 311–327.

Barrow, I. M., Collins, J. N., & Britt, L. D. (2006). The influence of an auditory distraction on rapid naming after a mild traumatic brain injury: A longitudinal study. *Journal of Trauma-Injury Infection and Critical Care, 61,* 1142–1149.

Barrow, I. M., Hough, M., Rastatter, M. P., Walker, M., Holbert, D., & Rotondo, M. F. (2006). The effects of mild traumatic brain injury on confrontation naming in adults. *Brain Injury, 20,* 845–855.

Bazarian, J. J. (2010). Preface. *Journal of Head Trauma Rehabilitation, 25,* 225–227.

Belanger, H. G., Curtiss, G., Demery, J. A., Lebowitz, B. K., & Vanderploeg, R. D. (2005). Factors moderating neuropsychological outcomes following mild traumatic brain injury: A meta-analysis. *Journal of the International Neuropsychological Society, 11,* 215–227.

Belanger, H. G., Scott, S. G., Scholten, J., Curtiss, G., & Vanderploeg, R. D. (2005). Utility of mechanism-of-injury-based assessment and treatment: Blast Injury Program case illustration. *Journal of Rehabilitation Research and Development, 42*(4), 403–412.

Belanger, H. G., Vanderploeg, R. D., Curtiss, G., & Warden, D. L. (2007). Recent neuroimaging techniques in mild traumatic brain injury. *Journal of Neuropsychiatry and Clinical Neurosciences, 19,* 5–20.

Bigler, E. D. (2008). Neuropsychology and clinical neuroscience of persistent postconcussive syndrome. *Journal of the International Neuropsychological Society, 14,* 1–22.

Blake, D. D., Weathers, F. W., Nagy, L. M., & Kaloupek, D. G. (1995). The development of a clinician-administered PTSD scale. *Journal of Traumatic Stress, 8,* 75–90.

Blanchard, E. B., Hickling, E. J., & Taylor, A. E. (1991). The psychophysiology of motor vehicle related posttraumatic stress disorder. *Biofeedback and Self Regulation, 16,* 449–458.

Bliese, P. D., Wright, K. M., Adler, A. B., Cabrera, O., Castro, C. A., & Hoge, C. W. (2008). Validating the Primary Care Posttraumatic Stress Disorder Screen and the Posttraumatic Stress Disorder Checklist with soldiers returning from combat. *Journal of Consulting and Clinical Psychology, 76,* 272–281.

Boake, C., McCauley, S. R., Levin, H. S., Contant, C. F., Song, J. X., Brown, S. A., et al. (2004). Limited agreement between criteria-based diagnoses of postconcussional syndrome. *Journal of Neuropsychiatry and Clinical Neurosciences, 16,* 493–499.

Bogner, J., & Corrigan, J. D. (2009). Reliability and predictive validity of the Ohio

State University TBI identification method with prisoners. *Journal of Head Trauma Rehabilitation, 24,* 279–291.

Bohnen, N., Jolles, J., & Twijnstra, A. (1992). Neuropsychological deficits in patients with persistent symptoms six months after mild head injury. *Neurosurgery, 30,* 692–695.

Borg, J., Holm, L., Cassidy, J. D., Peloso, P. M., Caroll, L. J., von Holst, H., et al. (2004). Diagnostic procedures in mild traumatic brain injury: Results of the WHO Collaborating Centre Task Force on Mild Traumatic Brain Injury. *Journal of Rehabilitation Medicine, 43,* 61–75.

Brenner, L. A., Vanderploeg, R. D., & Terrio, H. (2009). Assessment and diagnosis of mild traumatic brain injury, posttraumatic stress disorder, and other polytrauma conditions: Burden of adversity hypothesis. *Rehabilitation Psychology, 54,* 239–246.

Brewin, C. R. (2005). Systematic review of screening instruments for adults at risk of PTSD. *Journal of Traumatic Stress, 18,* 53–62.

Briere, J. (2001). *Detailed Assessment of Posttraumatic Stress (DAPS).* Odessa, FL: Psychological Assessment Resources.

Bryant, R. A. (2001). Posttraumatic stress disorder and traumatic brain injury: Can they co-exist? *Clinical Psychology Review, 21,* 931–948.

Bryant, R. A., & Harvey, A. G. (1998). Relationship between acute stress disorder and posttraumatic stress disorder following mild traumatic brain injury. *American Journal of Psychiatry, 155*(5), 625–629.

Bryant, R. A., O'Donnell, M. L., Creamer, M., McFarlane, A. C., Clark, C. R., & Silove, D. (2010). The psychiatric sequelae of traumatic injury. *American Journal of Psychiatry, 167,* 312–320.

Candel, I., & Merckelbach, H. (2004). Peritraumatic dissociation as a predictor of post-traumatic stress disorder: A critical review. *Comprehensive Psychiatry, 45,* 44–50.

Caplan, L. J., Ivins, B., Poole, J. H., Vanderploeg, R. D., Jaffee, M. S., & Schwab, K. (2010). The structure of postconcussive symptoms in 3 US military samples. *Journal of Head Trauma Rehabilitation.* (Online prepublication)

Carlson, K. F., Kehle, S. M., Meis, L. A., Greer, N., Macdonald, R., Rutks, I., et al. (2010). Prevalence, assessment, and treatment of mild traumatic brain injury and posttraumatic stress disorder: A systematic review of the evidence. *Journal of Head Trauma Rehabilitation.* (Online prepublication)

Carroll, L. J., Cassidy, J. D., Holm, L., Kraus, J., & Coronado, V. G. (2004). Methodological issues and research recommendations for mild traumatic brain injury: The WHO Collaborating Centre Task Force on Mild Traumatic Brain Injury. *Journal of Rehabilitation Medicine, 43*(Suppl.), 113–125.

Carroll, L. J., Cassidy, J. D., Peloso, P. M., Borg, J., von Holst, H., Holm, L., et al. (2004). Prognosis for mild traumatic brain injury: Results of the WHO Collaborating Centre Task Force on Mild Traumatic Brain Injury. *Journal of Rehabilitation Medicine, 43*(Suppl.), 84–105.

Cassidy, J. D., Carroll, L., Côté, P., Holm, L., & Nygren, A. (2004). Mild traumatic brain injury after traffic collisions: A population-based inception cohort study. *Journal of Rehabilitation Medicine, 43*(Suppl.), 15–21.

Cicerone, K. D., & Kalmar, K. (1995). Persistent postconcussion syndrome: The structure of subjective complaints after mild traumatic brain injury. *Journal of Head Trauma Rehabilitation, 10,* 1–17.

Corrigan, J. D., & Bogner, J. B. (2007). Screening and identification of TBI. *Journal of Head Trauma Rehabilitation, 22,* 315–317.

Crawford, S., Wenden, F. J., & Wade, D. T. (1996). The Rivermead Head Injury Follow Up Questionnaire: A study of a new rating scale and other measures to evaluate outcome after head injury. *Journal of Neurology, Neurosurgery, and Psychiatry, 60,* 510–514.

Davidson, J. R., Malik, M. A., & Travers, J. (1997). Structured interview for PTSD (SIP): Psychometric validation for DSM-IV criteria. *Depression and Anxiety, 5,* 127–129.

Dikmen, S., Machamer, J., Miller, B., Doctor, J., & Temkin, M. (2001). Functional status examination: A new instrument for assessing outcome in traumatic brain injury. *Journal of Neurotrauma, 18*(2), 127–140.

Dohrenwend, B. P., Turner, J. B., Turse, N. A., Adams, B. G., Koenen, K. C., & Marshall, R. (2006). The psychological risks of Vietnam for U.S. veterans: A revisit with new data and methods. *Science, 313,* 979–982.

Dunn, A. S., Julian, T., Formolo, L. R., Green, B. N., & Chicoine, D. R. (2011). Preliminary analysis of posttraumatic stress disorder screening within specialty clinic setting for OEF/OIFveterans seeking care for neck or back pain. *Journal of Rehabilitation Research and Development, 48,* 493–502.

First, M. B., Spitzer, R. L., Gibbon, M., & Williams, J. (1996). *Structured Clinical Interview for DSM-IV Axis I Disorders—Patient Edition (SCID-I/P, Version 2.0). New York: New York State Psychiatric Institute, Biometrics Research Department.*

Foa, E. B., Cashman, L., Jaycox, L., & Perry, K. (1997). The validation of a self-report measure of PTSD: The Posttraumatic Diagnostic Scale. *Psychological Assessment, 9,* 445–451.

Foa, E. B., Riggs, D. S., Dancu, C. V., & Rothbaum, B. O. (1993). Reliability and validity of a brief instrument for assessing post-traumatic stress disorder. *Journal of Traumatic Stress, 6,* 459–473.

Frencham, K. A., Fox, A. M., & Maybery, M. T. (2005). Neuropsychological studies of mild traumatic brain injury: A meta-analytic review of research since 1995. *Journal of Clinical and Experimental Neuropsychology, 27,* 334–351.

Frueh, B. C., Elhai, J. D., & Hamner, M. B. (2003). Post-traumatic stress disorder (combat). In M. Hersen & S. M. Turner (Eds.), *Diagnostic interviewing* (3rd ed., pp.321–343). New York: Kluwer Academic/Plenum.

Goldstein, F. C., Levin, H. S., Goldman, W. P., Clark, A. N., & Kenehan-Altonen, T. (2001). Cognitive and neurobehavioral functioning after mild and moderate traumatic brain injury. *Journal of the International Neuropsychological Society, 7,* 373–383.

Gouvier, W. D., Cubic, B., Jones, G., Brantley, P., & Cutlip, Q. (1992). Postconcussion symptoms and daily stress in normal and head-injured college populations. *Archives of Clinical Neuropsychology, 7,* 193–211.

Green, B. L. (1996). Trauma History Questionnaire. In B. H. Stamm & E. M. Varra (Eds.), *Measurement of stress, trauma, and adaptation* (pp. 366–368). Lutherville, MD: Sidran Press.

Gunstad, J., & Suhr, J. (2002). A Perception of illness: Nonspecificity of postconcussion syndrome symptom expectation. *Journal of the International Neuropsychological Society, 8*(1), 37–47.

Hall, K. M., Bushnik, T., Lakisic-Kazazic, B., Wright, J., & Cantagallo, A. (2001). Assessing traumatic brain injury outcome measures for long-term follow-up of community-based individuals. *Archives of Physical Medicine and Rehabilitation, 82*, 367–374.

Hall, R. C., Hall, R. C., & Chapman, M. J. (2005). Definition, diagnosis, and forensic implications of postconcussional syndrome. *Psychomatics, 46*, 195–202.

Hamilton, B. B., Granger, C. V., Sherwin, F. S., Zielezny, M., & Tashman, J. S. (1987). A uniform national data system for medical rehabilitation. In M. Fuhrer (Ed.), *Rehabilitation outcomes: Analysis and measurement* (pp. 137–147). Baltimore: Brookes.

Harvey, A. G., & Bryant, R. A. (2000). Two-year prospective evaluation of the relationship between acute stress disorder and posttraumatic stress disorder following mild traumatic brain injury. *American Journal of Psychiatry, 157*(4), 626–628.

Hoge, C. W., Castro, C. A., Messer, S. C., McGurk, D., Cotting, D. I., & Koffman, R. L. (2004). Combat duty in Iraq and Afghanistan, mental health problems, and barriers to care. *New England Journal of Medicine, 351*, 13–22.

Hoge, C. W., McGurk, D., Thomas, J. L., Cox, A. L., Engel, C. C., & Castro, C. A. (2008). Mild traumatic brain injury in U.S. Soldiers returning from Iraq. *New England Journal of Medicine, 358*(5), 453–463.

Holli, K. K., Wäljas, M., Harrison, L., Liimatainen, S., Luukkaala, T., Ryymin, P., et al. (2010). Mild traumatic brain injury: Tissue texture analysis correlated to neuropsychological and DTI findings. *Academic Radiology, 17*, 1096–1102.

Holowka, D. W., & Marx, B. P. (in press). Assessing PTSD-related functional impairment and quality of life. In G. Beck, & D. M. Sloan (Eds.), *Oxford handbook of traumatic stress disorders*. New York: Oxford University Press.

Institute of Medicine. (2007). A 21st century system for evaluating veterans for disability benefits. In M. Mcgeary, M. Ford, S. McCutchen, & D. Barnes (Eds.), *Institute of Medicine of the National Academies*, Washington DC: National Academies Press.

Iverson, G. L. (2006). Complicated vs uncomplicated mild traumatic brain injury: Acute neuropsychological outcome. *Brain Injury, 20*, 1335–1344.

Iverson, G. L., Brooks, B. L., Ashton, V. L., & Lange, R. T. (2010). Interview versus questionnaire symptom reporting in people with the postconcussion syndrome. *Journal of Head Trauma Rehabilitation, 25*, 23–30.

Iverson, G. L., & Lange, R. T. (2003). Examination of "postconcussion-like" symptoms in a healthy sample. *Applied Neuropsychology, 10*, 137–144.

Iverson, G. L., & McCracken, L. M. (1997). Postconcussive' symptoms in persons with chronic pain. *Brain Injury, 11*(11), 783–790.

Jennett, B., & Bond, M. (1975). Assessment of outcome after severe brain damage. *Lancet, 1*, 480–484.

Kashluba, S., Hanks, R. A., Casey, J. E., & Millis, S. R. (2008). Neuropsychologic and functional outcome after complicated mild traumatic brain injury. *Archives of Physical Medicine and Rehabilitation Medicine, 89,* 904–911.

Kaloupek, D. G., Chard, K. M., Freed, M. C., Peterson, A. L., Riggs, D. S., Stein, M. B., et al. (2010). Common data elements for posttraumatic stress disorder research. *Archives of Physical Medicine and Rehabilitation, 91,* 1684–1691.

Keane, T. M., Marx, B. P., Sloan, D. M., & Deprince, A. (2011). Trauma, dissociation and posttraumatic stress disorder. In D. H. Barlow (Ed.), *Handbook of Clinical Psychology* (pp. 359–386). New York: Oxford University Press.

Keane, T. M., Brief, D. J., Pratt, E. M., & Miller, M. W. (2007). Assessment of PTSD and its comorbidities in adults. In M. J. Friedman, T. M. Keane, & P. A. Resnick (Eds.), *Handbook of PTSD: Science and practice* (pp. 279–305). New York: Guilford Press.

Keane, T. M., Caddell, J. M., & Taylor, K. L. (1988). Mississippi Scale for Combat-Related Posttraumatic Stress Disorder: Three studies in reliability and validity. *Journal of Consulting and Clinical Psychology, 56,* 85–90.

Keane, T. M., Kolb, L. C., Kaloupek, D. G., Orr, S. P., Blanchard, E. B., Thomas, R. G., et al. (1998). Utility of psychophysiology measurement in the diagnosis of posttraumatic stress disorder: Results from a department of Veteran's Affairs cooperative study. *Journal of Consulting and Clinical Psychology, 66,* 914–923.

Keane, T. M., Fairbank, J. A., Caddell, J. M., Zimering, R. T., Taylor K. L., & Mora, C. A. (1989). Clinical evaluation of a measure to assess combat exposure. *Psychological Assessment, 1,* 53–55.

Kimerling, R., Ouimette, P., Prins, A., Nisco, P., Lawler, C., Cronkite, R., & Moos, R. H. (2006). Utility of a short screening scale for DSM-IV PTSD in primary care. *Journal of General Internal Medicine, 21,* 65–67.

King, D. W., King, L. A., Erickson, D. J., Huang, M. T., Sharkansky, E. J., & Wolfe, J. (2000). Posttraumatic stress disorder and retrospectively reported stressor exposure: A longitudinal prediction model. *Journal of Abnormal Psychology, 109,* 624–633.

King, D. W., King, L. A., Gudanowski, D. M., & Vreven, D. L. (1995). Alternative representation of war zone stressors: Relationships to posttraumatic stress disorder in male and female Vietnam veterans. *Journal of Abnormal Psychology, 104,* 184–196.

King, N. S., Crawford, S., Wenden, F. J., Moss, N. E., & Wade, D. T. (1995). The Rivermead Post Concussion Symptoms Questionnaire: A measure of symptoms commonly experienced after head injury and its reliability. *Journal of Neurology, 242,* 587–592.

Kreutzer, J. S., Marwitz, J. H., Seel, R., & Serio, C. D. (1996). Validation of a neurobehavioral functioning inventory for adults with traumatic brain injury. *Archives of Physical Medicine and Rehabilitation, 77,* 116–124.

Krinsley, K. E., Gallagher, J. G., Weathers, F. W., Kutter, C. J., & Kaloupek, D. G. (2003). Consistency of retrospective reporting about exposure to traumatic events. *Journal of Traumatic Stress, 16,* 399–409.

Kubany, E. S., Leisen, M. B., Kaplan, A. S., & Kelly, M. P. (2000). Validation of a brief measure of post-traumatic stress disorder: The Distressing Event Questionnaire (DEQ). *Psychological Assessment, 12,* 197–209.

Laffaye, C., Kennedy, C., & Stein, M. B. (2003). Post-traumatic stress disorder and health-related quality of life in female victims of intimate partner violence. *Violence and Victims, 18*, 227–238.

Lange, R. T., Iverson, G. L., & Rose, A. (2010). Post-concussion symptom reporting and the good-old days bias following mild traumatic brain injury. *Archives of Clinical Neuropsychology, 25*, 442–450.

Levin, H. S., Amparo, E., Eisenberg, H. M., Williams, D. H., High, W. M., Jr, McArdle, et al. (1987). Magnetic resonance imaging and computerized tomography in relation to the neurobehavioral sequelae of mild and moderate head injuries. *Journal of Neurosurgery, 66*, 706–713.

Maio, R. F., Kirsch, N. L., Tan-Schriner, C. U., Frederiksen, S., Breer, M. L., & Tanner, C. L. (2006). Outcome of minor traumatic brain injury. *Journal of Head Trauma Rehabilitation, 21*, 430–431.

Management of Concussion/mTBI Workgroup. (2009). VA/DoD Clinical Practice Guideline for Management of Concussion/Mild Traumatic Brain Injury. *Journal of Rehabilitation Research and Developjment, 46*, CP1–CP68.

Maruta, J., Suh, M., Niogi, S. N., Mukherjee, P., & Ghajar, J. (2010). Visual tracking synchronization as a metric for concussion screening. *Journal of Head Trauma Rehabilitation, 25*, 293–305.

McAllister, T. W., Flashman, L. A., McDonald, B. C., & Saykin, A. J. (2006). Mechanisms of working memory dysfunction after mild and moderate TBI: Evidence from functional MRI and neurogenetics. *Journal of Neurotrauma, 23*, 1450–1467.

McDonald, S. D., & Calhoun, P. S. (2010). The diagnostic accuracy of the PTSD checklist: A critical review. *Clinical Psychology Review, 30*, 976–987.

McNally, R. J. (2007). Revisiting Dohrenwend et al.'s revisit of the National Vietnam Veterans Readjustment Study. *Journal of Traumatic Stress, 20*, 481–486.

Meares, S., Shores, E. A., Taylor, A., Batchelor, J., Bryant, R., Baguley, I. J., et al. (2008). Mild traumatic brain injury does not predict acute postconcussion syndrome. *Journal of Neurology, Neurosurgery and Psychiatry, 8*, 300–306.

Orr, S. P., Pitman, R. K., Lashko, N. B., & Herz, L. R. (1993). Psychophysiological assessment of posttraumatic stress disorder imagery in World War II and Korean combat veterans. *Journal of Abnormal Psychology, 102*, 152–159.

Osterman, J. E., & de Jong, J. T. (2007). Cultural issues and trauma. In M. J. Friedman, T. M. Keane, & P. A. Resick (Eds.), *Handbook of PTSD: Science and practice* (pp. 425–446). New York: Guilford Press.

Paniak, C., Reynolds, S., Toller-Lobe, G., Melnyk, A., Nagy, J., & Schmidt, D. (2002). A longitudinal study of the relationship between financial compensation and symptoms after treated mild traumatic brain injury. *Journal of Clinical and Experimental Neuropsychology, 24*(2), 187–193.

Pertab, J., James, K., & Bigler, E. D. (2009). Limitations of mild traumatic brain injury meta-analyses. *Brain Injury, 23*, 498–508.

Pietrzak, R. H., Johnson, D. C., Goldstein, M. B., Malley, J. C., & Southwick, S. M. (2009). Posttraumatic stress disorder mediates the relationship between mild traumatic brain injury and health and psychosocial functioning in veterans of

Operations Enduring Freedom and Iraqi Freedom. *Journal of Nervous and Mental Disease, 197,* 748–753.

Ponsford, J., Willmott, C., Rothwell, A., Cameron, P., Kelly, A. M., Nelms, R., et al. (2000). Factors influencing outcome following mild traumatic brain injury in adults. *Journal of the International Neuropsychological Society, 6,* 568–579.

Porter, S., & Peace, K. A. (2007). The scars of memory: A prospective, longitudinal investigation of the consistency of traumatic and positive emotional memories in adulthood. *Psychological Science, 18*(7), 656.

Power, K., McGoldrick, T., Brown, K., Buchanan, R., Sharp, D., Swanson, V., et al. (2002). A controlled comparison of eye movement desensitization and reprocessing versus exposure plus cognitive restructuring versus waiting list in the treatment of post-traumatic stress disorder. *Clinical Psychology and Psychotherapy, 9,* 299–318.

Rosen, G. M., & Lilienfeld, S. O. (2008). Posttraumatic stress disorder: An empirical evaluation of core assumptions. *Clinical Psychology Review, 28,* 837–868.

Rubin, D. C., Berntsen, D., & Bohni, M. K. (2008). A memory-based model of posttraumatic stress disorder: Evaluating basic assumptions underlying the PTSD diagnosis. *Psychological Review, 115,* 985–1011.

Ruff, R. M. (2005). Two decades in understanding of mild traumatic brain injury. *Journal of Head Trauma Rehabilitation, 20,* 5–18.

Ruff, R. M., Iverson, G. L., Barth, J. T., Bush, S. S., Broshek, D. K., & NAN Policy and Planning Committee. (2009). Recommendations for diagnosing a mild traumatic brain injury: A National Academy of Neuropsychology education paper. *Archives of Clinical Neuropsychology, 24,* 3–10.

Ruff, R. M., & Jurica, P. (1999). In search of a unified definition for mild traumatic brain injury. *Brain Injury, 13,* 943–952.

Ruff, R. M., Levin, H. S., Mattis, S., High, W. M., Marshall, L. F., Eisenberg, H. M., et al. (1989). Recovery of memory after mild head injury: A three-center study. In H. Levin, H. Eisenberg, & A. Benton (Eds.), *Mild head injury* (pp. 176–188). New York: Oxford University Press.

Sayer, N. A., Rettmann, N. A., Carlson, K. F., Bernardy, N., Sigford, B. J., Hamblen, J. L., et al., (2009). Veterans with history of mild traumatic brain injury and posttraumatic stress disorder: Challenges from provider perspective. *Journal of Rehabilitation Research and Development, 46,* 703–715.

Schneiderman, A. I., Braver, E. R., & Kang, H. K. (2008). Understanding sequelae of injury mechanisms and mild traumatic brain injury incurred during the conflicts in Iraq and Afghanistan: Persistent postconcussive symptoms and posttraumatic stress disorder. *American Journal of Epidemiology, 167,* 1446–1452.

Schnurr, P. P., Lunney, C. A., Sengupta, A., & Waelde, L. C. (2003). A descriptive analysis of PTSD chronicity in Vietnam veterans. *Journal of Traumatic Stress, 16,* 545–553.

Schnurr, P. P., Vielhauer, M., Weathers, F., & Findler, M. (1999). *The Brief Trauma Questionnaire.* White River Junction, VT: National Center for PTSD.

Söderberg, P., Tungström, S., & Armelius, B. Å. (2005). Reliability of Global Assessment of Functioning ratings made by clinical psychiatric staff. *Psychiatric Services, 56*, 434–438.

Stein, M. B., & McAllister, T. W. (2009). Exploring the convergence of posttraumatic stress disorder and mild traumatic brain injury. *The American Journal of Psychiatry, 166*(7), 768–776.

Stulemeijer, M., van der Werf, S., Bleijenberg, G., Biert, J., Brauer, J., & Vos, P. E. (2006). Recovery from mild traumatic brain injury: A focus on fatigue. *Journal of Neurology, 253*, 1041–1047.

Temkin, N. R., Corrigan, J. D., Dikmen, S. S., & Machamer, J. (2009). Social functioning after traumatic brain injury. *Journal of Head Trauma Rehabilitation, 24*, 460–467.

Vasterling, J. J., Verfaellie, M., & Sullivan, K. D. (2009). Mild traumatic brain injury and posttraumatic stress disorder in returning veterans: Perspectives from cognitive neuroscience. *Clinical Psychology Review, 29*(8), 674–684.

Vanderploeg, R. D., Curtiss, G., & Belanger, H. G. (2005). Long-term neuropsychological outcomes following mild traumatic brain injury. *Journal of the International Neuropsychological Society, 11*, 228–236.

Vanderploeg, R. D., Curtiss, G., Luis, C. A., & Salazar, A. M. (2007). Long-term morbidity and quality of life following mild head injury. *Journal of Clinical and Experimental Neuropsychology, 29*, 585–598.

Wade, D. T., King, N. S., Wenden, F. J., Crawford, S., & Caldwell, F. E. (1998). Routine follow up after head injury: A second randomized controlled trial. *Journal of Neurology, Neurosurgery, and Psychiatry, 65*, 177–183.

Ware, J. E., Snow, K. K., Kosinski, M., & Gandek, B. (1993). *SF-36 health survey manual and interpretation guide.* Boston: New England Medical Center, The Health Institute.

Weathers, F. W., & Keane, T. M. (2007). The Criterion A problem revisited: Controversies and challenges in defining and measuring psychological trauma. *Journal of Traumatic Stress, 20*, 107–121.

Weathers, F. W., Keane, T. M., & Davidson, J. R. (2001). Clinician-Administered PTSD Scale: A review of the first ten years of research. *Depression and Anxiety, 13*, 132–156.

Weathers, F. W., Keane, T. M., & Foa, F. B. (2009). Assessment and diagnosis of adults. In E. Foa, M. J. Friedman, & J. A. Cohen (Eds.), *Effective treatments for PTSD: Practice guidelines from the International Society for Traumatic Stress Studies* (pp. 23–61). New York: Guilford Press.

Weathers, F. W., Litz, B. T., Herman, D. S., Huska, J. A., & Keane, T. M. (1993). *The PTSD Checklist: Reliability, validity, and diagnostic utility.* Paper presented at the annual meeting of the International Society for Traumatic Stress Studies, San Antonio, TX.

Weis, D. S. & Marmar, C. R. (1997). The Impact of Event Scale–Revised. In J. P. Wilson & T. M. Keane (Eds.), *Assessing psychological trauma and PTSD* (pp. 399–411). New York: Guilford Press.

Wilson, J., Jones, M., Hull, L., Hotopf, M., Wessely, S., & Rona, R. J. (2008). Does prior psychological health influence recall of military experiences?: A prospective study. *Journal of Traumatic Stress, 21*, 385–393.

Wolfe, J., Kimerling, R., Brown, P. J., Chrestman, K. R., & Levin, K. (1996). The Life-Stressor Checklist–Revised. In B. H. Stamm (Ed.), *Instrumentation in stress, trauma, and adaptation* (pp. 198–200). Northbrook, IL: SidranPress.

World Health Organization. (1994). The ICD-10 classification of mental and behavioral diseases. Retrieved from *apps.who.int/classifications/apps/icd/icd10online*.

World Health Organization. (2000). The World Health Organization Disability Assessment Schedule–II. Retrieved from *www.who.int/icidh/whodas/whodasversions/36sa.pdf*.

World Health Organization. (2001). International classification of functioning, disability and health: ICF. Retrieved from *whqlibdoc.who.int/publications/2001/9241545429.pdf*.

Zatzick, D. F., Kang, S., Muller, H., Russo, J. E., Rivara, F. P., Katon, W., et al. (2002). Predicting posttraumatic distress in hospitalized trauma survivors with acute injuries. *American Journal of Psychiatry, 159*, 941–946.

CHAPTER 9

Assessment in Contexts That Threaten Response Validity

Jon D. Elhai, Jerry J. Sweet, Leslie M. Guidotti Breting, and Danny Kaloupek

This chapter addresses threats to validity that may be present when evaluating people for posttraumatic stress disorder (PTSD) and/or mild traumatic brain injury (mTBI). In particular, it focuses on reasons why people may not accurately or truthfully report symptoms and underperform on cognitive tasks, and it outlines steps that can be taken to evaluate the accuracy of assessment and appropriately calibrate conclusions drawn from it.

Generally, inaccurate presentations during testing can involve several types of response styles that are not mutually exclusive, including careless or indifferent responding, random responding, yeah-saying, nay-saying, and overreporting or underreporting of symptoms. We focus on symptom overreporting or exaggeration and reduced cognitive effort and mTBI when PTSD and mTBI are evaluated in secondary gain contexts (i.e., those that have potential for providing external incentives). Such symptom overreporting can be evidenced by fabrication or exaggeration of hallmark symptoms and/or reduced cognitive effort during assessment that will lower scores and be interpreted as impairment. Similar exaggeration may occur regarding the triggering trauma or incident to which PTSD or mTBI is attributed.

Symptom overreporting could involve the complete fabrication of psychopathology in a person who is otherwise completely free from symptoms (referred to as "pure malingering") or could alternatively involve the exaggeration or amplification of bona fide symptoms by a person who has genuine-but-subclinical levels of psychopathology (referred to as "partial

174

malingering"; Rogers, 2008a). Thus, strong evidence of symptom over-reporting does not necessarily indicate a completely fabricated symptom presentation, but could involve a person in genuine need of mental health care—albeit with a questionable level of need. Within the broad category of response bias, the more specific conclusion of *malingering* is probabilistic, typically including the categories of *possible, probable,* and *definite* malingering (Slick, Sherman, & Iverson, 1999). Within this chapter we refer to the broader negative response bias that includes *exaggeration* and *overreporting.* Although we focus on intentional forms of symptom overreporting and reduced cognitive effort, it is important to acknowledge that alternative reasons to account for reduced cognitive effort could include such factors as the respondent being sick (e.g., the flu), enduring poor sleep, or suffering from acute medication effects.

The objectives of this chapter include (1) to describe important influences and contexts in which individuals may demonstrate biased reporting about psychological or cognitive symptoms on measures commonly used to assess PTSD and mTBI; (2) to review evidence-based psychological and neuropsychological assessment methods for detecting invalid presentations of PTSD and mTBI; and (3) to identify special assessment-related considerations in evaluating people presenting with comorbid PTSD and mTBI.

Motives for Symptom Exaggeration and Reduced Effort in PTSD and mTBI

There are several reasons that individuals might intentionally overreport symptoms or display reduced effort in an evaluation of PTSD and/or mTBI. These reasons primarily involve financial incentives, access to clinical services, avoiding criminal penalties, and receiving recognition or honor for surviving a traumatic event (Bianchini, Mathias, & Greve, 2001; Greiffenstein & Baker, 2008).

Financial Incentives

An individual may be able to obtain monetary disability benefits based on inability to work due to impairment that is secondary to PTSD and mTBI. In the United States, social security disability insurance (SSDI) can remunerate individuals who establish such a disability (Chafetz, Abrahams, & Kohlmaier, 2007). The U.S. Department of Veterans Affairs (VA) also provides disability benefits when impairment is tied to injury incurred during military service. Maximum disability benefits can provide a level of annual compensation that is commensurate with many part- or full-time jobs (Frueh et al., 2003), leading to concerns that these programs might provide a disincentive for individuals to return to work and recover from their condition (Frueh, Grubaugh, Elhai, & Buckley, 2007). In fact, PTSD is one of the most frequent conditions for which veterans apply for disability compensation (Department of Veterans Affairs, Office of Inspector General, 2005).

Worker's compensation benefits have similar financial incentives. These incentives might unintentionally encourage overreporting or exaggeration of symptoms when an employee files a worker's compensation claim against the employer for lost wages and damages incurred from PTSD or mTBI resulting from a job-related accident or trauma.

Finally, personal injury lawsuits are another context that provides potential incentives for reporting symptoms and impairment. For example, a person may file a civil lawsuit against another individual or business for damages incurred from PTSD or mTBI, resulting from an accident or from an assaultive incident such as interpersonal violence.

Obtaining Treatment

Individuals may also overreport PTSD or mTBI in order to secure mental health or medical treatment (e.g., Salloway, Southwick, & Sadowsky, 1990). Such treatment seeking can represent the so-called cry for help on the part of the patient who may be in genuine need of emotional support, but exaggerates his or her symptoms in order to assure access to treatment (e.g., hospital admission). However, a cry for help cannot be assumed as the motive, especially when the context involves secondary gain incentives such as future disability payments. In such a circumstance, a claimant's primary intention may be to establish a treatment record to provide support for a current or anticipated claim for disability or worker's compensation or for a personal injury lawsuit (Taylor, Frueh, & Asmundson, 2007).

Avoiding Criminal Penalties

PTSD has been cited as a mitigating factor in criminal sentencing. The typical approach is to introduce PTSD-related dysfunction as justification for reduction of criminal charges and mitigation of criminal penalty after conviction for a crime (Resnick, West, & Payne, 2008). Some military veterans in particular, when charged with a serious crime, have attempted to link their criminal behavior with PTSD as a defense (Burkett & Whitley, 1998). Resnick et al. (2008) described several ways in which combat PTSD can be successfully used to demonstrate that the defendant did not know that his or her criminal act was wrong (i.e., the insanity defense). Nonetheless, it is rare that PTSD has been the basis for an insanity defense (Applebaum et al., 1993).

Stolen Valor

Evidence indicates that some individuals fabricate a history of traumatic event exposure and/or PTSD in order to gain honor or recognition. Burkett and Whitley (1998) addressed this possibility by using Freedom of Information Act (FOIA) requests to obtain the official military records of individuals claiming to have served in Vietnam combat, but whose claims of war-zone service reported in the news media sounded exaggerated or suspicious. They discovered numerous examples of individuals who falsely claimed serving in Vietnam War combat, including public figures and celebrities, such as the actor Brian Dennehy.

The selective examination of records by Burkett and Whitley (1998) does not address the prevalence of such false claims of combat. A limited but systematic effort to examine the prevalence of false combat exposure claims was conducted by Frueh et al. (2005). This study was based on FOIA requests for the official military records of 100 veterans registered with the Charleston VA Medical Center, who were referred consecutively to the PTSD clinic for services based on combat-related PTSD. Experienced military records reviewers found that only 68% of those claiming combat exposure had documented evidence based on the locations in which they served in Vietnam and the awarding of decorations and medals related to combat. The difficulty associated with documenting war-zone experiences that meet the traumatic stressor criterion for PTSD has been highlighted by an expert panel (Institute of Medicine of the National Academies, 2006) and is now recognized in VA policy that eliminates the requirement of documenting the traumatic stressor (Department of Veterans Affairs, 2010). However, there appeared to be a relatively small subset of untruthful individuals, some of whom served in the military, but did not serve in Vietnam (3%), and some of whom never served in the military at all, despite being registered for VA services (2%). At minimum, this evidence suggests that it is warranted to make an effort to obtain available documentation.

Best Methods in Detecting Symptom Exaggeration of PTSD

Records-Based Confirmation

It is understandable that a clinician working in a nonforensic setting such as a medical center or private practice might generally accept a patient's report of previous trauma exposure. In this context, the incentives for false reporting are not prominent. In addition, betrayal of trust often is a clinical theme for individuals who have been exposed to interpersonal trauma; therefore therapists may be reluctant to pose questions that might imply distrust and undermine the therapeutic alliance with a patient who already has difficulty trusting authority figures such as mental health professionals (Herman, 1992). However, the context is different for a forensic evaluation that has potential to influence criminal penalties or financial compensation for injury or disability. The need for an empirical approach and concrete evidence is foremost in working with the person to document his or her traumatic event and symptom presentation. As such, it is extremely important to obtain records that confirm exposure to an index event that could cause PTSD and/or TBI, and that potentially corroborate behaviors that are relevant to the diagnosis. Relevant sources often include medical records, military records, police reports, and employment records. This approach is well suited to the rules of evidence in legal proceedings and increases the ability to withstand direct challenge during cross-examination by opposing counsel.

In addition, records can provide information about other potentially traumatic experiences and reactions that might be relevant to the current symptom presentation. This is broadly important because DSM-IV diagnostic rules require that the minimum qualifying set of symptom criteria are satisfied in relation to one specific trauma; meeting some PTSD symptom criteria based on one trauma and other symptom criteria based on a different trauma is not permissible (discussed in Elhai et al., 2009; Elhai, Ford, & Naifeh, 2010). This direct link between trauma exposure and adjustment is particularly relevant to forensic situations in which a specific event has been alleged as the cause of PTSD symptoms and disability. Records may help establish a timeline that is either consistent with or contrary to the claim that PTSD symptom presentation resulted from the traumatic event in question rather than from other events.

Overall Assessment Strategies

Elsewhere we describe in detail best practices for assessing trauma exposure history and PTSD (Elhai et al., 2010). In brief, assessment begins with an empathic explanation about the process and its aims. This is followed by administration of a psychometrically sound measure of lifespan trauma exposure that is supplemented with behaviorally specific follow-up questions, and, as necessary, interactive selection of an "index" traumatic event as the reference for PTSD symptom ratings. Subsequent information gathering about PTSD symptoms in relation to the index traumatic event uses a psychometrically sound instrument—preferably a structured diagnostic interview—that allows rating of symptoms on a continuum or multilevel scale rather than dichotomously (i.e., present vs. absent).

In a forensic context, the clinician should ask a respondent to elaborate on the index traumatic event sequentially and in detail. One aim is to provide opportunity to evaluate credibility. For example, some individuals who were found to have fabricated trauma exposure reported absurd event-related details only found in movies (Burkett & Whitley, 1998). Others may give the appearance that the report is being constructed rather than recollected, or their presentation may seem overly rehearsed. Suspicion about the validity of reporting may be raised by such behavior, but caution is still warranted and more supporting evidence is still needed before concluding that reporting is fabricated or selectively untrue.

In general, retrospective self-report about past psychological distress appears to be reasonably accurate in nonforensic samples (Brennan, Stewart, Jamhour, Businelle, & Gouvier, 2005), but can be problematic in litigants, including mTBI litigants (Iverson, Lange, Brooks, & Rennison, 2010). It is important to note that if an individual is questioned about trauma exposure on more than one occasion, there may be variation in the details being reported. Presumably this can reflect corrupting influences that involve secondary gain. However, it is quite plausible that individuals with PTSD can recall a traumatic experience in greater detail with later interviews (e.g., Southwick, Morgan, Nicolaou, & Charney, 1997; Wessely et al., 2003) due to factors such as repeated cuing or increases in symptoms that aid retrieval of trauma-related memories.

In querying the person about PTSD symptoms, preferably with a structured diagnostic interview for PTSD, the clinical interviewer should not only inquire about symptom frequency and intensity but should also probe that the circumstances in which symptoms occur and details of recent episodes. This information can help tease apart credible from noncredible reports of symptoms. Collateral informant interviews are a particularly valuable means for information gathering, especially when an informant has no incentive tied to the outcome of the situation (e.g., a spouse who might share the benefit of a financial award). Collateral information from those who might have secondary gain incentives is of interest (e.g., regarding sleep disturbance, social isolation), but the same cautions apply as when interviewing the target individual directly.

Psychological Testing

An extensive literature exists on detecting exaggerated PTSD symptom reports using psychological testing. Most studies have used multiscale, psychometric personality assessment instruments such as the Minnesota Multiphasic Personality Inventory–2 (MMPI-2; Butcher et al., 2001), the Personality Assessment Inventory (PAI; Morey, 1991), and the Trauma Symptom Inventory (TSI; Briere, 1995). Structured diagnostic interviews of malingering include the Structured Interview of Reported Symptoms (SIRS; Rogers, Bagby, & Dickens, 1992). These instruments have validity scales, including "fake bad" or overreporting scales, that assess response patterns including atypical responding about both symptom content and severity, obvious (vs. subtle) symptom responding, and inconsistency in symptom presentation (reviewed in Greene, 2008; Rogers, 2008c; Sellbom & Bagby, 2008). A special feature of the SIRS is that it calls for the evaluator to document behavioral indicators of symptom exaggeration. Other types of instruments that have been found ineffective in detecting exaggerated PTSD include projective personality tests and self-report checklists (Guriel & Fremouw, 2003).

Studies using a simulation research design typically instruct one group of participants to feign PTSD and then compare their scores with those from a group designated as honest reporters. Simulation designs offer the advantage of being tightly controlled, but they sacrifice real-world generalizability. Accordingly, Rogers (2008b) has stated that "the logical sequence is the development of an assessment method with simulation studies followed by known-groups comparisons" (p. 427). We focus on simulation studies that include genuine PTSD patients as the honest reporter comparison group because they offer the most realistic and forensically informative basis for comparison.

Most research on overreported PTSD has used the MMPI-2. Interestingly, meta-analytic findings demonstrate that effect sizes for detecting overreported PTSD are generally lower than for detecting other forms of overreported psychopathology (Rogers, Sewell, Martin, & Vitacco, 2003); high scores among genuine PTSD patients may account for the decreased effect sizes when compared to PTSD simulators (Elhai et al., 2010). Initial studies focused on the F (Infrequency) and F-K (Infrequency minus K Correction) scales of the MMPI-2. The scales were able to individually distinguish between PTSD simulators and patients with roughly 70–80% accuracy across men and women based on optimal cutoff scores (e.g., Elhai, Gold, Frueh, & Gold, 2000; Elhai, Gold, Sellers, & Dorfman, 2001). However, the F scale is arguably problematic because it is composed of infrequently endorsed items among healthy individuals, and these items are often endorsed by genuine mentally ill patients (Arbisi & Ben-Porath, 1995). Moreover, the F scale is highly correlated with forms of distress and psychopathology that are relatively common in trauma victims, including depression, dissociation, and PTSD (Klotz Flitter, Elhai, & Gold, 2003). Thus, extreme F-scale elevations may not indicate overreporting in trauma-exposed individuals.

Other variations of the MMPI-2's F scale have been recently developed, aiming to better discriminate genuine from exaggerated psychopathology. Among the most frequently studied in the psychological literature is the Fp (Infrequency Psychopathology) scale, composed of items that were infrequently endorsed among both psychiatric patients and nondisordered individuals. The Fp scale has evidenced good discrimination of PTSD simulators from patients, arguably better than scales from other psychological tests described here, as well as incremental validity over other MMPI-2 fake bad scales. Specifically, based on simulation studies, Fp has demonstrated detection accuracy in the 80–90% range based on a cutoff score for T between 85 and 100 (Arbisi, Ben-Porath, & McNulty, 2006; Efendov, Sellbom, & Bagby, 2008; Marshall & Bagby, 2006). The recently developed Fptsd (Infrequency PTSD) scale is composed of items infrequently endorsed by combat patients with PTSD. Fptsd seems to be more effective in detecting exaggerated PTSD when referenced to military PTSD comparison groups (Arbisi et al., 2006; Elhai et al., 2002) as opposed to civilian PTSD comparison groups (Elhai et al., 2004; Marshall & Bagby, 2006).

More recently, a large MMPI-2 literature has developed suggesting that the Response Bias Scale (RBS) or Symptom Validity Scale (FBS) may be more sensitive to detecting the impact of secondary gains than the traditional F-family validity scales. For example, meta-analytic techniques have demonstrated that FBS was more effective than traditional F-family validity scales when applied to forensic neuropsychology cases (Nelson, Hoelzle, Sweet, Arbisi, & Demakis, 2010; Nelson, Sweet, & Demakis, 2006).

The PAI also has been investigated in a few studies for overreported PTSD detection; however, the PAI validity scales have not proven as useful as the MMPI-2's validity scales. Specifically, the NIM (Negative Impression Management) scale and the MAL (Malingering Index) have been investigated, achieving no greater than 75% detection rates on average (e.g., Eakin, Weathers, Benson, Anderson, & Funderbunk, 2006; Lange, Sullivan, & Scott, 2010).

The TSI has also been investigated for its ability to detect overreported PTSD. The TSI is unique among other measures discussed here because it is specifically developed for assessing trauma-related psychopathology and it is one of the most widely used assessment scales in the traumatic stress field (Elhai, Gray, Kashdan, & Franklin, 2005). Although an early study found accuracy rates in the 80–90% range for an optimal T score threshold of 61 on the ATR (Atypical Response) scale (Edens, Otto, & Dwyer, 1998), that promising finding may have been due to the absence of a patient comparison group. Subsequent research with PTSD patient comparison groups has found less promising results for ATR and a lack of incremental contribution over relevant MMPI-2 scales (e.g., Efendov et al., 2008; Elhai, Gray, Naifeh, et al., 2005; Rogers, Payne, Correa, Gillard, & Ross, 2009). A revised version of the TSI, the TSI-2, will be published soon. One study that has used the TSI-2 to compare nonclinical PTSD simulators with nonclinical honest responders screening positive for PTSD found an overall correct classification rate of 75%, using a raw score of 7 (Gray, Elhai, & Briere, 2010).

The SIRS has been studied via simulation, but without PTSD comparison groups. Freeman, Powell, and Kimbrell (2008) assessed SIRS scores in a sample of veterans presenting for PTSD treatment and found substantial evidence of symptom exaggeration based on traditional cutoff scores from the SIRS. Rogers, Kropp, Bagby, and Dickens (1992) assessed how well SIRS scores could distinguish between simulators feigning PTSD, schizophrenia, and mood disorders, and general psychiatric inpatients. They found that SIRS scales distinguished between the disorders and several scales significantly distinguished between patients and PTSD simulators.

Future research may clarify the utility of the SIRS in distinguishing between overreported and genuine PTSD. A recent review of the newer edition by Rubenzer (2010) concluded that the SIRS-2 is the instrument of choice for assessing feigned psychosis and severe psychopathology, but that there is limited support for detection of malingering in conditions such as PTSD. Rubenzer also noted that there is little research to support use of SIRS-2 in detection of malingering of cognitive dysfunction.

Best Methods in Detecting Reduced Effort in mTBI

Overall Assessment Strategies

Since the early 1990s, clinical researchers have published an impressive number of peer-reviewed articles related to the increased risk of symptom exaggeration and malingering during forensic neuropsychological examinations. In fact, textbooks devoted to this topic have appeared (e.g., Larrabee, 2007; Morgan & Sweet, 2009), along with professional society position statements (Bush et al., 2005; Heilbronner et al., 2009) suggesting that neuropsychologists should evaluate motivation and effort using the multiple types of instruments described in this chapter when assessment occurs in a context involving potential secondary gain.

There is a large neuropsychology literature about methods for detecting reduced effort on ability measures or self-reported symptoms. In fact, from 1990 through 2000, 139 articles were published on forensic topics in the most popular journals read by clinical neuropsychologists, with 86% of these addressing the detection of malingering (Sweet, King, Malina, Bergman, & Simmons, 2002). This parallels a broad increase in the number of forensic cases in U.S. state and federal courts that have involved neuropsychological issues and the participation of clinical neuropsychologists as witnesses (Sweet & Guiffre Meyer, 2010). In large measure, this role for forensic neuropsychology has been stimulated by civil litigation alleging persistent effects of mTBI. This claim runs contrary to the majority of scientific studies that have found mTBI to be a time-limited neurological disturbance (see meta-analytic studies; e.g., Belanger, Curtiss, Demery, Lebowitz, & Vanderploeg, 2005; Carroll et al., 2004; Frencham, Fox, & Mayberry, 2005).

Factors implicated in the persistent report of symptoms following documented mTBI are baseline mental health characteristics (de Leon et al., 2009), headache and pain (Iverson & McCracken, 1997; Stovner, Schrader, Mickeviciene, Surkiene, & Sand, 2009), unrealistically positive appraisal of preinjury status (Gunstad & Suhr, 2001; Iverson et al., 2010), limitations on the accuracy of self-report (Barsky, 2002) that are amplified by the presence of depression (Zandi, 2004), and the nonspecific nature of most postconcussion symptoms (Hoge et al., 2004). In addition, being in litigation is itself one of the factors associated with persistent complaints after mTBI (Carroll et al., 2004). Likewise, meta-analytic studies have shown that being in litigation is associated with lack of recovery or worsening of symptoms across time (Belanger et al., 2005). Therefore, it is essential that a differential diagnosis in the context of a formal evaluation be carried out because the initial occurrence of mTBI is much less likely to create persistent symptom complaints and behavioral dysfunction than are nonbrain injury (e.g., psychosocial) factors (McCrea, 2008).

Neuropsychological Testing

Two categories of measures are typically used to assess symptom validity during a neuropsychological evaluation. One category is referred to as *stand-alone cognitive effort tests*, which were most often developed specifically to evaluate task performance validity. The format is either forced-choice like the Victoria Symptom Validity Test and the Test of Memory Malingering (e.g., Victoria Symptom Validity Test—Slick, Hopp, Strauss, & Thompson, 1997; Test of Memory Malingering—Tombaugh, 1997) or nonforced choice like the Dot Counting Test (e.g., The Dot Counting Test—Boone, Lu, & Herzberg, 2002; Vickery, Berry, Inman, Harris, & Orey, 2001). Forced-choice validity tests were first adopted by practitioners in the 1980s and have become widely used with both clinical and forensic referrals (Bianchini et al., 2001). The development of forced-choice tests is based on the binomial theorem, which recognizes that when there are only two available responses, chance alone will lead to a 50% response rate for each. Thus, the degree to which an examinee achieves less than 50% performance is indicative of intentional (nonchance) avoidance of correct answers (Frederick & Speed, 2007).

Most forced-choice validity tests use empirically derived cutoff scores based on the binomial theorem to define the levels of performance that are significantly below chance. Differently, many investigators have found that results of forced-choice tests can identify insufficient effort associated with invalid responding at levels that are well above chance. For example, research on some forced-choice tests has determined that a 90% rule, originally identified for digit-recognition procedures (Guilmette, Hart, & Giuliano, 1993), can effectively identify individuals whose effort is insufficient and therefore invalidates their cognitive performance results. This particular threshold as a line of demarcation between adequate and insufficient effort will not work on all forced-choice measures. Moreover, the effectiveness of specific cutoffs can vary based on context (i.e., secondary gain present or absent), type of disorder (e.g., feigned brain injury vs. feigned psychiatric disorder), and severity (e.g., mild vs. severe brain injury). Consideration of below-chance performances and additional indicators of invalid and noncredible test performance, as described below, can be used as an important part of the basis for establishing whether someone is exhibiting *definite, probable, or possible malingering* based on the Slick et al. (1999) criteria. For example, the criteria of Slick and colleagues states that *definite malingering* is characterized by an external incentive to malinger and definite negative response bias exhibited by below-chance performance on one or more forced-choice effort tests.

The non-forced-choice category consists of embedded indicators within neuropsychological tests of performance. The majority of embedded indicators were developed as a secondary step after the test was validated and released. Examples include the Wisconsin Card Sorting Test (King, Sweet, Sherer, Curtiss, & Vanderploeg, 2002) and the Category Test (Sweet & King, 2002). There are many embedded indicators of symptom validity, as summarized by Sweet (2009) and reviewed elsewhere (Larrabee, 2007). Embedded measures have the advantage of making it possible to evaluate effort repeatedly throughout the course of an evaluation (Boone, 2009) and to do so without administration of separate, time-consuming measures.

The American Academy of Clinical Neuropsychology (AACN) Consensus Conference Statement on Effort, Response Bias, and Malingering (Heilbronner et al., 2009) has recommended that neuropsychological evaluations conducted in contexts involving the potential for secondary gain include both stand-alone and embedded validity indicators whenever feasible, while embedded measures should be examined alone only when evaluation time is constrained. The AACN Consensus Conference also identified key topics that are in need of further investigation including cost–benefit analysis of response bias assessment and the need for examination of clinical populations at risk of failing effort and embedded validity indicators.

There is a long-standing and substantial body of published research studies that provide guidance to clinicians regarding assessment of mTBI, including literature reviews addressing response bias and malingering (e.g., Binder & Rohling, 1996; Nies & Sweet, 1994). Numerous individual studies, many of which have used forced-choice measures, have continued to appear in the literature (cf. Armistead-Jehle, 2010; Carone, 2008). A common finding among mTBI litigants is worse performance on effort measures than more severely injured nonlitigants. For example, Green, Rohling, Lees-Haley, and Allen (2001) found that effort has a greater effect on test scores than severe brain injury in compensation-seeking claimants.

Aside from the typical symptom validity tests, embedded validity indicators within neuropsychological assessment measures can be used to increase confidence when formulating conclusions. These include measures within tests of intelligence (Reliable Digit Span; Greiffenstein, Baker, & Gola, 1994), motor abilities (Grip Strength; Haaland, Temkin, Randahl, & Dikmen, 1994), standard memory measures (California Verbal Learning Test; Sweet et al., 2000), and numerous other domain-specific tests. It is also important to look for consistency across the clinical interview, assessment measures, and self-report because consistency is more difficult to feign, while discrepancies can often highlight malingering or poor effort.

Psychological Testing

Individuals who are being examined neuropsychologically in a secondary gain context can demonstrate response bias that is exclusively cognitive in nature, exclusively psychological in nature, or involves both types of bias. That is, reduced cognitive effort and psychiatric symptom overreporting may both be at play for a given individual. In a sample of forensic cases, a factor analysis by Nelson et al. (2007) demonstrated that an *insufficient cognitive effort* factor can be distinct from three other factors germane to *psychological* symptom reporting on the MMPI-2. Thus, it is essential that *both* cognitive and psychological response validity measures are utilized, as these are not redundant and will provide incremental value.

In the past, traditional validity scales on a personality test were considered sufficient to evaluate effort during an examination that included ability testing. In addition, elevated scores on personality tests were considered a typical outcome with TBI. However, a classic study by Youngjohn, Davis, and Wolf (1997) has challenged both of these beliefs. Figure 9.1 shows the three traditional MMPI-2 validity scales (L, F, and K) and the 10 clinical scales for nonlitigating and litigating groups with severe TBI and a group with mTBI. It is striking how the mTBI group has a very abnormal profile that contrasts with a profile entirely within the normal range for the nonlitigating severe TBI group. It also is of interest that the widely different clinical scale profiles of the groups were not reflected by the traditional validity scales.

Subsequent to the Youngjohn et al. (1997) article, a large MMPI-2 literature has developed relevant to neuropsychological cases. In part, this neuropsychological literature has provided evidence that newer validity

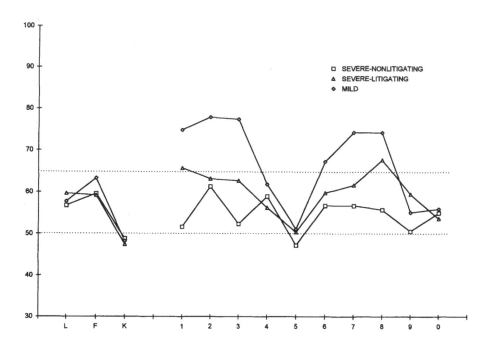

FIGURE 9.1. Paradoxical effects of mild versus more severe injury with and without litigation on the MMPI-2 basic scales and validity scales. From Youngjohn, Davis, and Wolf (1997). Copyright 1997 by the American Psychological Association. Reprinted by permission.

scales, such as the Response Bias Scale (RBS), which was specifically devised to be relevant to neuropsychological examinations, may be more useful in evaluating individuals with cognitive complaints. For example, among disability claimants, RBS has a greater relationship than traditional F-family validity scales with unverified memory complaints when cognitive effort is controlled (Gervais, Ben-Porath, Wygant, & Green, 2008). RBS also has a greater relationship to actual effort test failure than do the traditional F-family validity scales (Gervais, Ben-Porath, Wygant, & Sellbom, 2010), which was the original intent of RBS development. Previously, Nelson et al. (2006) had demonstrated via meta-analysis that FBS, also developed to have particular relevance to personal injury claimants, was more effective with forensic neuropsychological cases than traditional F-family validity scales. A graphic based on the updated meta-analysis of FBS and other MMPI-2 validity scales is shown as Figure 9.2, within which the composite effect sizes of the validity scales are shown, reflecting the effect of passing or failing cognitive effort tests.

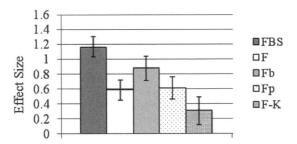

FIGURE 9.2. Symptom Validity Scale (FBS) and F-family composite effect sizes in published studies of neuropsychological examinees who passed or failed cognitive effort tests. k = the number of contributing effect sizes. For known insufficient effort, k was 33 for FBS, 31 for F, 28 for Fb, 30 for Fp, and 23 for F – K. Error bars reflect 95% confidence intervals.

Challenges of mTBI Assessment in the Context of Secondary Gain

The starting point for conducting a neuropsychological assessment of mTBI is knowledge of the diagnostic criteria and the natural course of recovery (cf. McCrea, 2008). The distinction between mTBI and postconcussion syndrome (PCS) also is important. As reviewed by Ulloa, Marx, Vanderploeg, and Vasterling (Chapter 8, this volume), diagnosis of mTBI is dependent upon initial injury criteria such as altered consciousness. An mTBI can take place without the subsequent lingering symptoms that constitute PCS. There are numerous definitions of PCS, but the DSM-IV requires a head trauma that caused a significant cerebral concussion with (1) three or more specific symptoms occurring shortly after the trauma and lasting for at least 3 months, (2) evidence from neuropsychological testing of difficulty in memory or attention, and (3) significant impairment in social or occupational functioning resulting from the cognitive symptoms (American Psychiatric Association, 2000).

As indicated earlier, aside from basic diagnostic issues, there are many challenges that arise when evaluating mTBI within the context of possible secondary gains. The issue of secondary gain is often raised when evaluating TBI, as head injury is a common reason for litigation and roughly 6% of plaintiff verdicts are associated with brain injury claims (Millis, 2008). The most common reason for neuropsychologists to become involved in litigation involving head injury is for assessment related to mTBI cases. Even outside of the forensic realm, this topic is of great concern for neuropsychologists, as a common reason to refer to a neuropsychologist in a clinical context is for assessment of cognitive and emotional sequelae of head injury. As with litigated cases, the majority of these clinical referrals concern mild injury (Sosin, Sniezek, & Thurman, 1996).

Assessment and diagnosis for moderate and severe TBIs are relatively straightforward on the basis of clinical signs and symptoms, neuroimaging abnormalities, and functional impairments, but there are no recognized markers for uncomplicated mTBI that persist over time. As described by Bigler and Maxwell (Chapter 2, this volume), some of the more common initial cognitive symptoms described among patients in the acute stage of mTBI include selective attention, short-term memory, processing speed, and executive functioning. Following the acute period after the head injury and within this 3-month window, no specific pattern of neurocognitive impairment detectable on currently available clinical neuropsychological tests exists that could be applied for neuropsychologists to help differentiate genuine from malingered deficits. It is also known that when evaluations occur within the context of secondary gain, there is a risk that examinee behavior will change (Hoge, Goldberg, & Castro, 2009), which can result in diagnostic error (McCrea et al., 2008). Therefore, assessment of mTBI in a secondary gain context, such as litigation, is unlikely to be sufficient without the inclusion of measures to detect malingering.

Research has shown that, in situations where secondary gain is a factor, effort has a greater impact on repeated test performance than does mTBI. Stevens, Friedel, Mehren, and Merten (2008) examined 233 adult patients, with the majority of referrals being for workers' compensation or personal injury claims, and found insufficient effort by 45% of the patients. This accounted for 35% of the variance in cognitive performance. After controlling for effort, Stevens and colleagues found there were no significant effects of brain injury on cognitive performance. Also related, Flaro, Green, and Robertson (2007) found that litigants with mTBI demonstrated a failure rate on symptom validity tests that was 23 times higher than litigants who were parents seeking custody of their children, suggesting the power of external incentives. These studies again reinforce the value of performing effort testing during mTBI evaluations.

With the increase in Operation Enduring Freedom (OEF)/Operation Iraqi Freedom (OIF) veterans returning with mTBI and reports of 15–20% prevalence among deployed service members, the question of mTBI and effort within the military population has recently become an area of interest. Several studies have found a relatively high prevalence of patients with mTBI scoring below symptom validity test cutoff scores. One study found that 58% of U.S. veterans who screened positive for mTBI in an outpatient VA neuropsychology clinic scored below the cutoff score on a symptom validity test suggestive of poor effort (Armistead-Jehle, 2010). A recent study of 119 OEF/OIF combat veterans found that the forensic concussion group exhibited significantly higher rates of insufficient effort relative to the OEF/OIF research concussion group, but a comparable rate of insufficient effort relative to the non-OEF/OIF forensic concussion group (Nelson, Hoelzle, McGuire, et al., 2010). These studies highlight the potential value of symptom validity tests when assessing brain injury within the military population.

Even when informed by tests of effort, the picture of what constitutes cognitive impairment due to mTBI versus malingering is not clear-cut. A recent study surveyed the validity concerns expressed by 40 providers of treatment to OEF/OIF veterans with mTBI/PTSD. Two of their main concerns were (1) uncertainty about the appropriate cutoff scores to apply when evaluating potential malingering by individuals with blast-related TBI via psychological testing and (2) how to evaluate and manage secondary gain issues (Sayer et al., 2009). It appears that both clinical and research efforts are moving toward gaining more knowledge about effort testing and mTBI in the military setting when secondary gain is an issue and in making movements toward educating clinicians on how to detect the difference between cognitive or psychological impairment in mTBI within the context of secondary gain.

Special Considerations for Assessing Comorbid PTSD and mTBI

Another layer of difficulty arises in the potential comorbidity of PTSD and mTBI given the numerous overlapping symptoms between the conditions. Most of the overlap involves nonspecific symptoms such as generalized depression and anxiety, insomnia, irritability and anger, concentration difficulty, and hyperarousal (Stein & McAllister, 2009). Much of the research to date regarding the comorbidity of PTSD and mTBI is limited by assessment focused on one condition or the other, and the use of self-report questionnaires without formal neuropsychological testing, collateral report, or measures of symptom validity.

Recent findings provide evidence for comorbidity between PTSD and mTBI in U.S. Veterans (Carlson et al., 2011; Kennedy et al., 2007; Schneiderman, Braver, & Kang, 2008; Stein & McAllister, 2009). Some studies have found that as many as 44% of service members with self-reported concussion may meet diagnostic criteria for PTSD when evaluated within 3–4 months after returning from deployment (Hoge et al., 2008). One study found that relative to mTBI symptoms assessed just prior to returning home from Iraq combat, PTSD assessed prior to returning home was a more potent predictor of mTBI symptoms assessed 1 year after returning home (Polusny et al., 2011). The conditions are so prevalent that the Department of Defense has prioritized research efforts devoted to PTSD and mTBI. In a review of 31 studies that included participants with a history of both PTSD and mTBI, Carlson et al. (2011) concluded that prevalence of TBI/PTSD varies widely and that prevalence estimates likely depend on patient characteristics, trauma etiology, disease definition, and ascertainment method. It is noteworthy that none of the studies cited by Carlson and colleagues appear to have examined the impact of secondary gain or administered measures of symptom validity. In fact, we have found only one empirical article to date that discusses the comorbidity issues of PTSD and mTBI within the context of secondary gain (Greiffenstein & Baker, 2008). Those authors found an "overendorsement continuum" in which "the more complex the post-traumatic presentation after mild neurological injury, the stronger the association with response bias" (p. 565).

It is clear that more outcome studies need to be carried out in examining how to appropriately assess for comorbid PTSD and mTBI, especially in the context of secondary gain. Long-term prospective observational studies are needed that use standardized, well-validated measures of symptoms to determine prevalence, severity, and long-term outcomes of comorbid PTSD and mTBI in individuals with a documented history of trauma and initial signs (not retrospective recall of possible symptoms) of mTBI. As stated previously, it will be important to use a combination of research designs, including studying the natural course of these comorbid conditions when well documented and outside of a secondary gain context, as well as use of simulations designs and known-groups comparisons (Rogers, 2008b) to evaluate response bias.

Conclusion

It is apparent that assessing the accuracy of both emotional symptom responding and cognitive effort in PTSD and mTBI is challenging in contexts in which there is potential for secondary gain. As we have documented, it is often difficult to distinguish between a genuine PTSD or mTBI symptom presentation from a malingered one in such contexts. We have provided background to elaborate on contextual factors that are relevant to assessing response validity among individuals evaluated for PTSD and/or mTBI. We have also offered suggested guidelines and strategies for assessing response validity in such cases. We hope that the reader is now better informed about the contributing factors, empirical findings, and methods for assessing response validity in these contexts.

References

American Psychiatric Association. (2000). *Diagnostic and statistical manual of mental disorders* (4th ed., text rev.). Washington, DC: Author.

Applebaum, P. S., Jick, R. Z., Grisso, T., Givelber, D., Silver, E., & Steadman, H. J. (1993). Use of posttraumatic stress disorder to support an insanity defense. *American Journal of Psychiatry, 150,* 229–234.

Arbisi, P. A., & Ben-Porath, Y. S. (1995). An MMPI-2 infrequent response scale for use with psychopathological populations: The Infrequency Psychopathology Scale, F(p). *Psychological Assessment, 7,* 424–431.

Arbisi, P. A., Ben-Porath, Y. S., & McNulty, J. (2006). The ability of the MMPI-2 to detect feigned PTSD within the context of compensation seeking. *Psychological Services, 3,* 249–261.

Armistead-Jehle, P. (2010). Symptom validity test performance in U.S. veterans referred for evaluation in mild TBI. *Applied Neuropsychology, 17,* 52–59.

Barsky, A. J. (2002). Forgetting, fabricating, and telescoping: The instability of the medical history. *Archives of Internal Medicine, 162,* 981–984.

Belanger, H. G., Curtiss, G., Demery, J., Lebowitz, B., & Vanderploeg, R. D. (2005). Factors moderating neuropsychological outcomes following mild traumatic brain injury: A meta-analysis. *Journal of the International Neuropsychological Society, 11,* 215–227.

Bianchini, K. J., Mathias, C. W., & Greve, K. W. (2001). Symptom validity testing: A critical review. *Clinical Neuropsychologist, 15,* 19–45.

Binder, L. M., & Rohling, M. L. (1996). Money matters: A meta-analytic review of the effects of financial incentive on recovery after closed-head injury. *American Journal of Psychiatry, 153,* 7–10.

Boone, K. B. (2009). The need for continuous and comprehensive sampling of effort/response bias during neuropsychological examination. *Clinical Neuropsychologist, 23,* 729–741.

Boone, K. B., Lu, P., & Herzberg, D. S. (2002). *The Dot Counting Test manual.* Los Angeles: Western Psychological Services.

Brennan, A. M., Stewart, H. A., Jamhour, N., Businelle, M. S., & Gouvier, W. D. (2005). An examination of the retrospective recall of psychological distress. *Journal of Forensic Neuropsychology, 4,* 99–110.

Briere, J. (1995). *Trauma Symptom Inventory professional manual.* Odessa, FL: Psychological Assessment Resources.

Burkett, B. G., & Whitley, G. (1998). *Stolen valor: How the Vietnam generation was robbed of its heroes and history.* Dallas, TX: Verity Press.

Bush, S. S., Ruff, R. M., Troster, A. I., Barth, J. T., Koffler, S. P., Pliskin, N. P., et al. (2005). Symptom validity assessment: Practice issues and medical necessity NAN policy and planning committee. *Archives of Clinical Neuropsychology, 20,* 419–426.

Butcher, J. N., Graham, J. R., Ben-Porath, Y. S., Tellegen, A., Dahlstrom, W. G., & Kaemmer, B. (2001). *MMPI-2 (Minnesota Multiphasic Personality Inventory–2): Manual for administration, scoring, and interpretation* (rev. ed.). Minneapolis: University of Minnesota Press.

Carlson, K. F., Kehle, S. M., Meis, L. A., Greer, N., Macdonald, R., Rutks, I., et al. (2011). Prevalence, assessment, and treatment of mild traumatic brain injury and posttraumatic stress disorder: A systematic review of the evidence. *Journal of Head Trauma and Rehabilitation, 26*, 103–115.

Carone, D. (2008). Children with moderate/severe brain damage/dysfunction outperform adults with mild-to-no brain damage on the Medical Symptom Validity Test. *Brain Injury, 22*, 960–971.

Carroll, L., Cassidy, J. D., Peloso, P., Borg, J., von Holst, J., Holm, L., et al. (2004). Prognosis for mild traumatic brain injury: Results of the WHO Collaborating Centre Task Force on Mild Traumatic Brain Injury. *Journal of Rehabilitation Medicine*, (Suppl. 43), 84–105.

Chafetz, M. D., Abrahams, J. P., & Kohlmaier, J. (2007). Malingering on the Social Security Disability Consultative Exam: A new rating scale. *Archives of Clinical Neuropsychology, 22*, 1–14.

de Leon, M. B., Kirsch, N., Maio, R., Tan-Schriner, C., Millis, S., Frederiksen, S., et al. (2009). Baseline predictors of fatigue 1 year after mild head injury. *Archives of Physical Medicine and Rehabilitation, 90*, 956–965.

Department of Veterans Affairs. (2010). New regulations on PTSD claims Retrieved November 30, 2010, from *www.va.gov/PTSD_QA.pdf*.

Department of Veterans Affairs, Office of Inspector General. (2005). Review of state variances in VA disability compensation payments (# 05-00765-137). Washington, DC: Department of Veterans Affairs Office of Inspector General. Available from *www4.va.gov/oig/52/reports/2005/VAOIG-05-00765-137.pdf*.

Eakin, D. E., Weathers, F. W., Benson, T. B., Anderson, C. F., & Funderbunk, B. (2006). Detection of feigned posttraumatic stress disorder: A comparison of the MMPI-2 and PAI. *Journal of Psychopathology and Behavioral Assessment, 28*, 145–155.

Edens, J. F., Otto, R. K., & Dwyer, T. J. (1998). Susceptibility of the Trauma Symptom Inventory to malingering. *Journal of Personality Assessment, 71*, 379–392.

Efendov, A. A., Sellbom, M., & Bagby, R. M. (2008). The utility and comparative incremental validity of the MMPI-2 and Trauma Symptom Inventory validity scales in the detection of feigned PTSD. *Psychological Assessment, 20*, 317–326.

Elhai, J. D., Engdahl, R. M., Palmieri, P. A., Naifeh, J. A., Schweinle, A., & Jacobs, G. A. (2009). Assessing posttraumatic stress disorder with or without reference to a single, worst traumatic event: Examining differences in factor structure. *Psychological Assessment, 21*, 629–634.

Elhai, J. D., Ford, J. D., & Naifeh, J. A. (2010). Assessing trauma exposure and posttraumatic morbidity. In G. M. Rosen & B. C. Frueh (Eds.), *Clinician's guide to posttraumatic stress disorder* (pp. 119–151). Hoboken, NJ: Wiley.

Elhai, J. D., Gold, P. B., Frueh, B. C., & Gold, S. N. (2000). Cross-validation of the MMPI-2 in detecting malingered posttraumatic stress disorder. *Journal of Personality Assessment, 75*, 449–463.

Elhai, J. D., Gold, S. N., Sellers, A. H., & Dorfman, W. I. (2001). The detection of malingered posttraumatic stress disorder with MMPI-2 fake bad indices. *Assessment, 8,* 221–236.

Elhai, J. D., Gray, M. J., Kashdan, T. B., & Franklin, C. L. (2005). Which instruments are most commonly used to assess traumatic event exposure and posttraumatic effects?: A survey of traumatic stress professionals. *Journal of Traumatic Stress, 18,* 541–545.

Elhai, J. D., Gray, M. J., Naifeh, J. A., Butcher, J. J., Davis, J. L., Falsetti, S. A., et al. (2005). Utility of the Trauma Symptom Inventory's Atypical Response Scale in detecting malingered post-traumatic stress disorder. *Assessment, 12,* 210–219.

Elhai, J. D., Naifeh, J. A., Zucker, I. S., Gold, S. N., Deitsch, S. E., & Frueh, B. C. (2004). Discriminating malingered from genuine civilian posttraumatic stress disorder: A validation of three MMPI-2 infrequency scales (F, Fp, and Fptsd). *Assessment, 11,* 139–144.

Elhai, J. D., Ruggiero, K. J., Frueh, B. C., Beckham, J. C., Gold, P. B., & Feldman, M. E. (2002). The Infrequency-Posttraumatic Stress Disorder scale (Fptsd) for the MMPI-2: Development and initial validation with veterans presenting with combat-related PTSD. *Journal of Personality Assessment, 79,* 531–549.

Flaro, L., Green, P., & Robertson, E. (2007). Word Memory Test failure 23 times higher in mild brain injury than parents seeking custody: The power of external incentives. *Brain Injury, 21,* 373–383.

Frederick, R. I., & Speed, F. M. (2007). On the interpretation of below-chance responding in forced-choice tests. *Assessment, 14,* 3–11.

Freeman, T., Powell, M., & Kimbrell, T. (2008). Measuring symptom exaggeration in veterans with chronic posttraumatic stress disorder. *Psychiatry Research, 158,* 374–380.

Frencham, K., Fox, A., & Mayberry, M. (2005). Neuropsychological studies of mild traumatic brain injury: A meta-analytic review of research since 1995. *Journal of Clinical and Experimental Neuropsychology, 27,* 334–351.

Frueh, B. C., Elhai, J. D., Gold, P. B., Monnier, J., Magruder, K. M., Keane, T. M., et al. (2003). Disability compensation seeking among veterans evaluated for posttraumatic stress disorder. *Psychiatric Services, 54,* 84–91.

Frueh, B. C., Elhai, J. D., Grubaugh, A. L. , Monnier, J., Kashdan, T. B., Sauvageot, J. A., et al. (2005). Documented combat exposure of U.S. veterans seeking treatment for combat-related posttraumatic stress disorder. *British Journal of Psychiatry, 186,* 467–472.

Frueh, B. C., Grubaugh, A. L., Elhai, J. D., & Buckley, T. C. (2007). U.S. Department of Veterans Affairs disability policies for posttraumatic stress disorder: Administrative trends and implications for treatment, rehabilitation, and research. *American Journal of Public Health, 97,* 2143–2145.

Gervais, R. O., Ben-Porath, Y. S., Wygant, D. B., & Green, P. (2008). Differential sensitivity of the RBS and MMPI-2 validity scales to memory complaints. *Clinical Neuropsychologist, 22,* 1061–1079.

Gervais, R. O., Ben-Porath, Y. S., Wygant, D. B., & Sellbom, M. (2010). Incremental validity of the MMPI-2-RF over-reporting scales and RBS in assessing the veracity of memory complaints. *Archives of Clinical Neuropsychology, 25,* 274–284.

Gray, M. J., Elhai, J. D., & Briere, J. (2010). Evaluation of the Atypical Response Scale of the Trauma Symptom Inventory-2 in detecting simulated posttraumatic stress disorder. *Journal of Anxiety Disorders, 24,* 447–451.

Green, P., Rohling, M. L., Lees-Haley, P. R., & Allen, L. M. (2001). Effort has a greater effect on test scores than severe brain injury in compensation claimants. *Brain Injury, 15,* 1045–1060.

Greene, R. L. (2008). Malingering and defensiveness on the MMPI-2. In R. Rogers (Ed.), *Clinical assessment of malingering and deception* (3rd ed., pp. 159–181). New York, New York: Guilford Press.

Greiffenstein, M. F., & Baker, W. J. (2008). Validity testing in dually diagnosed post-traumatic stress disorder and mild closed head injury. *Clinical Neuropsychologist, 22,* 565–582.

Greiffenstein, M. F., Baker, R., & Gola, T. (1994). Validation of malingered amnesia measures with a large clinical sample. *Psychological Assessment, 6,* 218–224.

Guilmette, T., Hart, K., & Giuliano, A. (1993). Malingering detection: The use of a forced-choice method in identifying organic versus simulated memory impairment. *Clinical Neuropsychologist, 7,* 59–69.

Gunstad, J., & Suhr, J. A. (2001). "Expectation as etiology" versus "the good old days": Postconcussion syndrome symptom reporting in athletes, headache sufferers, and depressed individuals. *Journal of the International Neuropsychological Society, 7,* 323–333.

Guriel, J., & Fremouw, W. (2003). Assessing malingered posttraumatic stress disorder: A critical review. *Clinical Psychology Review, 23,* 881–904.

Haaland, K. Y., Temkin, N., Randahl, G., & Dikmen, S. (1994). Recovery of simple motor skills after head injury. *Journal of Clinical and Experimental Neuropsychology, 16,* 448–456.

Heilbronner, R. L., Sweet, J. J., Morgan, J. E., Larrabee, G. J., Millis, S. R., & Conference Participants. (2009). American Academy of Clinical Neuropsychology consensus conference statement on the neuropsychological assessment of effort, response bias, and malingering. *Clinical Neuropsychologist, 23,* 1093–1129.

Herman, J. L. (1992). *Trauma and recovery: The aftermath of violence from domestic abuse to political terror.* New York: Basic Books.

Hoge, C. W., Castro, C. A., Messer, S. C., McGurk, D., Cotting, D. I., & Koffman, R. L. (2004). Combat duty in Iraq and Afghanistan: Mental health problems and barriers to care. *New England Journal of Medicine, 351,* 13–22.

Hoge, C. W., Goldberg, H. M., & Castro, C. A. (2009). Care of war veterans with mild traumatic brain injury-flawed perspectives. *New England Journal of Medicine, 360,* 1588–1591.

Hoge, C. W., McGurk, D., Thomas, J. L., Cox, A. L., Engel, C. C., & Castro, C. A. (2008). Mild traumatic brain injury in US soldiers returning from Iraq. *New England Journal of Medicine, 385,* 453–463.

Institute of Medicine of the National Academies. (2006). *Posttraumatic stress disorder: Diagnosis and assessment.* Washington, DC: National Academies Press.

Iverson, G. L., Lange, R., Brooks, B., & Rennison, V. L. (2010). "Good old days" bias following mild traumatic brain injury. *Clinical Neuropsychologist, 24*, 17–37.

Iverson, G. L., & McCracken, L. M. (1997). "Postconcussive" symptoms in persons with chronic pain. *Brain Injury, 11*, 783–790.

Kennedy, J. E., Jaffee, M. S., Leskin, G. A., Stokes, J. W., Leal, F. O., & Fitzpatrick, P. J. (2007). Posttraumatic stress disorder and posttraumatic stress disorder-like symptoms and mild traumatic brain injury. *Journal of Rehabilitation Research and Development, 44*, 895–920.

King, J., Sweet, J., Sherer, M., Curtiss, G., & Vanderploeg, R. D. (2002). Validity indicators within the Wisconsin Card Sorting Test: Application of new and previously researched multivariate procedures in multiple traumatic brain injury samples. *Clinical Neuropsychologist, 16*, 506–523.

Klotz Flitter, J. M., Elhai, J. D., & Gold, S. N. (2003). MMPI-2 F scale elevations in adult victims of child sexual abuse. *Journal of Traumatic Stress, 16*, 269–274.

Lange, R. T., Sullivan, K. A., & Scott, C. (2010). Comparison of MMPI-2 and PAI validity indicators to detect feigned depression and PTSD symptom reporting. *Psychiatry Research, 176*, 229–235.

Larrabee, G. J. (Ed.). (2007). *Assessment of malingered neuropsychological deficits*. New York: Oxford University Press.

Marshall, M. B., & Bagby, R. M. (2006). The incremental validity and clinical utility of the MMPI-2 Infrequency Posttraumatic Stress Disorder Scale. *Assessment, 13*, 417–429.

McCrea, M. (2008). *Mild traumatic brain injury and postconcussion syndrome: The new evidence base for diagnosis and treatment*. New York: Oxford University Press.

McCrea, M., Pliskin, N., Barth, J., Cox, D., Fink, J., French, L., et al. (2008). Official position of the military task force on the role of neuropsychology and rehabilitation psychology in the evaluation, management, and research of military veterans with traumatic brain injury. *Clinical Neuropsychologist, 22*, 10–26.

Millis, S. R. (2008). Assessment of incomplete effort and malingering in the neuropsychological examination. In J. E. Morgan & J. H. Ricker (Eds.), *Textbook of clinical neuropsychology* (pp. 891–904). New York: Taylor & Francis.

Morey, L. C. (1991). *Personality Assessment Inventory: Professional manual*. Lutz, FL: Psychological Assessment Resources.

Morgan, J., & Sweet, J. (Eds.). (2009). *Neuropsychology of malingering casebook*. New York: Psychology Press.

Nelson, N., Hoelzle, J. B., McGuire, K. A., Ferrier-Auerbach, A. G., Charlesworth, M. J., & Sponheim, S. R. (2010). Evaluation context impacts neuropsychological performance of OEF/OIF veterans with reported combat-related concussion. *Archives of Clinical Neuropsychology, 25*, 713–723.

Nelson, N., Hoelzle, J. B., Sweet, J. J., Arbisi, P. A., & Demakis, G. J. (2010). Updated meta-analysis of the MMPI-2 Fake Bad Scale: Verified utility in forensic practice. *Clinical Neuropsychologist, 24*, 701–724.

Nelson, N., Sweet, J., Berry, D., Bryant, F., & Granacher, R. P. (2007). Response validity in forensic neuropsychology: Exploratory factor analytic evidence of distinct cognitive and psychological constructs. *Journal of the International Neuropsychological Society, 13,* 440–449.

Nelson, N., Sweet, J., & Demakis, G. (2006). Meta-analysis of the MMPI-2 Fake Bad Scale: Utility in forensic practice. *Clinical Neuropsychologist, 20,* 39–35.

Nies, K. J., & Sweet, J. J. (1994). Neuropsychological assessment and malingering: A critical review of past and present strategies. *Archives of Clinical Neuropsychology, 9,* 501–552.

Polusny, M. A., Kehle, S. M., Nelson, N. W., Erbes, C. R., Arbisi, P. A., & Thuras, P. (2011). Longitudinal effects of mild traumatic brain injury and posttraumatic stress disorder comorbidity on postdeployment outcomes in National Guard soldiers deployed to Iraq. *Archives of General Psychiatry, 68,* 79–89.

Resnick, P. J., West, S., & Payne, J. W. (2008). Malingering of posttraumatic disorders. In R. Rogers (Ed.), *Clinical assessment of malingering and deception* (3rd ed., pp. 109–127). New York: Guilford Press.

Rogers, R. (2008a). An introduction to response styles. In R. Rogers (Ed.), *Clinical assessment of malingering and deception* (3rd ed., pp. 3–13). New York: Guilford Press.

Rogers, R. (2008b). Researching response styles. In R. Rogers (Ed.), *Clinical assessment of malingering and deception* (3rd ed., pp. 411–434). New York: Guilford Press.

Rogers, R. (2008c). Structured interviews and dissimulation. In R. Rogers (Ed.), *Clinical assessment of malingering and deception* (3rd ed., pp. 301–322). New York: Guilford Press.

Rogers, R., Bagby, R. M., & Dickens, S. E. (1992). *Structured Interview of Reported Symptoms: Professional manual.* Tampa, FL: Psychological Assessment Resources.

Rogers, R., Kropp, P. R., Bagby, R. M., & Dickens, S. E. (1992). Faking of specific disorders: A study of the Structured Interview of Reported Symptoms (SIRS). *Journal of Clinical Psychology, 48,* 643–648.

Rogers, R., Payne, J. W., Correa, A. A., Gillard, N. D., & Ross, C. A. (2009). A study of the SIRS with severely traumatized patients. *Journal of Personality Assessment, 91,* 429–438.

Rogers, R., Sewell, K. W., Martin, M. A., & Vitacco, M. J. (2003). Detection of feigned mental disorders: A meta-analysis of the MMPI-2 and malingering. *Assessment, 10,* 160–177.

Rubenzer, S. (2010). Review of the Structured Inventory of Reported Symptoms–2 (SIRS-2). *Journal of Forensic Psychology, 2,* 273–286.

Salloway, S., Southwick, S., & Sadowsky, M. (1990). Opiate withdrawal presenting as posttraumatic stress disorder. *Hospital and Community Psychiatry, 41,* 666–667.

Sayer, N. A., Rettmann, N. A., Carlson, K. F., Bernardy, N., Sigford, B. J., Hamblen, J. L., et al. (2009). Veterans with history of mild traumatic brain injury and posttraumatic stress disorder: Challenges from provider perspective. *Journal of Rehabilitation and Research Development, 46,* 703–716.

Schneiderman, A. I., Braver, E. R., & Kang, H. K. (2008). Understanding sequelae of injury mechanisms and mild traumatic brain injury incurred during the conflicts in Iraq and Afghanistan: Persistent postconcussive symptoms and posttraumatic stress disorder. *American Journal of Epidemiology, 167,* 1446–1452.

Sellbom, M., & Bagby, R. M. (2008). Response styles on multiscale inventories. In R. Rogers (Ed.), *Clinical assessment of malingering and deception* (3rd ed., pp. 182–206). New York: Guilford Press.

Slick, D. J., Hopp, G., Strauss, E., & Thompson, G. B. (1997). *Victoria Symptom Validity Test version 1.0 professional manual.* Odessa, FL: Psychological Assessment Resources.

Slick, D. J., Sherman, E. M., & Iverson, G. L. (1999). Diagnostic criteria for malingered neurocognitive dysfunction: Proposed standards for clinical practice and research. *Clinical Neuropsychologist, 13,* 545–561.

Sosin, D. M., Sniezek, J. E., & Thurman, D. J. (1996). Incidence of mild and moderate brain injury in the United States. *Brain Injury, 10,* 47–57.

Southwick, S. M., Morgan, C. A., Nicolaou, A. L., & Charney, D. S. (1997). Consistency of memory for combat-related traumatic events in veterans of Operation Desert Storm. *American Journal of Psychiatry, 154,* 173–177.

Stein, M. B., & McAllister, T. W. (2009). Exploring the convergence of posttraumatic stress disorder and mild traumatic brain injury. *American Journal of Psychiatry, 166,* 768–776.

Stevens, A., Friedel, E., Mehren, G., & Merten, T. (2008). Malingering and uncooperativeness in psychiatric and psychological assessment: Prevalence and effects in a German sample of claimants. *Psychiatry Research, 157,* 91–200.

Stovner, L., Schrader, H., Mickeviciene, D., Surkiene, D., & Sand, T. (2009). Headache after concussion. *European Journal of Neurology, 16,* 112–120.

Sweet, J. J. (2009). Appendix. Forensic bibliography: Effort/malingering and other common forensic topics encountered by clinical neuropsychologists. In J. E. Morgan & J. J. Sweet (Eds.), *Neuropsychology of malingering casebook* (pp. 566–630). New York: Psychology Press.

Sweet, J. J., & Guiffre Meyer, D. (2010). Well documented, serious brain dysfunction followed by malingering. In J. Morgan, I. S. Baron, & J. Ricker (Eds.), *Casebook of clinical neuropsychology* (pp. 200–212). New York: Oxford University Press.

Sweet, J. J., & King, J. (2002). Category test validity indicators: Overview and practice recommendations. *Journal of Forensic Neuropsychology, 3,* 241–274.

Sweet, J. J., King, J., Malina, A., Bergman, M., & Simmons, A. (2002). Documenting the prominence of forensic neuropsychology at national meetings and in relevant professional journals from 1990–2000. *Clinical Neuropsychologist, 16,* 481–494.

Sweet, J. J., Wolfe, P., Sattlberger, E., Numan, B., Rosenfeld, J. P., Clingerman, S., et al. (2000). Further investigation of traumatic brain injury versus insufficient effort with the California Verbal Learning Test. *Archives of Clinical Neuropsychology, 15,* 105–113.

Taylor, S., Frueh, B. C., & Asmundson, G. J. G. (2007). Detection and management of malingering in people presenting for treatment of posttraumatic stress disorder: Methods, obstacles, and recommendations. *Journal of Anxiety Disorders, 21,* 22–41.

Tombaugh, T. (1997). The Test of Memory Malingering (TOMM): Normative data from cognitively intact and cognitively impaired individuals. *Psychological Assessment, 9,* 260–268.

Vickery, C. D., Berry, D. T. R., Inman, T. H., Harris, M. J., & Orey, S. A. (2001). Detection of inadequate effort on neuropsychological testing: A meta-analytic review of selected procedures. *Archives of Clinical Neuropsychology, 16,* 45–73.

Wessely, S., Unwin, C., Hotopf, M., Hull, L., Ismail, K., Nicolaou, V., et al. (2003). Stability of recall of military hazards over time: Evidence from the Persian Gulf War of 1991. *British Journal of Psychiatry, 183,* 314–322.

Youngjohn, J., Davis, D., & Wolf, I. (1997). Head injury and the MMPI-2: Paradoxical severity effects and the influence of litigation. *Psychological Assessment, 9,* 177–184.

Zandi, T. (2004). Relationship between subjective memory complaints, objective memory performance, and depression among older adults. *American Journal of Alzheimer's Disease and Other Dementias, 19,* 353–360.

CHAPTER 10

Treatment of Mild
Traumatic Brain Injury

Jennie Ponsford

Despite the high frequency of mild traumatic brain injury (mTBI), effective methods of treating this condition have not yet been established. This is at least partly the result of continuing controversy regarding the relative contributions of organic brain injury, physical factors, or psychological factors to continuing symptoms. This chapter discusses the nature of postconcussive symptoms and associated factors. Following from this, it outlines approaches to management of mTBI and discusses review studies evaluating their efficacy. Interventions include provision of information/psychoeducation; routine early assessment and multidisciplinary follow-up treatment addressing physical, cognitive, and psychological issues as needed; cognitive remediation; the provision of cognitive-behavioral therapy (CBT) to assist in management of symptoms; and the use of medications or homeopathy. Bryant and Litz (Chapter 11, this volume) present a more detailed discussion of the use of CBT to treat PTSD occurring in conjunction with mTBI.

What Is mTBI?

mTBI has been defined as "an acute brain injury resulting from mechanical energy to the head from external physical forces" (Carroll, Cassidy, Holm, Kraus, & Coronado, 2004a, p. 115). The issues in establishing operational criteria for mTBI have been outlined in several prior chapters in this volume. The World Health Organization uses the following operational criteria for clinical identification: (1) one or more of the following: confusion or disorientation, loss of consciousness for 30 minutes or less, posttraumatic amnesia for less than 24 hours and/or other transient neurological abnormalities such as focal signs, seizure, and intracranial lesion not requiring surgery; (2) a Glasgow Coma Scale score of 13–15 after 30 minutes postinjury or later upon presentation for health care. These manifestations must not be due to drugs, alcohol, or medications; not be caused by other injuries or treatment for other injuries (e.g., systematic injuries, facial injuries, or intubation); not be caused by other problems (e.g., psychological trauma, language barrier, or coexisting medical conditions), or caused by penetrating craniocerebral injury (Carroll et al., 2004a, p. 115). This definition makes reference to the numerous factors that may complicate the diagnosis of mTBI. These factors may also complicate its management.

In civilian settings, mTBI occurs most commonly in young males, with falls and motor vehicle accidents the most frequent causes; followed by sports injuries, most frequently in football, rugby, soccer, hockey, and boxing; and assaults (Cassidy et al., 2004a). mTBI also occurs as a consequence of military combat (see Bryant, Castro, & Iverson, Chapter 12, this volume). The circumstances in which an injury was sustained also have some bearing on management of mTBI. For example, the issues in managing a professional football player who has sustained a concussion differ somewhat from those where the injury was one of multiple injuries sustained in a potentially fatal motor vehicle accident. Football players and other athletes are highly motivated to return to their sport. They are less likely to have other injuries or to perceive the injury as a life-threatening event and also arguably less likely to have a history of psychiatric disorder and other life stressors.

Postconcussion Symptoms

People with mTBI commonly experience a range of so-called postconcussion symptoms (PCS) in the days or weeks after injury, including headache, nausea, dizziness, sensitivity to noise and/or bright lights, tinnitus, blurred or double vision, restlessness, insomnia, slowed thinking, concentration and memory problems, fatigue, irritability, anxiety, and depression (Carroll et al., 2004b; Ponsford, Cameron, Fitzgerald, Grant, & Mikocka-Walus, 2011). Impaired performances on tests of attention, information-processing speed, and/or memory are also frequently evident on neuropsychological assessment within the first week after injury and may persist in some cases (Carroll et al., 2004b; Malojcic, Mubrin, Coric, Susnic, &

Spilich, 2008; Ponsford et al., 2000; Ponsford et al., 2011; Vanderploeg, Curtis, & Belanger, 2005), although there is not necessarily a strong association between presence of PCS and neuropsychological test performance (Landre, Poppe, Davis, Schmaus, & Hobbs, 2006; Meares et al., 2008; Ponsford, Cameron, Fitzgerald, Grant, & Mikocka-Walus, et al., in press). Most individuals appear to make a full recovery from mTBI, both in terms of symptoms and cognitive performance. However, a proportion of cases, varying between 15 and 25%, report significant ongoing symptoms (Carroll et al., 2004b; Ponsford et al., 2000).

There is continuing debate concerning the causes of these ongoing symptoms. Preinjury psychiatric history is one of the strongest predictors of ongoing PCS (Meares et al., 2008; Ponsford et al., in press). However, there is also strong evidence that mTBI in itself is a strong contributor to these symptoms, at least in the early stages after injury (Ponsford et al., in press), while pain, concurrent anxiety, and other life stressors contribute to symptoms in the longer term. While psychiatric factors undoubtedly play a role in chronic PCS, it seems most likely that *both* cognitive and other neurological deficits and emotional distress contribute to continuing PCS after mTBI (Tiersky et al., 2005). Both of these aspects of the disorder therefore need to be addressed in treatment.

Interventions in the Emergency Department

Before interventions are applied, it is very important to the initial management of mTBI to conduct a thorough assessment while in the emergency department (ED) or when first seen by a doctor. This involves gathering information as to the cause, duration of any loss of consciousness, and posttraumatic confusion and other symptoms experienced. It is crucial to establish whether the injured person is still in posttraumatic amnesia (PTA). Ponsford and colleagues (2004) revised the Westmead PTA Scale for assessment of patients with mTBI at hourly intervals. Patients need to be monitored to ascertain whether they are able to lay down new memories. If they are not able to do so, this is indicative that they are still in PTA. Patients who remain in PTA should not be sent home, as the longer PTA persists the more likely it is that they may have more serious injuries. PTA is a significant predictor of the severity of a TBI (Sherer, Struchen, & Yablon, 2008).

Ponsford and colleagues (2002) found that the presence of ongoing PCS was associated with high levels of anxiety and that levels of anxiety were higher in patients who had not been given information about what symptoms to expect and how best to cope with these. This finding highlights the need for provision of information to patients early after injury.

Interventions provided in the early stages after injury have comprised either early information provision/education or the provision of more intensive therapeutic intervention.

Information Provision: Early Education

Interventions in the acute stages after injury focus on the alleviation of PCS. Detailed information may be provided that outlines the nature of expected symptoms and provides suggestions as to how best to cope with these. This information is provided with reassurance that symptoms are likely to resolve, in order to maximize the injured person's ability to manage the symptoms he or she experiences. It also aims to minimize his or her anxiety concerning these symptoms, which may in turn exacerbate them. A number of studies have shown that the provision of such information enhances reduction in reported symptoms 3–6 months postinjury (Gronwall, 1986; Minderhoud, Boelens, Huizenga, & Saan, 1980; Ponsford et al., 2002).

Ponsford and colleagues (2002) developed a booklet based on one originally created by Gronwall (1986), which describes the symptoms of mTBI (headaches, dizziness, tiredness, problems with concentration, forgetting, clumsiness, slowness, irritability, vision problems, and coping with noise), including guidelines as to how best to manage these. For example, it is suggested that activity levels and engagement in mentally demanding activities be reduced, that the injured person avoids crowded or noisy situations for a while, gets more rest, and paces his or her return to activities of a physically and mentally demanding nature, such as work or school. It is indicated that symptoms are likely to lessen over time, and that activity levels may be gradually increased accordingly. The person with mTBI is encouraged to seek further medical assistance if this does not occur. Ponsford et al. (2002) found that people who received the booklet reported fewer symptoms and were less anxious 3 months postinjury than those who did not receive the booklet.

Given that PCS commonly resolve within the first week after mTBI and most people return to work within a week (Paniak, Toller-Lobe, Durand, & Nagy, 1998; Ponsford et al., 2011), psychoeducational information is best delivered in the ED, in the acute care doctor's office, or in the acute stages of recovery. However, it is desirable to draw the attention of any accompanying relatives or others to the psychoeducational information to ensure that it is read subsequently and not left in the back seat of a taxi. Based on study findings by Alves and colleagues (Alves, Macciocchi, & Barth, 1993), it appears that patient reassurance that recovery is expected to be uncomplicated may be an important component of education. They found that such reassurance combined with education resulted in a lower relative risk of PCS than education alone or no intervention.

Despite the emerging evidence in support of information provision following mTBI, the extent to which such interventions are used remains unclear. While the majority of EDs provide some information (Moore & Leathem, 2004), there is considerable inconsistency in the content and a lack of detail regarding management strategies (Fung, Willer, Moreland, & Leddy, 2006). General practitioners are far less likely to provide information than specialists (Moore & Leathem, 2004). There is a need for implementation of more universal guidelines for mTBI management, incorporating provision of educational material.

Patients with mTBI may be given other instructions in the ED, such as whether or not to rest, to drive, or to return to work. Only one study has examined the efficacy of such instructions. De Kruijk, Leffers, Meerhoff, Rutten, and Twijnstra (2002) compared outcomes when instructions were given to have no bed rest versus advice to take 6 days of full bed rest in people presenting to the ED with mTBI. While the full bed rest group reported less dizziness 2 weeks after injury, there were no significant group differences in symptoms reported or health-related quality of life at 2 weeks, 3 months, or 6 months postinjury. In the absence of an evidence base to guide advice as to when to return to work or driving it seems most appropriate to encourage a graduated approach, with avoidance of these activities while symptoms persist in the early days after injury. However, from the study of Ponsford et al. (2011), it appears that many people have returned to work within a week of uncomplicated mTBI and are able to sustain employment over time.

Provision of Early Therapeutic Intervention

A number of studies have examined the efficacy of more intensive assessment and intervention procedures following mTBI. Provision of a full neuropsychological assessment with availability of additional treatment if necessary was found to be no more effective than provision of information either in booklet form (the National Head Injury Foundation's minor head injury brochure; Kay, 1986) or with additional single-session explanation within the first 3 weeks after injury, as measured both in terms of symptom reduction and reported patient satisfaction assessed at 3 and 12 months postinjury (Paniak, Toller-Lobe, Durand, & Nagy, 1998; Paniak, Toller-Lobe, Reynolds, Melnyk, & Nagy, 2000). There was no untreated control group in this study.

Relander, Troupp, and Bjorkesten (1972) showed that when patients hospitalized for mTBI were encouraged to get up early, and provided with physiotherapy as well as educational information, regular physician follow-up, and encouragement to resume normal activities, they had fewer days off work than patients receiving conventional management and information only as requested. However there were no significant group differences in symptom reporting or disability at 12 months postinjury.

Wade and colleagues (Wade, Crawford, Wenden, King, & Moss 1997; Wade, King, Wenden, Crawford, & Caldwell, 1998) evaluated an intervention in which patients with mild, moderate, and severe TBI were contacted 7–10 days postinjury, mostly in person, and offered information, reassurance, and advice on strategies for coping with specific symptoms, cognitive problems, posttraumatic stress and the impact of stress on PCS, taking a graduated approach to returning to activities, with further intervention for specific symptoms as needed. If participants in the intervention group could not be contacted by telephone or in person, they were sent an information leaflet with contact details for further help. Controls received standard treatment. Following a less successful trial with a low follow-up rate (Wade et al., 1997), Wade et al. (1998) conducted a second trial with a better follow-up rate (69%) and in which 40% of participants had mTBI. The intervention resulted in a significant overall reduction in reported frequency and severity of PCS 6 months postinjury and less disruption of social activities. The effects were greatest in patients with mTBI and those with PTA less than 7 days. Patients with severe injuries were underrepresented but such an intervention could arguably not be expected to alleviate their more significant ongoing disabilities.

Bell et al. (2008) conducted a randomized controlled trial (RCT) examining the efficacy of scheduled follow-up telephone counseling, comprising five calls during the first 3 months after uncomplicated mTBI, addressing individual patient concerns and providing "education, reassurance, and reactivation." The intervention also resulted in significantly reduced reporting of mTBI-related symptoms at 6 months postinjury and less negative impact of symptoms on daily activities such as work or leisure, but no difference in general health outcomes.

Two other studies have evaluated the efficacy of more intensive interventions. Ghaffar, McCullagh, Ouchterlony, and Feinstein (2006) evaluated provision of initial medical assessment one week postinjury; provision of information by an occupational therapist and regular medical appointments with both a rehabilitation physician and a neuropsychiatrist to assess and treat physical symptoms (e.g., pain, headache, dizziness) or psychiatric problems (depression, anxiety, sleep disturbance); and provision of pharmacological therapy, psychotherapy, physiotherapy, and occupational therapy as needed. A control group was offered no follow-up or treatment. There were no significant overall group differences in outcome measured in terms of severity of symptoms, psychosocial functioning, or psychological distress. However, the intervention did have a relatively beneficial outcome for participants with a history of psychiatric illness. Ghaffar et al. (2006) concluded that it may be appropriate to identify these individuals on initial assessment and target them for more intensive intervention. Given the association between mTBI and preinjury psychiatric illness that has emerged in recent studies (Meares et al., 2008; Ponsford et al., in press), this finding is potentially significant.

In a similar well designed study by Elgmark Andersson, Emanuelson, Bjorklund, and Stalhammar (2007), patients with uncomplicated mTBI and no significant previous neurological or psychiatric disease were randomly allocated to an intervention or a control group. Participants assigned to the intervention group ($n = 264$) were contacted by telephone 2–8 weeks postinjury and, if experiencing any PCS or problems in daily activities, they were referred to a rehabilitation specialist ($n = 96$). They were offered information; counseling; encouragement; assessment for pharmacotherapy for pain, depression, and sleep disturbances; and referred to relevant health professionals (mainly occupational therapy, but also social work, physiotherapy, other medical specialists). Intervention group participants were reassured that the symptoms were common and were likely to resolve over time, and provided with strategies to manage their symptoms and to structure their daily activities to cope with them. For example, people with memory problems were encouraged to use a diary. The intervention also included visits to work, school, or home as needed; ergonomic counseling; and relaxation exercises. Participants received an average of five weekly sessions (range = 1–15) followed by an average of 10 telephone contacts (range = 1–20). Controls received "regular care." Results showed no significant differences between intervention and control groups in terms of PCS, life satisfaction, health-related quality of life, and community integration in the domains of home and family life, occupational, social, and leisure activities assessed at 1 year postinjury on the Community Integration Questionnaire (CIQ). Participants who had declined the intervention because they were experiencing few PCS early after injury were functioning as well as preinjury and as well as the general population at 1 year, whereas those who had required and received the intervention had not recovered. There was statistically significant improvement in only a single item: satisfaction with physical health on the Life Satisfaction Questionnaire.

The lack of significant findings might reflect limitations in the measures used to assess outcome in this study. For example the CIQ has shown limited sensitivity to change in the mTBI population. Moreover, the exclusion of individuals with previous psychiatric or substance use problems excluded one-third of the mTBI population. Notwithstanding this, it would appear that individuals who displayed symptoms 2–8 weeks postinjury did not benefit from the interventions provided in this study. A range of interventions were used, so it is not possible to say which aspects may and may not have been effective. This is true of most of the studies offering comprehensive therapy as necessary. More controlled studies of the efficacy of specific aspects of each intervention are needed.

Treating Physical or Other Associated Problems

Increasing evidence in recent years indicates that symptoms of mTBI overlap significantly with symptoms associated with pain due to physical injury to the neck, back, or other bodily parts; medication; posttraumatic stress disorder (PTSD); anxiety; depression; preaccident psychiatric disturbance; individual coping styles; or the presence of other stressors and/or litigation/compensation (Carroll et al., 2004a, 2004b; Mateer, Sira, & O'Connell, 2005; Rose, 2005; Ruff, 2005; Wood, 2004). These factors have been shown to contribute to the likelihood of the presence of continuing PCS (Ponsford et al., 2000; Ponsford et al., in press; Meares et al., 2008). McKerral et al. (2005) have appropriately argued that they need to be considered an intrinsic part of the complex clinical picture of mTBI. There is, however, a need for further exploration and differentiation of the relative influence of these factors in relation to TBI-related factors in order to guide treatment.

In proposing a model for managing mTBI sustained in the workplace, Rose (2005) emphasized the importance of both minimizing overreaction to or misattribution of symptoms, but also addressing comorbid physical injuries. Thus, referral needs to be made to the relevant medical specialists, with conduct of scans or x-rays as appropriate, physiotherapy and/or pharmacological treatment for musculoskeletal pain, and investigation and treatment for headache, balance problems, vertigo, dizziness, hearing loss or tinnitus, and sleep disturbance, which commonly exacerbate stress levels.

Dealing with Cognitive Impairments

It is neither realistic nor necessary to undertake a full neuropsychological assessment in all cases of mTBI (Peloso et al., 2004). Rather, it is preferable to provide information and advise patients to make an appointment for further review if they are still experiencing symptoms 4 weeks postinjury. The exceptions to this may be certain groups identified as most vulnerable, namely, students, individuals in extremely demanding occupations (Ponsford et al., 2000), or other situations where there are specific questions regarding fitness to return to work or study. As described in more detail by Ulloa, Marx, Vanderplueg, and Vasterling (Chapter 8, this volume), during the assessment process it is most important to take a very careful history regarding PTA, symptom evolution, other physical injuries, medication, previous history of head injury, other neurological or learning difficulties, preinjury psychiatric disorders, symptoms of PTSD, other forms of anxiety or depression, and other life stressors. Presence of cognitive impairments may be due to the injury but may also be exacerbated by any of these factors, which in turn need to be addressed in treatment. In the context of litigation it is also necessary to consider the possibility of malingering, using appropriate assessment tools (see Elhai, Sweet, Guidotti Breting, & Kaloupek, Chapter 9, this volume).

The most common cognitive impairments documented are reduced information-processing speed, which limits attentional capacity and particularly affects the capacity to take in, process, and manipulate complex material in working memory, as well as to divide and switch attention. These difficulties may also affect memory functions (Cicerone, 1996; Malojcic et al., 2008; Ponsford et al., 2000). Fatigue is particularly common, so that the injured person may have difficulty sustaining effort or attention to complex tasks over the course of a day (Ponsford et al., 2011). He or she may also have reduced tolerance for noise or bustle. Two approaches may be taken to the remediation of cognitive impairments, namely, cognitive retraining, aimed at restoring impaired function, and functional compensation, which enhances performance through the use of compensatory strategies.

Numerous studies have examined the effectiveness of computerized interventions for retraining of attentional dysfunction following mild, moderate, and severe TBI (for a detailed review, see Ponsford & Willmott, 2004). These involve repeated practice on hierarchically organized attentional tasks generally delivered via a computer. One example is Attention Process Training, developed by Sohlberg and colleagues (Palmese & Raskin, 2000; Sohlberg & Mateer, 1987; Sohlberg, McLaughliin, Pavese, Heidrich, & Posner, 2000). Several meta-analytic reviews have concluded that there is modest evidence in support of the efficacy of attentional training following TBI (Cicerone et al., 2005; Rohling, Beverly, Faust, & Demakis, 2009). However, in another meta-analysis Park and Ingles (2001) found that significant performance improvements were evident only in the pre- to poststudies of individuals with TBI, but not in the studies that included controls. They concluded that specific-skills training resulted in gains or practice effects on tests of attention similar to the training tasks, but did not have a significant impact on functional outcomes in those treated. Indeed, there is little evidence of generalization of such attentional training to real-world activities (Ponsford & Willmott, 2004). Moreover in a large RCT involving over 11,000 uninjured people, Owen et al. (2010) found that improved performance on trained computerized cognitive tasks did not generalize to untrained tasks.

These criticisms apply to a study by Laatsch, Thulborn, Krisky, Sho-bat, and Sweeney (2004), who provided 12–25 hours of training in visual scanning and language processing skills to five people with mTBI, of whom three had a significant neurological history. All participants exhibited post-training improvement on some neuropsychological measures of visual processing and/or language processing, and changes in the pattern and extent of activation were evident on two functional MRI (fMRI) block activation tasks, a reading comprehension task, and a visually guided saccade task. While these findings are interesting and should form the basis for more controlled studies, the study had significant limitations, including the lack of a control group to control for practice effects on the measures used and to examine changes in fMRI activation in response to repeated performance of such tasks in an uninjured brain, as well as the lack of a randomized treatment alternative. The neuropsychological measures were similar to the training tasks and there was no objective assessment of generalization to everyday activities. In a similar vein, Kapoor, Ciuffreda, and Han (2004) reported improvement in response to oculomotor training on basic versional ocular motility and reading eye movements in a single mTBI case, but again no control condition was included.

In terms of compensatory approaches, Cicerone (2002) evaluated a compensatory approach to the remediation of "working attention" in four individuals with mTBI, comparing outcomes with those of four untreated individuals. Treatment involved developing and practicing strategies for more effective allocation of attentional resources and management of the pace of information while performing complex tasks of relevance to their daily lives. Therapy had a particular focus on improving capacity to focus and sustain attention, shift attentional priority between several tasks or aspects of a task at a time, maintain task performance in the presence of background noise and distractions, and monitor and correct errors. An additional focus of therapy was on reducing "secondary emotional reactions" or "frustration response" when participants experienced difficulty, so that effective task performance could be maintained. Compensatory strategies for dealing with memory and communication problems were also taught. Participants also received a cognitive-behavioral intervention aimed at management of other PCS including dizziness, sensitivity to noise or light, fatigue and affective symptoms, with encouragement to resume activities despite their symptoms. Physical and occupational therapy provided exercises to reduce problems with dizziness, balance, and vision, and vocational support, including graded work trials. These four people showed significantly better functional outcomes in terms of improved cognitive performance, reduced PCS, and return to work than four untreated comparison participants. However, given the multifaceted nature of the intervention it is not possible to ascertain what specific benefit was attributable to the compensatory attentional strategy training.

Another example of a compensatory approach applicable to mTBI is Time Pressure Management (TPM, Fasotti, Kovacs, Eling, & Brouwer, 2000). This is a method of training in awareness of situations where mental slowness is affecting task performance and using compensatory self-instructional strategies before or during the task to slow down the delivery of information (e.g., asking for repetition or asking another person to slow down his or her delivery of information). Implementation of the steps is taught initially with overt demonstration, then overt self-instruction with written prompts, gradually withdrawn, and finally the application and generalization of strategies under more distracting conditions (e.g., with a radio playing in the background). Relative to a control group, those who received TPM took more managing steps, resulting in greater and more lasting gains, which generalized to other measures of attention and memory. Those who benefited more showed greater awareness of the need for the strategies and were more assertive in applying the steps in social situations. This technique has recently been applied with some success to reduce mental slowness in an RCT involving stroke patients (Winkens, Van Heugten, Wade, & Fasotti, 2009a; Winkens, Van Heugten, Wade, Habets, & Fasotti, 2009b). It has not been specifically evaluated in mTBI populations. Ultimately these forms of intervention hold greatest promise in terms of their capacity to alleviate attentional difficulties following mTBI. However, as Winkens et al. (2009b) have noted, their success will depend on the level of awareness and motivation of the injured person.

Other compensatory strategies that might be applied include using mnemonic strategies, such as visualization; external memory aids such as a diary, daily planner and/ or handheld PDF or mobile phone to assist with structuring the day and remembering things; using a tape recorder to tape meetings or telephone conversations to allow for review of their contents; undertaking cognitively demanding tasks only when feeling alert; working in a quiet area free from noise and distraction; taking frequent rest breaks; and taking a graduated approach to engagement in activities. However, there has been very limited controlled evaluation of interventions of this nature.

One recent uncontrolled study by Huckans et al. (2010) assessed the impact of a six to eight session group-based cognitive strategy training intervention in 21 combat veterans with a history of mTBI and documented cognitive impairments. As they were referred from a mental health program, they also had psychiatric symptoms. They were provided with training and practice in the use of strategies, including use of a daily planner, visual imagery mnemonics, problem-solving strategies, mindfulness exercises to focus attention, removing environmental distractions, and the use of external aids (e.g., timers, visual reminders, daily planners). Sixteen participants completed pre–posttreatment self-report measures. They reported significantly increased strategy use and an increased perception that strategies were helpful to them, increased life satisfaction, and decreased severity of depression, memory, and cognitive symptoms. This study is limited by the fact that positive outcomes were evident only on self-report measures. There was no significant change in functional outcomes on the Community Integration Questionnaire and no follow-up. Nevertheless the study suggests that at least some individuals with mTBI who are experiencing ongoing cognitive difficulties find instruction in compensatory strategies helpful. They may also have been supported by the group interactions. It is arguable, however, that individualized compensatory strategies applied according to the individual's needs and abilities may be more effective.

The only RCT addressing cognitive difficulties has been conducted by Tiersky et al., (2005), who evaluated the impact of a combined cognitive remediation and CBT intervention for persistent PCS in 20 people with mild-to-moderate TBI. Weekly individual 1-hour sessions were devoted to cognitive remediation with a focus on attentional, information-processing, and memory difficulties, using retraining exercises from the Attention Process Training program, with additional encouragement to develop compensatory strategies to remove distractions or allow for planning and problem solving, and homework assignments to facilitate generalization of skills. Notebook use, note taking, and environmental modification were encouraged to compensate for memory difficulties. Separate weekly 1-hour sessions were devoted to CBT to increase effective coping behaviors for managing PCS, reduce stress levels, teach skills for preventing relapse, and help participants cope with their sense of loss over decreased cognitive and physical functioning. This intervention resulted in lower levels of endorsement of anxiety and depression symptoms and improved performance on one measure of auditory divided attention, the Paced Auditory Serial Addition Test (Gronwall, 1977), relative to wait-list controls, but no differences in functional outcome. This study involved a relatively high proportion of well-educated women. The findings, while promising, need to be replicated in a larger and broader sample. Moreover, as with the Cicerone (1996) study, it is not possible to separate the effects of the cognitive remedial interventions and the cognitive-behavioral interventions.

Psychological Therapy

As mentioned at the beginning of this chapter, the majority of studies suggest that PCS, including cognitive impairments, are experienced by most people in the early days or weeks after mTBI but generally resolve. Individuals with persistent PCS show high levels of anxiety. They are also more likely to have a history of previous psychiatric disorder (Meares et al., 2008; Ponsford et al. 2000; Ponsford et al., in press). This suggests that the injured person's appraisal or attribution of symptoms plays a role in perpetuating them. Based on the premise that individuals with mTBI tend to overestimate PCS change in a manner consistent with their symptom expectations, Mittenberg and colleagues developed and evaluated their cognitive-behavioral education manual, entitled *Recovering from Mild Head Injury: A Guide From Patients* (Mittenberg, Zielinski, & Fichera, 1993). The therapist guides the patient through the cognitive-behavioral model of symptom maintenance and treatment, discussing techniques for minimizing their particular symptoms. The aim is for the person with mTBI to change his or her inner dialogue, develop a sense of mastery over symptoms, and take control of his or her lifestyle. Instructions for thought stopping, replacing negatively biased thoughts, and encouragement to return to rewarding activities are provided. This manual was delivered in a single session intervention (Mittenberg, Tremont, Zielinski, Fichera, & Rayls, 1996). Participant knowledge of the content of the manual was assessed, and they were provided with an opportunity for rehearsal. Patients receiving intervention reported significantly shorter overall symptom duration, fewer symptoms, and lower symptom severity levels (Mittenberg et al., 1996).

Cognitive-behavioral approaches may also be used to alleviate anxiety and depression. When the injury has been sustained under psychologically traumatic circumstances, the possibility of PTSD should also be considered, and presence of PTSD symptoms is common in those with persistent PCS (Ponsford et al., 2011). For individuals with PTSD symptoms, there will be a need to incorporate techniques for addressing these symptoms as discussed by Bryant and Litz (Chapter 11, this volume). Only a small number of studies have evaluated the impact of CBT for anxiety following mTBI. Hodgson, McDonald, Tate, and Gertler (2005) conducted a RCT of a CBT intervention for managing social anxiety following predominantly mild brain injury in 12 people. Their CBT program included components such as relaxation training, cognitive restructuring, assertiveness skills, and graded exposure. Participants' cognitive limitations were accommodated using various strategies including the use of external aids, repeated repetitions of treatment materials, and shorter sessions. They reported a significant improvement on measures of general anxiety, depression, and transient mood for the treatment group compared to wait-list control, which was maintained at 1-month follow-up. As discussed by Bryant and Litz (Chapter 11, this volume), Bryant, Moulds, Guthrie, and Nixon (2003) evaluated the efficacy of a 5-week group CBT program to treat acute stress disorder in 24 participants with mTBI. Upon treatment completion, fewer participants in the CBT group (17%) still met the diagnostic criteria for PTSD compared to participants who received nondirective supportive counseling (58%), and treatment gains were maintained at 6-month follow-up. No group studies to date have evaluated the impact of CBT on depression following mTBI. Sleep disturbance associated with mTBI has been treated with success using CBT focused on sleep problems, including stimulus control, restricting daytime sleep, cognitive restructuring, sleep hygiene education, and fatigue management (Ouellet & Morin, 2007).

As Ruff (2005) has pointed out, the experience of mTBI may bring to the surface the impact of previous psychologically traumatic experiences, for which much more intensive psychotherapy may be required. Although there have been several published case studies, together with the above-mentioned interventions incorporating CBT with or without other interventions, there is a need for more comprehensive evaluative studies and examination of the impact of other psychotherapeutic approaches.

Management of Sports-Related mTBI

An important issue in the management of sports-related injuries is the development and implementation of guidelines for return to play. According to Peloso et al. (2004), most guidelines recommend no return to play until there is full recovery from symptoms, although this recommendation is not based on clear scientific evidence. The impact of repeated concussions on cognitive function remains controversial, with studies showing mixed findings, but some evidence of greater cognitive impairment associated with multiple head injuries (Belanger, Spiegel, & Vanderploeg, 2010). There are no consistent guidelines relating to the number of concussions sustained before the athlete should be given advice to retire (Peloso et al., 2004).

Although there is a widely held view that athletes are less likely to experience psychological or social problems because of their strong motivation to return to play and lack of traumatic circumstances surrounding injury, they face unique stressors and this aspect of their management tends to be neglected (Bloom, Horton, McCrory, & Johnston, 2004). Horton, Bloom, and Johnston (2002) conducted a study showing that participation in a social support group resulted in an improvement in mood and a reduction in anger, confusion, frustration, anxiety, depression, and isolation in concussed athletes. The components of rehabilitation following sports-related concussion proposed by this research group include graded return to activity following resolution of symptoms; adequate rest; engagement in less physically demanding fitness activities, such as yoga or pilates; using strategies to manage cognitive changes, balance and vestibular problems, and headache; keeping up contact with the team, but also having time out at home; and receiving psychological interventions as needed (Johnston et al., 2004). The evidence base for these and all other guidelines relating to the management of sports-related concussion has yet to be established.

Treatment with Medication or Homeopathy

Because patients generally experience multiple symptoms, the use of a number of medications to treat PCS at one time, including anti-inflammatory agents, narcotics, muscle relaxants, antivertigo agents, psychostimulants, and antidepressants, is common. Pharmacological treatment of one symptom may potentially exacerbate other deficits. There is limited evidence in support of the efficacy of any pharmacological treatment following mTBI. A nonrandomized single cohort study by Fann, Uomoto, and Katon (2001) revealed a positive impact of an selective serotonin reuptake inhibitor (SSRI), sertraline, on depressive symptoms and cognitive function. However, two more recent trials of SSRIs (citalopram and sertraline) in depressed patients with mild-to-moderate injuries (Rapoport et al., 2008) and in depressed patients with mild, moderate, and severe injuries (Ashman et al., 2009) have not shown significantly greater response to SSRIs than in controls. An RCT by Chapman and colleagues (Chapman, Weintraub, Milburn, Pirozzi, & Woo, 1999) demonstrated a positive impact of a range of homeopathic remedies on functional outcome in people with mTBI and persistent PCS, treated a mean of 2.9 years postinjury. A single medicine was selected by consensus of two physicians, based on the individual characteristics of the patient, and administered over a 1-month period. However, as treatments varied across participants, it is not clear how they could be replicated. These study findings suggest he need for further controlled research in this area.

Summary and Conclusions

Despite the high frequency of mTBI, there has been limited research evaluating treatment effectiveness. Developing uniform screening procedures is an important initial step, particularly given the evidence in support of early intervention. MTBI is a complex and multifaceted condition that therefore requires multifaceted treatment, best initiated soon after injury. There is evidence that provision of information, reassurance, and coping strategies, including a graded return to activities early after injury, ideally in the ED or doctor's office as soon as possible after the injury, may reduce reported symptoms. More consistent use of such information is to be encouraged. The evidence in support of more intensive interventions is mixed. It appears that individuals with a history of psychiatric disorder may be most vulnerable, possibly because they are most likely to become anxious over symptoms. They may benefit from more intensive intervention addressing their physical, cognitive, and psychiatric symptoms, again commencing early after injury. Further studies identifying the effective elements of multifaceted interventions would provide further guidance as to the specific nature of therapies to be delivered. CBT has demonstrated usefulness in helping individuals with PCS to reframe symptoms and regulate activity levels to manage symptoms, while remaining engaged with daily activities. CBT may also be helpful in managing sleep disturbance, as well as PTSD. It is also important to assess and treat vestibular symptoms, headache, and physical injuries, which may exacerbate PCS and stress levels, and to prevent misattribution of symptoms to the mTBI. There is a need for more evidence-based guidelines for return to play following sports-related concussion and to address psychological and social issues in management of the concussed athlete. Given the limited efficacy of pharmacotherapy, these interventions hold greatest promise for enhancing outcome following mTBI, but further controlled studies identifying what specific aspects of therapy are helpful, and for whom, are sorely needed.

References

Alves, W. M., Macciocchi, S. N., & Barth, J. T. (1993). Postconcussive symptoms after uncomplicated mild head injury. *Journal of Head Trauma Rehabilitation, 8*, 48–59.

Ashman, T. A., Cantor, J. B., Gordon, W. A., Spielman, L., Flanagan, S., Ginsberg, A., (2009). A randomized controlled trial of sertraline for the treatment of depression in persons with traumatic brain injury. *Archives of Physical Medicine and Rehabilitation, 90*(5), 733–740.

Belanger, H. G., Spiegel, E., & Vanderploeg, R. D. (2010). Neuropsychological performance following a history of multiple self-reported concussions. *Journal of the International Neuropsychological Society, 16*, 262–267.

Bell, K. R., Hoffman, J. M., Temkin, N. R., Powell, J. M., Fraser, R. T., Esselman, P. C., et al. (2008). The effect of telephone counselling on reducing posttraumatic symptoms after mild traumatic brain injury: a randomised trial. *Journal of Neurology, Neurosurgery and Psychiatry, 79*(11), 1275–1281.

Bloom, G. A., Horton, A. S. McCrory, P., & Johnston, K. M. (2004). Sport psychology and concussion: New impacts to explore. *British Journal of Sports Medicine, 38*(5), 519–521.

Bryant, R. A., Moulds, M., Guthrie, R., & Nixon, R. D. V. (2003). Treating acutre stress disorder following mild traumatic brain injury. *American Journal of Psychiatry, 160*, 585–587.

Carroll, L. J., Cassidy, J. D., Holm, L., Kraus, J., & Coronado, V. (2004a). Methodological issues and research recommendations for mild traumatic brain injury: The WHO Collaborating Centre Task Force on Mild Traumatic Brain Injury. *Journal of Rehabilitation Medicine, 37* (Suppl. 43), 113–125.

Carroll, L. J., Cassidy, J. D., Peloso, P. M., Borg, J., von Holst, H., Holm, L., et al. (2004b). Prognosis for mild traumatic brain injury: Results of the WHO Collaborating Centre Task Force on Mild Traumatic Brain Injury. *Journal of Rehabilitation Medicine, 37* (Suppl. 43), 84–105.

Cassidy, J. D., Carroll, L. J., Peloso, P. M., Borg, J., von Holst, H., Holm, L., et al. (2004). Incidence, risk factors and prevention of mild traumatic brain injury: Results of the WHO Collaborating Centre Task Force on Mild Traumatic Brain Injury. *Journal of Rehabilitation Medicine, 37* (Suppl. 43), 28–60.

Chapman, E. H., Weintraub, R. J., Milburn, M. A, Pirozzi, T. O., & Woo, E. (1999). Homeopathic treatment of mild traumatic brain injury: A randomized double-blind, placebo-controlled clinical trial. *Journal of Head Trauma Rehabilitation, 14*, 521–542.

Cicerone, K. D. (1996). Attention deficits and dual task demands after mild traumatic brain injury. *Brain Injury, 10*(2), 79–89.

Cicerone, K. D. (2002). Remediation of "working attention" in mild traumatic brain injury. *Brain Injury, 16*(3), 185–195.

Cicerone, K. D., Dahlberg, C., Malec, J. F., Langenbaum, D. M., Felicetti, T., Kneipp, S., et al. (2005). Evidence-based cognitive rehabilitation: Updated review of the literature from 1998 through 2002. *Archives of Physical Medicine and Rehabilitation, 86*, 1681–1692.

de Kruijk, J. R., Leffers, P., Meerhoff, S., Rutten, J., & Twijnstra, A. (2002). Effectiveness of bed rest after mild traumatic brain injury: A randomised trial of no versus six days of bed rest. *Journal of Neurology, Neurosurgery, and Psychiatry, 73*(2), 167–172.

Elgmark Andersson, E., Emanuelson, I., Bjorklund, R., & Stalhammar, D. A. (2007). Mild traumatic brain injuries: The impact of early intervention on late sequelae. A randomized controlled trial. *Acta Neurochirurgica, 149*(2), 151–159; discussion, 160.

Fann, J. R., Uomoto, J. M., & Katon, W. J. (2001). Cognitive improvement with treatment of depression following mild traumatic brain injury. *Psychosomatics, 42*, 48–54.

Fasotti, L., Kovacs, F., Eling, P. A. T. M., & Brouwer, W. H. (2000). Time pressure management as a compensatory strategy training after closed head injury. *Neuropsychological Rehabilitation, 10*, 47–65.

Fung, M., Willer, B., Moreland, D., & Leddy, J. J. (2006). A proposal for an evidence-based emergency department discharge form for mild traumatic brain injury. *Brain Injury, 20*(9), 889–894.

Ghaffar, O., McCullagh, S., Ouchterlony, D., & Feinstein, A. (2006). Randomized treatment trial in mild traumatic brain injury. *Journal of Psychosomatic Research, 61*(2), 153–160.

Gronwall, D. M. (1977). Paced auditory serial-addition task: A measure of recovery from concussion. *Perceptual and Motor Skills, 44*(2), 367–373.

Gronwall, D. M. (1986). Rehabilitation programs for patients with mild head injury: Components, problems and evaluation. *Journal of Head Trauma Rehabilitation, 1*, 53–63.

Hodgson, J., McDonald, S., Tate, R., & Gertler, P. (2005). A randomised controlled trial of a cognitive behavioural therapy program for managing social anxiety after acquired brain injury. *Brain Impairment, 6*, 169–180.

Horton, A. S., Bloom, G. A., & Johnston, K. M. (2002). The impact of support groups on the psychological state of athletes experiencing concussion. *Medicine and Science in Sports and Exercise, 34*, 99.

Huckans, M., Pavawalla, S., Demadura, T., Kolessar, M., Seelye, A., Roost, N., et al. (2010). A pilot study examining effects of group-based cognitive strategy training treatment on self-reported cognitive problems, psychiatric symptoms, functioning, and compensatory strategy use in OIF/OEF combat veterans with persistent mild cognitive disorder and history of traumatic brain injury. *Journal of Rehabilitation Research and Development. 47*(1), 43–60.

Johnston, K. M., Bloom, G. A., Ramsay, J., Kissick, J., Montgomery, D., Foley, D., et al. (2004). Current concepts in concussion rehabilitation. *Current Sports Medicine Reports, 3*, 316–323.

Kapoor, N., Ciuffreda, K. J., & Han, Y. (2004). Oculomotor rehabilitation in acquired brain injury: A case series. *Archives of Physical Medicine and Rehabilitation, 85*, 1667–1678.

Kay, T. (1986). *The unseen injury: Minor head trauma: An introduction for patients and families.* Washington, DC: National Head Injury Foundation.

Laatsch, L. K., Thulborn, K. R., Krisky, C. M., Shobat, D. M., & Sweeney, J. A. (2004). Investigating the neurobiological basis of cognitive rehabilitation therapy with fMRI. *Brain Injury, 18*(10), 957–974.

Landre, N., Poppe, C. J., Davis, N., Schmaus, B., & Hobbs, S. E. (2006). Cognitive functioning and postconcussive symptoms in trauma patients with and without mild TBI. *Archives of Clinical Neuropsychology, 21*(4), 255–273.

Malojcic, B., Mubrin, Z., Coric, B., Susnic, M., & Spilich, G. J. (2008). Consequences of mild traumatic brain injury on information processing assessed with attention and short-term memory tasks. *Journal of Neurotrauma, 25*, 30–37.

Mateer, C. A., Sira, C. S., & O'Connell, M. E. (2005). Putting Humpty Dumpty together again: The importance of integrating cognitive and emotional interventions. *Journal of Head Trauma Rehabilitation, 20*(1), 62–75.

McKerral, M., Guerin, F., Kennepohl, S., Dominique, A., Honore, W., Leveille, G., et al. (2005). Comments on the Task Force Report on Mild Traumatic Brain Injury. *Journal of Rehabilitation Medicine, 37*, (Suppl. 43), 61–62.

Meares, S., Shores, E., Taylor, A., Batchelor, J., Bryant, R., Baguley, I., et al. (2008). Mild traumatic brain injury does not predict acute postconcussion syndrome. *Journal of Neurology, Neurosurgery, and Psychiatry, 79*(3), 300–306.

Minderhoud, J. M., Boelens, M. E., Huizenga, J., & Saan, R. J. (1980). Treatment of minor head injuries. *Clinical Neurology and Neurosurgery, 82*, 127–140.

Mittenberg, W., Tremont, G., Zeilinski, R. E., Fichera, S., & Rayls, K. R. (1996). Cognitive-behavioural prevention of postconcussion syndrome. *Archives of Clinical Neuropsychology, 11*, 139–145.

Mittenberg, W., Zielinski, R. E., & Fichera, S. (1993). Recovery from mild head injury: A treatment manual for patients. *Psychotherapy in Private Practice, 12*, 37–52.

Moore, C., & Leathem, J. (2004). Information provision after mild traumatic brain injury. *New Zealand Medical Journal, 117*(1201), U1046.

Ouellet, M. C., & Morin, C. M. (2007). Efficacy of cognitive-behavioural therapy for insomnia associated with traumatic brain injury: A single case experimental design. *Archives of Physical Medicine and Rehabilitation, 88*(12), 1581–1592.

Owen, A. M., Hampshire, A., Grahn, J. A., Stenton, R., Dajani, S., Burns, A. S., et al. (2010). Putting brain training to the test. *Nature, 465,* 775–779.

Palmese, C. A., & Raskin, S. A. (2000). The rehabilitation of attention in individuals with mild traumatic brain injury, using the APT-II programme. *Brain Injury, 14*(6), 535–548.

Paniak, C., Toller-Lobe, G., Durand, A., & Nagy, J. (1998). A randomized trial of two treatments for mild traumatic brain injury. *Brain Injury, 12,* 1011–1023.

Paniak, C., Toller-Lobe, G., Reynolds, S., Melnyk, A., & Nagy, J. A. (2000). A randomized trial of two treatments for mild traumatic brain injury: 1 year follow-up. *Brain Injury, 14,* 219–226.

Park, N. W., & Ingles, J. L. (2001). Effectiveness of attention rehabilitation after an acquired brain injury: A meta-analysis. *Neuropsychology, 15*(2), 199–210.

Peloso, P. M., Carroll, L. J., Cassidy, J. D., Borg, J., von Holst, H., Holm, L., et al. (2004). Critical evaluation of the existing guidelines on mild traumatic brain injury. *Journal of Rehabilitation Medicine, 37* (Suppl. 43), 106–112.

Ponsford, J., Cameron, P., Fitzgerald, M., Grant, M., Mikocka-Walus, A. (2011) Long-term outcomes after uncomplicated mild traumatic brain injury: A comparison with trauma controls. *Journal of Neurotrauma 28*(6), 937–948.

Ponsford, J., Cameron, P., Fitzgerald, M., Grant, M., Mikocka-Walus, A., & Schönberger, M. (in press). Predictors of post-concussive symptoms three months after mild TBI. *Neuropsychology.*

Ponsford, J., Cameron, P., Willmott, C., Rothwell, A., Kelly, A. M., Nelms, R., et al. (2004). Use of the Westmead PTA Scale to monitor recovery of memory after mild head injury. *Brain Injury, 18*(4), 603–614.

Ponsford, J., & Willmott, C. (2004). Rehabilitation of non-spatial attention. In J. Ponsford (Ed.), *Cognitive and behavioural rehabilitation: From neurobiology to clinical practice* (pp. 299–342). New York: Guilford Press.

Ponsford, J., Willmott, C., Rothwell, A., Cameron, P., Kelly, A. M., Nelms, R., et al. (2000). Factors influencing outcome following mild traumatic brain injury in adults. *Journal of the International Neuropsychological Society, 6*(5), 568–579.

Ponsford, J., Willmott, C., Rothwell, A., Cameron, P., Nelms, R., & Curran, C. (2002). Impact of early intervention on outcome after mild traumatic brain injury in adults. *Journal of Neurology, Neurosurgery and Psychiatry, 73,* 330–332.

Rapoport, M., Chan, F., Lanctot, K., Herrmann, N., McCullagh, S., & Feinstein, A. (2008). An open-label study of citalopram for major depression following traumatic brain injury. *Journal of Psychopharmacology, 22,* 860–864.

Relander, M., Troupp, H., & Bjorkesten, G. (1972). Controlled trial of treatment for cerebral concussion. *British Medical Journal, 4,* 777–779.

Rohling, M. L., Beverly, B., Faust, M. E., & Demakis, G. (2009). Effectiveness of cognitive rehabilitation following acquired brain injury: A meta-analytic re-examination of Cicerone et al.'s (2000, 2005) systematic reviews. *Neuropsychology, 23*(1), 20–39.

Rose, J. M. (2005). Continuum of care model for managing mild traumatic brain injury in a workers' compensation context: A description of the model and its development. *Brain Injury, 19*(1), 29–39.

Ruff, R. (2005). Two decades of advances in understanding of mild traumatic brain injury. *Journal of Head Trauma Rehabilitation, 20*(1), 5–18.

Sherer, M., Struchen, M., & Yablon, S. A. (2008). Comparison of indices of traumatic brain injury severity: Glasgow Coma Scale, length of coma and posttraumatic amnesia. *Journal of Neurology, Neurosurgery and Psychiatry, 79*, 678–685.

Sohlberg, M. M., & Mateer, C. A. (1987). Effectiveness of an attention-training program. *Journal of Clinical and Experimental Neuropsychology, 9*, 117–130.

Sohlberg, M. M., McLaughliin, K. A., Pavese, A., Heidrich, A., & Posner, A. I. (2000). Evaluation of attention process training and brain injury education in persons with acquired brain injury. *Journal of Clinical and Experimental Neuropsychology, 22*, 656–676.

Tiersky, L. A., Anselmi, V., Johnston, M. V., Kurtyka, J., Roosen, E., Schwartz, T., et al. (2005). A trial of neuropsychologic rehabilitation in mild-spectrum traumatic brain injury. *Archives of Physical Medicine and Rehabilitation, 86*, 1565–1574.

Vanderploeg, R. D., Curtiss, G., & Belanger, H. G. (2005). Long-term neuropsychological outcomes following mild traumatic brain injury. *Journal of the International Neuropsychological Society, 11*, 228–236.

Wade, D. T., Crawford, S., Wenden, F. J., King, N. S., & Moss, N. E. (1997). Does routine follow-up after head injury help?: A randomized controlled trial. *Journal of Neurology, Neurosurgery, and Psychiatry, 62*(5), 478–484.

Wade, D. T., King, N. S., Wenden, F. J., Crawford, S., & Caldwell, F. E. (1998). Routine follow-up after head injury: A second randomized controlled trial. *Journal of Neurology, Neurosurgery, and Psychiatry, 65*(2), 177–183.

Winkens, I., Van Heugten, C. M., Wade, D. T., & Fasotti, L. (2009a). Training patients in time pressure management: A cognitive strategy for mental slowness. *Clinical Rehabilitation, 23*, 79–90.

Winkens, I., Van Heugten, C. M., Wade, D. T., Habets, E., & Fasotti, L. (2009b). Efficacy of time pressure management in stroke patients with slowed information processing: A randomized controlled trial. *Archives of Physical Medicine and Rehabilitation, 90*(10), 1672–1679.

Wood, R. L. (2004). Understanding the "miserable minority": A diasthesis–stress paradigm for post-concussional syndrome. *Brain Injury, 18*(11), 1135–1153.

CHAPTER 11

Treatment of Posttraumatic Stress Disorder Following Mild Traumatic Brain Injury

Richard A. Bryant and Brett T. Litz

As many chapters in this volume have indicated, traumatic brain injury (TBI) can occur in the context of an experience that is perceived as highly threatening and anxiety-producing. Accordingly, it is not surprising that a proportion of people who sustain a TBI also develop posttraumatic stress disorder (PTSD). Indeed, as recent evidence has indicated, suffering a mild TBI (mTBI) may even increase the risk for developing PTSD (Bryant et al., 2010). This pattern raises the important clinical issue of appropriate treatment strategies for assisting people with PTSD that occurs in the context of TBI. TBI can either predate the occurrence of PTSD, be sustained in the course of the event that triggers the PTSD, or possibly be sustained after PTSD has developed. This chapter initially provides an overview of current evidence of how to treat PTSD generally, and then turns to discuss the specific modifications that one may need to include to address specific needs of PTSD patients who have sustained a TBI.

Determining the Presence of PTSD Following mTBI

The first step in treating PTSD is to determine if the person suffers the condition. Ulloa, Marx, Vanderploeg, and Vasterling (Chapter 8 this volume) provide a more comprehensive discussion of considerations in assessing

PTSD in the context of comorbid TBI. It is particularly important if one is considering early intervention for acute stress reactions following mTBI. The diagnostic criteria for acute stress disorder (ASD) places much emphasis on dissociative symptoms, such as depersonalization, derealization, reduced awareness, emotional numbing, and dissociative amnesia. These reactions may be associated with the loss of consciousness or concussion rather than psychological responses that arise in the context of intense fear and arousal. In terms of identifying people who may be suffering ASD or PTSD following TBI, it is useful to focus on the presence of reexperiencing symptoms. The predictive power of reexperiencing in mTBI populations is comparable to that observed in no-TBI populations (Bryant & Harvey, 1998). Accordingly, assessing patients with PTSD who may be eligible for treatment after mTBI can usually rely on normal PTSD criteria.

Evidence-Based Treatment of PTSD

There is overwhelming evidence that trauma-focused psychotherapy, and particularly cognitive-behavioral therapy (CBT), is the treatment of choice for PTSD (Foa, 2000, 2006; Foa & Meadows, 1997; Harvey, Bryant, & Tarrier, 2003; van Etten & Taylor, 1998). Consensus on this conclusion is seen in a range of recent treatment guidelines, including the International Society of Traumatic Stress Studies Treatment Guidelines (Foa, Keane, Friedman, & Cohen, 2009), the Australian National Health and Medical Research Council Treatment Guidelines (Forbes et al., 2007), and the United Kingdom's National Institute of Clinical Excellence (National Collaborating Centre for Mental Health, 2005). Accordingly, this review focuses on the role of CBT in managing PTSD following TBI.

CBT usually involves psychoeducation, anxiety management, cognitive restructuring, imaginal and *in vivo* exposure, and relapse prevention (Foa & Meadows, 1997; Harvey et al., 2003). Psychoeducation provides information about common symptoms following a traumatic event, normalizes the trauma reactions, and establishes a rationale for treatment. Anxiety management techniques include breathing retraining, muscle relaxation strategies, and self-talk. These techniques aim to assist the patient to gain a sense of mastery over his or her fear and to reduce arousal levels. Prolonged imaginal exposure requires the individual to vividly imagine the trauma for prolonged periods. Prolonged exposure typically occurs for at least 40 minutes, and is usually supplemented by daily homework exercises. Variants of imaginal exposure may require patients to write down detailed descriptions of the experience (Resick & Schnicke, 1993) or implement exposure with the assistance of virtual reality paradigms implemented via computer-generated imagery (Rothbaum, Ruef, Litz, Han, & Hodges, 2003). Most exposure treatments supplement imaginal exposure with *in vivo* exposure. This form of exposure is comparable to treating phobic reactions in other disorders, and involves live graded exposure to the feared stimuli. Cognitive restructuring is based on the premise that maladaptive appraisals underpin the maintenance of PTSD (Ehlers & Clark, 2000), and involves teaching patients to identify and evaluate the evidence for negative automatic thoughts, as well as helping patients to evaluate their beliefs about the trauma, the self, the world, and the future in an evidence-based manner. Across most randomized controlled trials, the length of treatment is usually between 8 and 12 weekly individual sessions.

Over the past two decades, there have been many well-controlled trials that attest to the efficacy of CBT, and arguably of the role of exposure in reducing PTSD symptom (Foa et al., 2009). Although there is evidence that cognitive restructuring can be efficacious (Resick, Galovski, O'Brien, Scher, Clum, & Young-Xu, 2008), and even augment the effects of exposure (Bryant, Moulds, Guthrie, Dang, & Nixon, 2003), most studies have employed exposure as a central strategy. The efficacy of treating PTSD with CBT has resulted in efforts toward secondary prevention by applying CBT to high-risk trauma survivors shortly after trauma exposure. Some studies have focused on individuals who meet criteria for acute stress disorder (ASD). By providing abridged forms of CBT that include the same components as with chronic PTSD to patients with ASD, there is strong evidence that CBT can limit development of PTSD in the majority of cases relative to supportive counseling (Bryant, Harvey, Dang, Sackville, & Basten, 1998; Bryant et al., 2008; Bryant, Sackville, Dang, Moulds, & Guthrie, 1999). Similar results have been found by applying CBT strategies to patients with elevated PTSD in the initial months after trauma exposure (Bisson, Shepherd, Joy, Probert, & Newcombe, 2004; Ehlers et al., 2003; Sijbrandij et al., 2007).

A range of variants of trauma-focused therapy have proven efficacy. One variant, eye movement desensitization and reprocessing (EMDR), requires the patient to focus his or her attention on a traumatic memory while simultaneously visually tracking the therapist's finger as it is moved across his or her visual field, and then to engage in restructuring of the memory (Shapiro, 1995). The patient identifies more adaptive or positive thoughts related to the memory or traumatic experience, and to again track the therapist's fingers; in this sense, EMDR includes both exposure and cognitive restructuring components. Across a series of trials it has shown to be as effective as CBT, especially when it is combined with *in vivo* exposure guidelines (Australian Centre for Posttraumatic Mental Health, 2007; Spates, Koch, Cusack, Pagoto, & Waller, 2009). Another variant is cognitive processing therapy (CPT), in which attention is focused on reframing unrealistic beliefs about safety, trust, control, esteem, and intimacy; CPT also engages trauma memories by requiring the patient to write detailed accounts of the trauma and relating these accounts to the therapist (Resick & Schnicke, 1993). Interestingly, a recent trial indicated that the effects of CPT can be achieved by focusing on modification of cognitive factors in the absence of writing about the traumatic experience (Resick et al., 2008). There have also been recent modifications to CBT that attempt to prepare patients with poor emotion tolerance capacity to manage the distress of exposure—this form of CBT has been shown to result in fewer dropouts and better outcomes than standard CBT (Cloitre et al., 2010).

In terms of the evidence base for treating MTBI-related PTSD, there is currently only one controlled trial. In this study patients with ASD following MTBI were provided with five 1.5-hour weekly individual therapy sessions (Bryant, Moulds, Guthrie, & Nixon, 2003b). Patients were randomized to either CBT or supportive counseling. CBT included education about posttraumatic reactions, relaxation training, cognitive restructuring, and imaginal and *in vivo* exposure to the traumatic event. Imaginal exposure focused on those aspects of the trauma memory that patients could recall. The supportive counseling condition included trauma education and more general problem-solving skills training in the context of an unconditionally supportive relationship. Fewer participants receiving CBT (8%) met criteria for PTSD at 6-months follow-up than those receiving supportive counselling (58%). At this point in time, there are no controlled trials of treating mTBI-related chronic PTSD.

Mechanisms of CBT

Two major classes of models can account for CBT: (1) fear conditioning and (2) cognitive models. Both approaches have specific relevance to treating patients with PTSD following TBI. Fear conditioning models posit that a traumatic event (the unconditioned stimulus) leads to a fear reaction (the unconditioned response), which becomes conditioned to many stimuli associated with the traumatic event. Accordingly, when people are exposed to reminders of the trauma (conditioned stimuli), they experience a strong fear reaction (conditioned response) (Milad, Rauch, Pitman, & Quirk, 2006). Supporting this proposal is a large body of evidence that patients with PTSD have strong conditioned responses to trauma reminders (Orr et al., 2000; Orr, Solomon, Peri, Pitman, & Shalev, 1997; Pitman, Orr, Forgue, de Jong, & Claiborn, 1987). According to this model, successful recovery from trauma, including application of CBT, involves extinction learning, in which repeated exposure to trauma reminders or memories results in new learning that these reminders no longer signal threat (Milad et al., 2006). As exposure therapy involves repeated exposures to memories and reminders until the patient masters their anxiety, CBT is conceptualized as a form of extinction learning in which conditioned fear responses are inhibited by new learning of safe associations.

The other major class of models that account for change in CBT adopts a cognitive perspective (Ehlers & Clark, 2000). Cognitive models posit that PTSD responses are influenced by (1) maladaptive appraisals of the trauma and its aftermath, and (2) disturbances in autobiographical memory that involve impaired retrieval and strong associative memory. In these models, it is proposed that mental representations of the traumatic experience are encoded at the time of trauma under conditions of extreme stress, and accordingly are often encoded in fragmented ways. This results in these memories not being adequately integrated into one's normal autobiographical memory base, which contributes to intrusive memories and ongoing disorder. It is argued that these memories need to be integrated into normal autobiographical memory because this permits mastery of the memory and associated anxiety (similar to extinction learning). It is for this reason that cognitive models support the use of exposure therapy because it facilitates the integration of trauma memories into a coherent narrative of the event.

Cognitive models also place considerable emphasis on how people appraise the event, one's role in the experience, how one is responding to the event, and the likelihood of future harm. Supporting this position is a large body of evidence that catastrophic appraisals about oneself or one's future in the period after trauma exposure predict subsequent PTSD (Dunmore, Clark, & Ehlers, 1999; Ehlers, Mayou, & Bryant, 1998; Warda & Bryant, 1998). Similarly, patients who adopt a cognitive style that catastrophizes about the likelihood of recovery also respond poorly to treatment (Ehlers, Clark, et al., 1998).

The change mechanisms operating in CBT are apparently multifaceted, and particularly those underpinning exposure therapy (Jaycox & Foa, 1996; Rothbaum & Schwartz, 2002). Patients may benefit from CBT because it (1) promotes habituation to feared stimuli, (2) promotes correction of the belief that anxiety remains unless avoidance occurs, (3) impedes the negative reinforcement associated with fear reduction that leads to cognitive avoidance, (4) facilitates integration of corrective information into the trauma memory, (5) promotes establishment of a coherent narrative of the traumatic memory, (6) establishes the trauma as a discrete event that is not indicative of the world being globally threatening, and (7) enhances self-mastery through management of therapy exercises.

Potential Treatment Issues Arising from TBI

Fear Conditioning after TBI

Can fear conditioning explain PTSD following TBI? Earlier commentators proposed that PTSD would not develop after TBI because the absence of conscious memories precludes associations of fear (Sbordone & Liter, 1995). Consistent with this notion, there is evidence that the strength of fear conditioning partially depends on the individual's awareness of the contingency between the unconditioned stimulus and the response (Shanks & Lovibond, 2002). In contrast, patients with severe TBI who are amnesic of their trauma can develop PTSD; these patients tend to not have actual intrusive memories of the event but suffer reexperiencing in the form of distress or physiological reactivity to reminders of the trauma (Bryant, Marosszeky, Crooks, & Gurka, 2000). This pattern suggests that some form of conditioning can occur. Further support for this notion comes from evidence that severe TBI patients who do eventually develop PTSD have higher resting heart rates immediately after the traumatic injury than those patients who do not develop PTSD (Bryant, Marosszeky, Crooks, & Gurka, 2004). This finding is consistent with many studies of non-TBI patients (Bryant, 2006), and suggests that the strength of the unconditioned response (reflected by increased heart rate) may reflect stronger conditioning.

Exposure-based therapy is founded on the premise that extinction learning occurs when the conditioned stimulus is repeatedly presented in the absence of an aversive outcome, thereby facilitating new learning that the stimulus is no longer signaling threat. In the context of CBT, presenting memories or reminders of the trauma to the patient in the safety of therapy normally leads to symptom reduction. On the premise that fear conditioning and extinction still occurs in the context of TBI, this would suggest that exposure-based therapy is an indicated intervention for PTSD following TBI. Supporting this conclusion is evidence that patients with acute stress disorder following mTBI that CBT effectively treated PTSD symptoms to a similar extent as when applied to non-TBI samples (Bryant et al., 2003b).

Related to the process of extinction learning is recent work conducted on the neural circuitry of extinction. The amygdala is central to the development and expression of conditioned fear reactions, and human and animal studies have shown that learning to inhibit these fear reactions (i.e., extinction learning) involves inhibition by the medial prefrontal cortex (Milad, et al., 2007). Prevailing biological models of PTSD propose that PTSD involves exaggerated amygdala response and impaired regulation by the medial prefrontal cortex (Charney, Deutch, Krystal, Southwick, & Davis, 1993). Consistent with this model, patients with PTSD have diminished medial prefrontal cortex during processing of fear (Lanius, Bluhm, Lanius, & Pain, 2006). Recent neuroimaging studies indicate that the capacity of PTSD patients to respond to CBT is associated with the size of their rostral anterior cingulate, which is a critical region associated with the medial prefrontal cortex (Bryant, Felmingham, Whitford, et al., 2008). Further, poor CBT response is predicted by reactivity of the amygdala to fearful faces prior to treatment, suggesting that inadequate regulation of fear may hinder treatment response (Bryant, Felmingham, Kemp, et al., 2008). TBI often involves damage to the prefrontal cortex, and so it is possible that an individual's capacity to regulate his or her's fear reaction may be impaired after TBI because the neural networks involved in regulation of anxiety may be damaged as a result of the mTBI (Bryant, 2008). This possibility suggests that exposure-based therapies may need to be modified to accommodate the impaired capacity of TBI patients to regulate distress and learn that previously conditioned stimuli are no longer threatening.

Developing a Coherent Narrative

As noted above, cognitive models posit that recovery from a traumatic experience involves integrating the trauma memory into one's autobiographical memory base in a way that promotes a coherent narrative of the experience (Ehlers & Clark, 2000). This perspective holds that one reason trauma memories are difficult to integrate into memory is the manner in which they are encoded—experiences are often fragmented because they are encoded under conditions of extreme arousal. It is important to note that fragmented memories of the traumatic experience can also occur in the context of TBI because of the impaired consciousness secondary to the injury. It has been documented that patients with TBI can reconstruct the traumatic experience in the period after the injury in a way that includes the period during which they were unconscious. One longitudinal study found that 40% of patients with mTBI reported direct memories of the trauma 2 years after the injury even though they reported amnesia of these events at an assessment shortly after the event (Harvey & Bryant, 2001). This tendency is consistent with much research that trauma survivors tend to reconstruct their trauma over time, such that the content often changes: people tend to recall events more negatively when they experience more severe PTSD, and conversely they recall initial events more positively when they are enjoying good mental health (Harvey & Bryant, 2000; Southwick, Morgan, Nicolaou, & Charney, 1997). One of the challenges for treating PTSD after TBI is the patient's ability to reconstruct events in a coherent way because cognitive models argue that this is an important mechanism to facilitate adaptation.

The extent to which a person with TBI needs to reconstruct the trauma narrative to recover from PTSD has yet to be empirically determined. Several large-scale studies have recently reported that mTBI may be associated with increased risk for PTSD, including studies of combat troops returning from Iraq or Afghanistan (Hoge et al., 2008; Schneiderman, Braver, & Kang, 2008) and civilians who suffer traumatic injuries (Bryant et al., 2010). One possibility for this observation may be that people who sustain an mTBI do not have a coherent narrative of their traumatic experience because of the impaired consciousness secondary to the brain injury, and this may impede their capacity to contextualize the experience in their autobiographical memory base.

On the other hand, there is evidence that the fewer details one recalls of the traumatic experience (Gil, Caspi, Ben-Ari, Koren, & Klein, 2005) and the longer one experiences posttraumatic amnesia (Bryant et al., 2009), then the less likely one will experience PTSD symptoms. Other studies have found that amnesia is linearly related to reduced rates of PTSD (Bombardier et al., 2006; Glaesser, Neuner, Lutgehetmann, Schmidt, & Elbert, 2004; Levin et al., 2001; Sbordone & Liter, 1995; Warden & Labbate, 2005). This evidence suggests that having a full narrative of the trauma experience may not be necessary for successful adaptation to a traumatic experience. On the contrary, not being able to recall particularly distressing aspects of the event may serve a protective function because one does not have certain anxiety-producing memories.

There is also evidence that TBI patients can reconstruct the traumatic experience in ways that can exacerbate their anxiety. Case studies indicate that even patients with severe TBI with no memory of their traumatic experience can reconstruct their experience, and this is influenced strongly by current mood. For example, one patient who sustained a severe TBI in a motor vehicle accident presented with delayed-onset PTSD a year after his accident when he was required to commence driving again—this patient reported compelling intrusive "memories" that were based on newspaper pictures that he had subsequently seen of his mangled car (Bryant, 1996). As time progressed, he was encouraged to drive with his children in the car—at that time his intrusive images included his children (who were not in the accident) being injured in his accident. This case reflects the tendency for people to reconstruct their autobiographical memories in the context of current concerns and emotional states. Prevailing models of memory propose that people constantly reconstruct their memories in ways that are consistent with their current self-construct (Conway & Pleydell-Pearce, 2000). Accordingly, a TBI patient who is highly anxious about future trauma or one who feels very guilty about his or her role in the traumatic event may re-create events in ways that highlight fear or guilt. In this sense, therapy with patients with TBI need to be cognizant of advantages of reconstructing events in ways that are adaptive rather than reconstructions that highlight extreme threat or other maladaptive emotional responses.

Adapting Trauma-Focused Therapy for Patients with mTBI

Psychoeducation

All trauma-focused therapy requires a clear rationale at the commencement to ensure that the patient understands the treatment framework and enters therapy with a sense of optimism and mastery. This is especially important in the case of mTBI because of the potential for the patient to attribute symptoms to neurological insult. In the wake of the attention given to mTBI in military and civilian contexts in recent years, some agencies have promoted awareness of "mTBI symptoms," including postconcussive symptoms—deficits in memory and concentration, impaired balance, ringing in the ears, sensitivity to light or sound, and irritability. This policy has the potential to result in mTBI patients seeking treatment for PTSD to have expectations that stress-related symptoms may be a function of organic brain injury rather than a traumatic stressor. That is, some patients with mTBI may have a low expectation of treatment success because they do not expect brain damage-related symptoms to resolve. There is now very strong evidence that stress factors are a major determinant of mTBI-related symptoms, including postconcussive symptoms (Meares et al., 2008). Treatment of PTSD with mTBI patients should emphasize at the outset that some of their postacute symptoms may be attributable to PTSD reactions rather than to neurological insult, and that they can be treated through proven techniques. Encouraging a sense of expectancy is important at the outset of treatment and dispelling any misconceptions about the role of mTBI as the cause of symptoms can assist the patient to embark on treatment in a positive manner.

Exposure Therapy

The use of imaginal exposure in TBI patients depends on the severity of TBI, and the extent to which patients have memories of the experience. Most patients with a mTBI have islands of memory that involve the period after resumption of a few minutes of impaired consciousness. For many patients with PTSD, these memories may involve transport in an ambulance or experiencing painful medical procedures in an emergency room setting. These experiences can form the basis of the traumatic memories that can be consolidated in the same manner as memories in patients who do not sustain a TBI. Imaginal exposure with mTBI patients will typically focus on the aspects of the trauma memory that they do recall. Patients should understand that the goal of imaginal exposure is to retain focus of the feared memory so they learn to master it *rather* than being able to retrieve the entire episode. Accordingly, patients need to understand that one does not need to have full memory of the experience in order to enjoy treatment gains.

Imaginal exposure will not be as relevant to patients with more severe TBI because they are largely amnesic of their trauma. Some severe TBI patients can have nightmares or can develop intrusive memories or even flashbacks on the basis of reconstructions of their trauma (e.g., on the basis of police reports, media accounts, or photographs of their traumatic event).

In these cases, one can administer imaginable exposure to those mental representations that are causing anxiety. In most cases of moderate/severe TBI, however, it is more useful to employ *in vivo* exposure because reminders of the trauma may elicit anxiety in the absence of actual memories or images. A survivor of a motor vehicle accident who sustained a severe TBI may experience marked fear when watching film footage of traffic; in such a case, the patient could complete exposure by repeatedly watching traffic footage. Additionally, therapy can systematically expose the patient to increasingly anxiety-provoking situations that elicit fear, ensuring that each situation is mastered prior to commencing the next step. In this way extinction learning can be achieved, even though the patient may never have memories of the traumatic event.

Cognitive Restructuring

The other major strategy of CBT is cognitive restructuring. Several modifications may be warranted in delivery of this strategy to patients with TBI. In terms of the content or themes that often arise in patients with TBI is the issue that they cannot recall some pivotal aspect of the experience. It is understandable to want to make sense of an experience that has had some impact on one's life, and this is difficult when one cannot recall the details of it. Cognitive restructuring often needs to assist the patient to accept the reality that he or she did not encode the information during periods of impaired consciousness. It also can assist the patient to reconstruct the experience in an adaptive way. Some patients may experience guilt, anger, shame, or excessive fear because of the manner in which they interpret events that occurred during loss of consciousness. For example, a patient may accuse himself of killing his partner because he erred in his driving and he may exacerbate his mistakes in his reconstruction of events. Therapy can assist him to use available information to reconstruct events in a way that does not catastrophize the event. Even if this patient was at fault and did cause the accident in which his partner died, therapy can encourage a reconstruction that does not exacerbate aspects of the event that cause greater guilt than is appropriate.

In terms of delivery mode, some mTBI patients may present with cognitive impairments. Although cognitive impairment is typically observed following moderate/severe TBI, as described by Iverson (Chapter 3, this volume), some mTBI patients can present with attentional and memory deficits. These may be attributed to a combination of pain, stress, sleep disturbance, and some neurological factors interacting in the postinjury phase. Limitations in attentional capacity may require more directive cognitive restructuring than normal in ways that do not rely entirely on the patient's ability to (1) engage in abstract reasoning or probabilistic thinking, or (2) to remember to engage in thought monitoring or challenging outside therapy sessions. In cases where one suspects cognitive deficits, it can be useful to use directive cognitive restructuring that informs the patient about specific thoughts to rehearse, and possibly provide written cards to remind the patient to rehearse specific thoughts.

Postconcussive Symptoms

Although postconcussive symptoms are not symptoms of PTSD, it is worth noting that there is considerable overlap between the two constructs. Moreover, PTSD is a major predictor of postconcussive reactions. Although data are lacking on this point, it can be useful to adapt cognitive restructuring to also include maladaptive appraisals about any postconcussive symptoms. Specifically, patients who are overly concerned, for example, about the adverse outcomes of dizziness or sensitivity to light can be taught to normalize these reactions in ways that minimize distress about these sensations. In this way, cognitive restructuring can be adapted in a way comparable to treating panic disorder. In panic disorder, one induces the feared somatic sensation (e.g., making the patient dizzy by spinning in a chair) and having him or her practice appraisals that dizziness is not harmful. Focusing on any postconcussive symptoms that causes distress to the patient and teaching patients to interpret the sensations more adaptively may alleviate the significance of the target symptom. It is also possible that the alleviation of stress reactions via exposure may also contribute to reduced postconcussive symptoms. This outcome may potentially be achieved by reducing (1) arousal, (2) attention to negative symptoms, or (3) cognitive load that depletes one's capacity to manage symptoms.

Conclusions

Recent studies highlight that a significant proportion of PTSD patients have experienced an mTBI. Accordingly, there is a need to better understand how a history of mTBI may impact on treating PTSD symptoms. Overall, there are few marked treatment-relevant differences between most mTBI and no-TBI PTSD patients, with the exception that people who experience an mTBI may have only partial memory of the traumatic experience that resulted in both PTSD and brain injury. More importantly, when the TBI and psychologically traumatic event are one in the same, treatment is optimally presented in a way that minimizes the role of the brain injury and normalizes that aspect of the trauma. Subtle differences may exist in PTSD patients with mTBI but further research is needed to clarify if these factors substantially impact on treatment delivery.

References

Australian Centre for Posttraumatic Mental Health. (2007). *Australian guidelines for the treatment of adults with acute stress disorder and posttraumatic stress disorder: Practitioner guide.* Melbourne, Victoria: Author.

Bedard-Gilligan, M., & Zoellner, L. A. (2008). The utility of the A1 and A2 criteria in the diagnosis of PTSD. *Behaviour Research and Therapy, 46*(9), 1062–1069.

Bisson, J. I., Shepherd, J. P., Joy, D., Probert, R., & Newcombe, R. G. (2004). Early cognitive-behavioural therapy for post-traumatic stress symptoms after physical injury: Randomised controlled trial [see comment]. *British Journal of Psychiatry, 184* (Suppl.), 63–69.

Bombardier, C. H., Fann, J. R., Temkin, N., Esselman, P. C., Pelzer, E., Keough, M., et al. (2006). Posttraumatic stress disorder symptoms during the first six months after traumatic brain injury. *Journal of Neuropsychiatry and Clinical Neurosciences, 18*(4), 501–508.

Breslau, N., & Kessler, R. C. (2001). The stressor criterion in DSM-IV posttraumatic stress disorder: An empirical investigation. *Biological Psychiatry, 50*(9), 699–704.

Bryant, R. A. (1996). Posttraumatic stress disorder, flashbacks, and pseudomemories in closed head injury. *Journal of Traumatic Stress, 9*(3), 621–629.

Bryant, R. A. (2001). Posttraumatic stress disorder and traumatic brain injury: Can they co-exist? *Clinical Psychology Review, 21*(6), 931–948.

Bryant, R. A. (2006). Longitudinal psychophysiological studies of heart rate: Mediating effects and implications for treatment. In R. Yehuda (Ed.), *Psychobiology of posttraumatic stress disorder: A decade of progress* (Vol. 1071, pp. 19–26). New York: New York Academy of Science.

Bryant, R. A. (2008). Disentangling mild traumatic brain injury and stress reactions. *New England Journal of Medicine, 358*(5), 525–527.

Bryant, R. A., Creamer, M., O'Donnell, M., Silove, D., Clark, C. R., & McFarlane, A. C. (2009). Post-traumatic amnesia and the nature of post-traumatic stress disorder after mild traumatic brain injury. *Journal of the International Neuropsychological Society, 15*(6), 862–867.

Bryant, R. A., Creamer, M., O'Donnell, M., Silove, D., Clark, C. R., & McFarlane, A. C. (2010). The psychiatric sequelae of traumatic injury. *American Journal of Psychiatry, 167,* 312–320.

Bryant, R. A., Felmingham, K. L., Kemp, A., Das, P., Hughes, G., Peduto, A., et al. (2008a). Amygdala and ventral anterior cingulate activation predicts treatment response to cognitive behaviour therapy for post-traumatic stress disorder. *Psychological Medicine, 38,* 555–561.

Bryant, R. A., Felmingham, K. L., Whitford, T., Kemp, A., Hughes, G., Peduto, A., et al. (2008b). Rostral anterior cingulate volume predicts treatment response to cognitive behavior therapy for posttraumatic stress disorder. *Journal of Psychiatry and Neuroscience, 33,* 142–146.

Bryant, R. A., & Harvey, A. G. (1998). Relationship between acute stress disorder and posttraumatic stress disorder following mild traumatic brain injury. *American Journal of Psychiatry, 155*(5), 625–629.

Bryant, R. A., Harvey, A. G., Dang, S. T., Sackville, T., & Basten, C. (1998). Treatment of acute stress disorder: A comparison of cognitive-behavioral therapy and supportive counseling. *Journal of Consulting and Clinical Psychology, 66*(5), 862–866.

Bryant, R. A., Marosszeky, J. E., Crooks, J., & Gurka, J. A. (2000). Posttraumatic stress disorder after severe traumatic brain injury. *American Journal of Psychiatry, 157*(4), 629–631.

Bryant, R. A., Marosszeky, J. E., Crooks, J., & Gurka, J. A. (2004). Elevated resting heart rate as a predictor of posttraumatic stress disorder after severe traumatic brain injury. *Psychosomatic Medicine, 66*(5), 760–761.

Bryant, R. A., Mastrodomenico, J., Felmingham, K. L., Hopwood, S., Kenny, L., Kandris, E., et al. (2008). Treatment of acute stress disorder: A randomized controlled trial. *Archives of General Psychiatry, 65*(6), 659–667.

Bryant, R. A., Moulds, M. L., Guthrie, R. M., Dang, S. T., & Nixon, R. D. (2003). Imaginal exposure alone and imaginal exposure with cognitive restructuring in treatment of posttraumatic stress disorder. *Journal of Consulting Clinical Psychology, 71*(4), 706–712.

Bryant, R. A., Moulds, M., Guthrie, R., & Nixon, R. D. (2003b). Treating acute stress disorder following mild traumatic brain injury. *American Journal of Psychiatry, 160*(3), 585–587.

Bryant, R. A., Sackville, T., Dang, S. T., Moulds, M., & Guthrie, R. (1999). Treating acute stress disorder: An evaluation of cognitive behavior therapy and supportive counseling techniques. *American Journal of Psychiatry, 156*(11), 1780–1786.

Charney, D. S., Deutch, A. Y., Krystal, J. H., Southwick, S. M., & Davis, M. (1993). Psychobiologic mechanisms of posttraumatic stress disorder. *Archives of General Psychiatry, 50*, 294–305.

Cloitre, M., Stovall-McClough, K. C., Nooner, K., Zorbas, P., Cherry, S., Jackson, C. L., et al. (2010). Treatment for PTSD related to childhood abuse: A randomized controlled trial. *American Journal of Psychiatry, 167*(8), 915–924.

Conway, M. A., & Pleydell-Pearce, C. W. (2000). The construction of autobiographical memories in the self-memory system. *Psychological Review, 107*(2), 261–288.

Dunmore, E., Clark, D. M., & Ehlers, A. (1999). Cognitive factors involved in the onset and maintenance of posttraumatic stress disorder (PTSD) after physical or sexual assault. *Behaviour Research and Therapy, 37*(9), 809–829.

Ehlers, A., & Clark, D. M. (2000). A cognitive model of posttraumatic stress disorder. *Behaviour Research and Therapy, 38*(4), 319–345.

Ehlers, A., Clark, D. M., Dunmore, E., Jaycox, L. H., Meadows, E. A., & Foa, E. B. (1998). Predicting response to exposure treatment in PTSD: The role of mental defeat and alienation. *Journal of Traumatic Stress, 11*(3), 457–471.

Ehlers, A., Clark, D. M., Hackmann, A., McManus, F., Fennell, M., Herbert, C., et al. (2003). A randomized controlled trial of cognitive therapy, a self-help booklet, and repeated assessments as early interventions for posttraumatic stress disorder. *Archives of General Psychiatry, 60*(10), 1024–1032.

Ehlers, A., Mayou, R. A., & Bryant, B. (1998). Psychological predictors of chronic posttraumatic stress disorder after motor vehicle accidents. *Journal of Abnormal Psychology, 107*(3), 508–519.

National Collaborating Centre for Mental Health. (2005). *Posttraumatic stress disorder: The management of PTSD in adults and children in primary and secondary care.* Volume 26. London: National Centre for Clinical Excellence.

Foa, E. B. (2000). Psychosocial treatment of posttraumatic stress disorder. *Journal of Clinical Psychiatry, 61*(Suppl. 5), 43–48; discussion 49–51.

Foa, E. B. (2006). Psychosocial therapy for posttraumatic stress disorder. *Journal of Clinical Psychiatry, 67*(Suppl. 2), 40–45.

Foa, E. B., Keane, T. M., Friedman, M. J., & Cohen, J. A. (Eds.). (2009). *Effective treatments for PTSD: Practice guidelines from the International Society of Traumatic Stress Studies* (2nd ed.). New York: Guilford Press.

Foa, E. B., & Meadows, A. (1997). Psychosocial treatments for posttraumatic stress disorder: A critical review. *Annual Review of Psychology, 48,* 449–480.

Forbes, D., Creamer, M., Phelps, A., Bryant, R., McFarlane, A., Devilly, G. J., et al. (2007). Australian guidelines for the treatment of adults with acute stress disorder and post-traumatic stress disorder. *Australian and New Zealand Journal of Psychiatry, 41*(8), 637–648.

Friedman, M. J., Resick, P. A., Bryant, R. A., Brewin, C. R. (in press). Considering PTSD for DSM-V. *Depression and Anxiety.*

Gil, S., Caspi, Y., Ben-Ari, I. Z., Koren, D., & Klein, E. (2005). Does memory of a traumatic event increase the risk for posttraumatic stress disorder in patients with traumatic brain injury?: A prospective study. *American Journal of Psychiatry, 162*(5), 963–969.

Glaesser, J., Neuner, F., Lutgehetmann, R., Schmidt, R., & Elbert, T. (2004). Post-traumatic stress disorder in patients with traumatic brain injury. *BMC Psychiatry, 4,* 5.

Harvey, A. G., & Bryant, R. A. (2000). Memory for acute stress disorder symptoms—A two-year prospective study. *Journal of Nervous and Mental Disease, 188*(9), 602–607.

Harvey, A. G., & Bryant, R. A. (2001). Reconstructing trauma memories: A prospective study of "amnesic" trauma survivors. *Journal of Traumatic Stress, 14*(2), 277–282.

Harvey, A. G., Bryant, R. A., & Tarrier, N. (2003). Cognitive behaviour therapy for posttraumatic stress disorder. *Clinical Psychology Review, 23*(3), 501–522.

Hoge, C. W., McGurk, D., Thomas, J. L., Cox, A. L., Engel, C. C., & Castro, C. A. (2008). Mild traumatic brain injury in US Soldiers returning from Iraq. *New England Journal of Medicine, 358*(5), 453–463.

Jaycox, L. H., & Foa, E. B. (1996). Obstacles in implementing exposure therapy for PTSD: Case discussions and practical solutions. *Clinical Psychology and Psychotherapy, 3,* 176–184.

Lanius, R. A., Bluhm, R., Lanius, U., & Pain, C. (2006). A review of neuroimaging studies in PTSD: Heterogeneity of response to symptom provocation. *Journal of Psychiatric Research, 40*(8), 709–729.

Levin, H. S., Brown, S. A., Song, J. X., McCauley, S. R., Boake, C., Contant, C. F., et al. (2001). Depression and posttraumatic stress disorder at three months after mild to moderate traumatic brain injury. *Journal of Clinical and Experimental Neuropsychology, 23*(6), 754–769.

Meares, S., Shores, E. A., Taylor, A. J., Batchelor, J., Bryant, R. A., Baguley, I. J., et al. (2008). Mild traumatic brain injury does not predict acute postconcussion syndrome. *Journal of Neurology, Neurosurgery and Psychiatry, 79*(3), 300–306.

Milad, M. R., Rauch, S. L., Pitman, R. K., & Quirk, G. J. (2006). Fear extinction in rats: Implications for human brain imaging and anxiety disorders. *Biological Psychology, 73*(1), 61–71.

Milad, M. R., Wright, C. I., Orr, S. P., Pitman, R. K., Quirk, G. J., & Rauch, S. L. (2007). Recall of fear extinction in humans activates the ventromedial prefrontal cortex and hippocampus in concert. *Biological Psychiatry, 62*(5), 446–454.

O'Donnell, M. L., Creamer, M., Bryant, R. A., Schnyder, U., & Shalev, A. (2003). Posttraumatic disorders following injury: An empirical and methodological review. *Clinical Psychology Review, 23*(4), 587–603.

Orr, S. P., Metzger, L. J., Lasko, N. B., Macklin, M. L., Peri, T., & Pitman, R. K. (2000). De novo conditioning in trauma-exposed individuals with and without posttraumatic stress disorder. *Journal of Abnormal Psychology, 109*(2), 290–298.

Orr, S. P., Solomon, Z., Peri, T., Pitman, R. K., & Shalev, A. Y. (1997). Physiologic responses to loud tones in Israeli veterans of the 1973 Yom Kippur War. *Biological Psychiatry, 41*(3), 319–326.

Pitman, R. K., Orr, S. P., Forgue, D. F., de Jong, J. T., & Claiborn, J. (1987). Psychophysiologic assessment of posttraumatic stress disorder imagery in Vietnam combat veterans. *Archives of General Psychiatry, 44*(11), 970–975.

Resick, P. A., Galovski, T. E., O'Brien U., M., Scher, C. D., Clum, G. A., & Young-Xu, Y. (2008). A randomized clinical trial to dismantle components of cognitive processing therapy for posttraumatic stress disorder in female victims of interpersonal violence. *Journal of Consulting and Clinical Psychology, 76*(2), 243–258.

Resick, P. A., & Schnicke, M. K. (1993). *Cognitive processing therapy for sexual assault victims: A treatment manual.* Newbury Park, CA: Sage.

Rothbaum, B. O., Ruef, A. M., Litz, B. T., Han, H., & Hodges, L. (2003). Virtual reality exposure therapy of combat-related PTSD: A case study using psychophysiological indicators of outcome. *Journal of Cognitive Psychotherapy, 17*, 163–177.

Rothbaum, B. O., & Schwartz, A. C. (2002). Exposure therapy for posttraumatic stress disorder. *American Journal of Psychotherapy, 56*(1), 59–75.

Sbordone, R. J., & Liter, J. C. (1995). Mild traumatic brain injury does not produce post-traumatic stress disorder. *Brain Injury, 9*(4), 405–412.

Schneiderman, A. I., Braver, E. R., & Kang, H. K. (2008). Understanding sequelae of injury mechanisms and mild traumatic brain injury incurred during the conflicts in Iraq and Afghanistan: persistent postconcussive symptoms and posttraumatic stress disorder. *American Journal of Epidemiology, 167*(12), 1446–1452.

Shanks, D. R., & Lovibond, P. F. (2002). Autonomic and eyeblink conditioning are closely related to contingency awareness: reply to Wiens and Ohman (2002) and Manns et al. (2002). *Journal of Experimental Psychology Animal Behavior Processes, 28*(1), 38–42.

Shapiro, F. (1995). *Eye movement desensitization and reprocessing: Basic principles, protocols, and procedures.* New York: Guilford Press.

Sijbrandij, M., Olff, M., Reitsma, J. B., Carlier, I. V. E., de Vries, M. H., & Gersons, B. P. R. (2007). Treatment of acute posttraumatic stress disorder with brief cognitive behavioral therapy: A randomized controlled trial. *American Journal of Psychiatry, 164*(1), 82–90.

Southwick, S. M., Morgan, A., Nicolaou, A. L., & Charney, D. S. (1997). Consistency of memory for combat-related traumatic events in veterans of Operation Desert Storm. *American Journal of Psychiatry, 154*(2), 173–177.

Spates, C. R., Koch, E., Cusack, K., Pagoto, S., & Waller, S. (2009). Eye movement desensitization and reprocessing. In E. B. Foa, T. M. Keane, M. J. Freidman, & J. A. Cohen (Eds.), *Effective treatments for PTSD: Practice guidelines from the International Society for Traumatic Stress Studies* (pp. 279–305). New York: Guilford Press.

van Etten, M. L., & Taylor, S. (1998). Comparative efficacy of treatments for posttraumatic stress disorder: A meta-analysis. *Clinical Psychology and Psychotherapy, 5*, 126–144.

Warda, G., & Bryant, R. A. (1998). Cognitive bias in acute stress disorder. *Behaviour Research and Therapy, 36*(12), 1177–1183.

Warden, D. L., & Labbate, L. A. (2005). Posttraumatic stress disorder and other anxiety disorders. In J. M. Silver, T. W. McAllister, & S. C. Yudofsky (Eds.), *Textbook of traumatic brain injury* (pp. 231–243). Arlington, VA: American Psychiatric Publishing.

CHAPTER 12

Implications for Service Delivery in the Military

Richard A. Bryant, Carl A. Castro, and Grant L. Iverson

During the recent wars in Iraq and Afghanistan, tremendous attention has been given to mild traumatic brain injury (mTBI) and posttraumatic stress disorder (PTSD). This chapter reviews the current evidence concerning the prevalence of mTBI in military personnel, differential diagnosis issues, the potential overlap between mTBI and PTSD, and implications for current practices in managing mTBI and PTSD.

Current Military Policies on mTBI

Most militaries have employed policies and programs aimed at identifying service members who may have experienced an mTBI. In the U.S. military, for example, there are two types of screening programs: acute and postdeployment. An obvious objective of screening for mTBI is to identify as early as possible service members who may have sustained an mTBI so they can either be rested or receive medical care.

In the U.S. military, service members who are within 100 meters of a blast are required to be screened for mTBI using the Military Acute Concussion Assessment (MACE; Coldren, Kelly, Parish, Dretsch, & Russell, 2010; Galetta et al., 2011), a three-part screening evaluation that includes the Standardized Assessment of Concussion (Barr & McCrea, 2001). If the service member is deemed to have suffered a concussion, he or she is placed on temporary profile for 72 hours to prevent him or her from being exposed to another blast. After his or her symptoms abate, he or she is returned to duty. A clinical practice guideline sets out the procedures for managing an mTBI during deployment. Interested readers can download this practice guideline from *www.healthquality.va.gov/mtbi/concussion_mtbi_full_1_0.pdf.*

Early upon returning home, all service members are screened for an mTBI that may have occurred during the deployment, and for which symptoms might still exist. Concerns have been expressed that this method for identifying service members with mTBI is flawed and that screening estimates are inflated (see Golding, Bass, Percy, & Goldberg, 2009; Hoge, Goldberg, & Castro, 2009).

Prevalence of mTBI in the Military

mTBIs in the military can occur before, during, or after operational deployment. In the recent and current conflicts, arguably the most common cause of mTBI comes in the form of an explosive device, which can result in exploded fragments striking the head, the force throwing a soldier through space, or blast injuries. Emotional consequences of the effects of the blast are also possible, either as a result of the injury or because of witnessing other military personnel and/or civilians sustaining injuries. These injuries can result in serious short-term physical, emotional, and cognitive symptoms that sometimes evolve into long-term changes in functioning. During deployment, many service members can experience a combination of physical injuries, psychological trauma, and mTBI. An mTBI and traumatic stress reaction can occur as a result of the same event or of separate events. Service members who are wounded in combat are at increased risk for PTSD (Ramchand et al., 2010), depression (Grieger et al., 2006), and/or chronic pain (Dobscha et al., 2009). These comorbidities make it challenging to determine if a service member does or does not suffer from residual symptoms associated with the original injury. Further, there is doubt over the exact neural effects of mTBI. Recent diffusion tremor imaging studies of troops exposed to blast injuries suggests that these injuries may result in axonal injury (MacDonald et al., 2011), although the current evidence is limited by methodological factors that do not allow firm conclusions to be drawn (Ropper, 2011). At this point we are limited by the dearth of strong neuroimaging evidence to clarify the specific effects of mTBI on military personnel.

The Defense and Veterans Brain Injury Center (DVBIC) released official surveillance numbers for medically diagnosed TBI in the military. The surveillance numbers represent individual service members who sustained

TABLE 12.1. TBI in the Military: 2000–2009

	2000	2001	2002	2003	2004	2005	2006	2007	2008	2009	2010
Total	10,963	11,830	12,470	12,898	13,312	12,192	16,946	23,160	28,555	29,252	30,703
Mild	6,333	7,771	8,989	9,790	10,556	9,894	13,998	18,786	21,964	22,696	24,846
Moderate	4,145	3,543	3,067	2,628	2,267	1,858	2,396	3,592	3,117	3,705	3,683
Severe	176	186	148	170	146	155	191	205	226	320	201
Penetrating	272	291	227	274	311	244	309	362	423	484	254
Not classifiable	37	39	39	36	32	41	52	215	2,825	2,047	1,719

Note. Data from Defense and Veterans Brain Injury Center (retrieved May 17, 2011, from *www.dvbic. org/TBI-Numbers.aspx*).

a TBI of any severity, anywhere in the world, between 2000 and 2010 (see Table 12.1). Injured service members were counted only once in order to represent the total number of injured people, not the total number of injuries (i.e., some service members have been injured more than once). The number of recorded TBIs increased significantly between 2006 and 2008. The reasons for this increase are unclear, and multiple factors could have contributed to the upswing, including possible changes to the methodology by which service members were screened and then clinically diagnosed. Over the years, there generally has been a gradual increase in the percentage of all injuries classified as mild.

Compared to the official DVBIC surveillance numbers, postdeployment screening studies have yielded far greater estimates for mTBI in military personnel returning from Iraq and Afghanistan (e.g., 11.2–22.8%; Hudon, Belleville, & Gauthier, 2008; Mental Health Advisory Team V, 2008; Schwab et al., 2007; Tanielian & Jaycox, 2008; Terrio et al., 2009), although these estimates have methodological limitations that limit their accuracy (Golding et al., 2009; Iverson, 2010; Iverson, Langlois, McCrea, & Kelly, 2009). As discussed in the next section, however, it is essential to appreciate that screening positive for a deployment-related mTBI on a questionnaire is not definitive evidence that the injury actually occurred or whether any residual symptoms or cognitive deficits are directly attributable to a brain injury (Iverson, 2010; Iverson et al., 2009).

Postdeployment Assessment of mTBI

Post-deployment health assessments occur at the end of deployment, while in theater, in transit, or shortly after return to the United States. The vast majority occur stateside. All U.S. service members complete a self-report questionnaire called the *Post-Deployment Health Assessment* (PDHA). The Department of Defense (DoD) TBI screening questions are reprinted in Table 12.2 and illustrated in Figure 12.1. The DoD and VA have harmonized their methodologies for TBI screening. Screening positive for a TBI results in a referral for a follow-up interview with a clinician. If the clinician believes the service member has ongoing symptoms and problems attributable to an mTBI, referrals are made for specialty evaluations, treatment, and rehabilitation services.

To screen positive for a deployment-related TBI, the service member or veteran must answer yes on all four screening questions (Table 12.2 and Figure 12.1). In practice, the screening questions will fail to identify those who were injured and fully recovered. Moreover, the screening

TABLE 12.2. DoD Post-Deployment Health Assessment

9.a. During this deployment, did you experience any of the following events? *(Mark all that apply)*
(1) Blast or explosion *(IED, RPG, land mine, grenade, etc.)*
☐ No ☐ Yes
(2) Vehicular accident/crash *(any vehicle, including aircraft)*
☐ No ☐ Yes
(3) Fragment wound or bullet wound above your shoulders
☐ No ☐ Yes
(4) Fall ☐ No ☐ Yes
(5) Other event *(for example, a sports injury to your head).*
☐ No ☐ Yes
Describe:

9.b. Did any of the following happen to you, or were you told happened to you, IMMEDIATELY after any of the event(s) you just noted in question 9.a.?
(Mark all that apply)
(1) Lost consciousness or got "knocked out" ☐ No ☐ Yes
(2) Felt dazed, confused, or "saw stars" ☐ No ☐ Yes
(3) Didn't remember the event ☐ No ☐ Yes
(4) Had a concussion ☐ No ☐ Yes
(5) Had a head injury ☐ No ☐ Yes

9.c. Did any of the following problems begin or get worse after the event(s) you noted in question 9.a.?
(Mark all that apply)
(1) Memory problems or lapses ☐ No ☐ Yes
(2) Balance problems or dizziness ☐ No ☐ Yes
(3) Ringing in the ears ☐ No ☐ Yes
(4) Sensitivity to bright light ☐ No ☐ Yes
(5) Irritability ☐ No ☐ Yes
(6) Headaches ☐ No ☐ Yes
(7) Sleep problems ☐ No ☐ Yes

9.d. In the past week, have you had any of the symptoms you indicated in 9.c.?
(Mark all that apply)
(1) Memory problems or lapses ☐ No ☐ Yes
(2) Balance problems or dizziness ☐ No ☐ Yes
(3) Ringing in the ears ☐ No ☐ Yes
(4) Sensitivity to bright light ☐ No ☐ Yes
(5) Irritability ☐ No ☐ Yes
(6) Headaches ☐ No ☐ Yes
(7) Sleep problems ☐ No ☐ Yes

Note. Questions from a U.S. Government survey that is completed by returning service members.

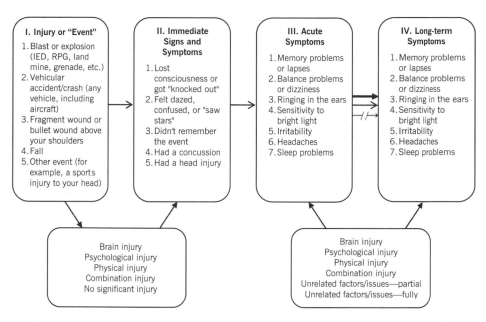

I. Injury or "Event"	II. Immediate Signs and Symptoms	III. Acute Symptoms	IV. Long-term Symptoms
1. Blast or explosion (IED, RPG, land mine, grenade, etc.) 2. Vehicular accident/crash (any vehicle, including aircraft) 3. Fragment wound or bullet wound above your shoulders 4. Fall 5. Other event (for example, a sports injury to your head)	1. Lost consciousness or got "knocked out" 2. Felt dazed, confused, or "saw stars" 3. Didn't remember the event 4. Had a concussion 5. Had a head injury	1. Memory problems or lapses 2. Balance problems or dizziness 3. Ringing in the ears 4. Sensitivity to bright light 5. Irritability 6. Headaches 7. Sleep problems	1. Memory problems or lapses 2. Balance problems or dizziness 3. Ringing in the ears 4. Sensitivity to bright light 5. Irritability 6. Headaches 7. Sleep problems

Brain injury
Psychological injury
Physical injury
Combination injury
No significant injury

Brain injury
Psychological injury
Physical injury
Combination injury
Unrelated factors/issues—partial
Unrelated factors/issues—fully

FIGURE 12.1. Challenges associated with postdeployment screening for mTBI. At step III (i.e., item 9.c. in Table 12.2), the acute symptoms, retrospectively endorsed following deployment, can relate to different types of injuries, different types of injuries plus unrelated factors such as sleep deprivation or general deployment-related stress, or unrelated factors entirely. In the transition from step III to step IV (i.e., item 9.d. in Table 12.2): (1) the symptoms can continue, strongly causally related, mostly unabated (dark arrow); (2) the symptoms can continue to a lesser degree and/or be less causally related to the original event (middle arrow), or (3) there can be a break in the chain of causation, indicating that the symptoms have improved or that later symptoms are likely attributable to something else (e.g., other events or conditions). From Iverson (2010). Copyright 2010 by Wolters Kluwer Health. Reprinted by permission.

questionnaire applies to the current deployment only. Therefore, injuries occurring during previous deployments, prior to the implementation of this screening program, might not be documented. Another concern regarding the screening questions is false positives. Each question in the screening process carries risk for false positive identification of mTBI. Question 9a refers to an "event" not an "injury." Therefore, it is possible that a person will endorse experiencing one or more of those events without actually being injured during the event. The events in 9a could represent an mTBI, traumatic stress reaction, physical injury, polytrauma, or no injury.

Question 9b attempts to document classic signs and symptoms of mTBI. The challenge at this step is that a service member who is psychologically traumatized, physically injured, or both could experience one or more of these signs and symptoms—especially feeling dazed, confused, or having poor memory for events immediately following the event. Alterations in mental status and poor memory for the event are associated with acute traumatic stress in civilians (Birmes et al., 2003; Cardeña & Spiegel, 1993; Freinkel, Koopman, & Spiegel, 1994; Harvey & Bryant, 1999; Madakasira & O'Brien, 1987). Thus, the immediate signs and symptoms in question 9b can be associated with an mTBI or occur for other reasons.

For question 9c, the service member is required to retrospectively rate symptoms experienced after an event that occurred weeks or months prior. These symptoms, if accurately recalled, could represent the acute consequences of an mTBI. They could also relate in whole or in part to other factors, such as acute traumatic stress, chronic stress, mild depression, sleep deprivation and fatigue, or bodily injuries. Similarly, for question 9d, the symptoms listed are nonspecific. It is well documented in the civilian literature that these symptoms are associated with chronic pain (Gasquoine, 2000; Iverson & McCracken, 1997; Radanov, Dvorak, & Valach, 1992; Smith-Seemiller, Fow, Kant, & Franzen, 2003) and depression (Iverson, 2006). Researchers have reported that service members and veterans with posttraumatic stress endorse some of these symptoms (Hudon et al., 2008; Schneiderman, Braver, & Kang, 2008). It has been found that high rates of symptoms reported by service members who screen positive for mTBI are mediated, in large part, by PTSD or depression (Hoge et al., 2008). In contrast, it has also been found that mTBI is independently related to symptom reporting in veterans (Vanderploeg, Belanger, & Curtiss, 2009).

One of the fundamental problems with military screening and follow-up assessments of TBI is comorbidity. In the presence of comorbidity, it is virtually impossible to determine the underlying cause, or more likely *causes*, of these symptoms using the existing tools. Symptom endorsement or reporting can be causally related to a past mTBI and/or be influenced by personality characteristics, life stress, psychiatric problems, substance abuse, symptom expectations, misattribution, and external incentives/secondary gains.[1] There is a tremendous effort underway within the Depart-

---

[1]PTSD is also screened postdeployment with the PDHA and Post-deployment Health Re-assessment (PDHRA). Like TBI, there are also methodological challenges associated with postdeployment screening for PTSD, including (1) preexisting PTSD symptoms not attributable to deployment; (2) risk of false positive and false negatives in the absence of a multimethod evaluation, including clinical diagnostic interviews; and (3) self-report bias, for which there is no established method of detecting on the PDHA/PDHRA.

ment of Defense (DoD) to better identify and document mTBI in-theater. Follow-up clinical evaluations are also necessary to determine more accurately whether an injury occurred and whether the person experiences residual symptoms and/or a comorbid condition. Even in-depth clinical evaluations, however, can result in false-positive or false-negative diagnoses of long-term problems associated with mTBI. More detailed discussion of assessment issues can be found in other chapters of this volume (Ulloa, Marx, Vanderploeg, & Vasterling, Chapter 8, and Elhai, Sweet, Guidotti Breting, & Kaloupek, Chapter 9, this volume).

Combat Exposure and Traumatic Stress

Large-scale surveys of service members and veterans have confirmed the relation between combat experiences and posttraumatic stress symptoms (Hoge et al., 2004; Hoge, Terhakopian, Castro, Messer, & Engel, 2007; Kang, Natelson, Mahan, Lee, & Murphy, 2003; Rona et al., 2009; Toomey et al., 2007). For example, in a survey of four U.S. combat infantry units, the prevalence of mental health disorders after deployment to Iraq was 27.9% (Hoge et al., 2004). In this study, 11.5–19.9% screened positive for PTSD using a liberal definition, and 6.2–12.9% screened positive using a strict definition. Service members reported a high frequency of contact with the enemy and high rates of potentially traumatic combat experiences (e.g., seeing dead bodies or human remains [95%], knowing someone who was seriously injured or killed [43%], or being responsible for the death of an enemy combatant [48%]). There was a strong relationship between the number of combat experiences and the rate of PTSD. For example, 9.3% of military personnel who were involved in one or two firefights screened positive for PTSD, compared to 19.3% of those involved in five or more firefights (Hoge et al., 2004).

mTBI and PTSD

The nature of traumatic experiences suffered during combat has been well documented (for a review, see Shephard, 2001). It is not surprising that rates of screening positive for PTSD following the Iraq and Afghanistan conflicts have been reported as high as 50% in service members and veterans who are seeking treatment (compared to 5–20% in those who are not seeking treatment; Ramchand et al., 2010). A key question facing the military is whether sustaining an mTBI impacts on risk of, and/or recovery from, PTSD. Some researchers have reported that injuries to the brain that result in loss of consciousness and posttraumatic amnesia are protective against PTSD because of the limited encoding of the traumatic experience (Bombardier et al., 2006; Levin et al., 2001; Sbordone & Liter, 1995). Low rates of PTSD have been reported in individuals who have sustained TBI with loss of consciousness in both military (Warden & French, 2005) and civilian populations (Gil, Caspi, Ben-Ari, Koren, & Klein, 2005; Glaesser, Neuner, Lutgehetmann, Schmidt, & Elbert, 2004).

Other researchers, however, have reported that PTSD can exist as a comorbid condition with TBI, especially mTBI (Harvey & Bryant, 2000; Hickling, Gillen, Blanchard, Buckley, & Taylor, 1998; Mather, Tate, & Hannan, 2003; Mayou, Black, & Bryant, 2000). Some evidence suggests that mTBI may exacerbate the risk for PTSD and other psychiatric disorders (Fann et al., 2004). For example, Fann and colleagues reported from a large-scale study of 939 civilian health plan members that patients with a history of mTBI were 2.8 times more likely to develop a psychiatric disorder than patients with no TBI history (Fann et al., 2004). In terms of the military, a seminal survey study by Hoge and colleagues (2008) reported that whereas 16% of troops who sustained a bodily injury screened positive for PTSD, 44% of those with mTBI-related loss of consciousness screened positive for PTSD. These findings are important for the military because occurrence of mTBI in the context of psychologically traumatic experiences may increase the risk for PTSD, and potentially other mental health problems. We note that these studies were limited by reliance on self-report of brain injury or retrospective reporting rather than prospective assessments at the time of injury. Supporting these conclusions, however, was a longitudinal study of over 1,000 polytrauma civilian patients with and without mTBI; this study found that sustaining an mTBI was associated with an increased risk for PTSD (Bryant et al., 2010).

The possible mechanisms for increased PTSD risk following a traumatic stressor and co-occurring mTBI in the military are unknown. Obviously, sustaining an mTBI in combat can be disorienting and highly stressful. An acute disruption of one's mental faculties can render a soldier unable to function effectively in a combat situation, which can compound the psychological stress associated with the unfolding events. Physiologically,[2] an mTBI, acutely, is associated with a complex, dynamic, and multilayered cascade of neurochemical and neurometabolic events (Barkhoudarian, Hovda, &

---

[2] The acute pathobiological effects of mTBI in humans are difficult to study. Most of our knowledge is translational (Giza & Hovda, 2001, 2004; Iverson, 2005; Iverson, Lange, Gaetz, & Zasler, 2007), from animal and *in vitro* experimental models and should be considered an evidence-supported theoretical conceptualization of acute pathophysiology in the human brain.

Giza, 2011). Initially, there is likely a disruption of the neuronal cell membranes and axonal stretching, causing a large and indiscriminate flux of ions through previously regulated ion channels. This initiates widespread release of neurotransmitters compounding the ionic flux. Neurons are overworked (e.g., the sodium–potassium ATP-dependent pump) to reestablish ionic balance, depleting energy stores. These factors contribute to a state of hypermetabolism, which occurs in tandem with decreased cerebral blood flow, further compounding the hypermetabolism. The sustained influx of Ca^{2+} can result in mitochondrial accumulations of this ion and contribute to metabolic dysfunction and energy failure. The energy production of the cell is compromised further by overutilization of anaerobic energy pathways and elevated lactate as a by-product. The potential beneficial or detrimental effects of this complex neurobiology on fear conditioning and processing are not understood.

Theoretically, the neural networks implicated in mastering fear following trauma could be compromised by mTBI. One neurobiological model posits that PTSD involves exaggerated amygdala response resulting in impaired regulation by the medial prefrontal cortex (Rauch, Shin, & Phelps, 2006). The amygdala appears to be pivotal to the development and expression of conditioned fear reactions in human and animal studies, and learning to inhibit these fear reactions (extinction learning) involves inhibition by the ventral medial prefrontal cortex (Milad, Rauch, Pitman, & Quirk, 2006). Consistent with this model, researchers have reported that patients with PTSD have diminished medial prefrontal cortex activation during processing of fear (Lanius, Bluhm, Lanius, & Pain, 2006). It is possible that mTBI results in damage or dysfunction to the neural networks implicated in regulation of anxiety (Bryant, 2008; see also Verfaellie, Amick, & Vasterling, Chapter 5, this volume).

Delayed-Onset PTSD

Acute stress symptoms following exposure to a traumatic event typically occur in the initial days and weeks. For example, the onset of PTSD symptoms in the survivors of the Oklahoma City bombing was swift, with 76% reporting symptoms on the day of the event (North et al., 1999). Some researchers have reported that delayed-onset PTSD is rare. Following the Oklahoma City bombing, no cases of delayed-onset PTSD were identified (North, 2001; North et al., 2004). In a sample of former prisoners of war, 53.4% had a lifetime history of PTSD—and only 1.4% were noted to have delayed-onset type (Engdahl, Dikel, Eberly, & Blank, 1998). Onset of PTSD delayed by decades has been reported in elderly veterans, especially in those with neurological disorders (Grossman, Levin, Katzen, & Lechner, 2004; Ruzich, Looi, & Robertson, 2005).

If delayed-onset PTSD is reliably diagnosed, it might better reflect an individual who was distressed and symptomatic, but undetected or subsyndromal in the weeks following the trauma. Although uncommon following civilian trauma, it has been reported to occur more frequently in troops returning home from deployment (Solomon, Shklar, Singer, & Mikulincer, 2006; Southwick et al., 1995). Based on a review of the literature (Andrews, Brewin, Philpott, & Stewart, 2007), if delayed-onset PTSD is defined as an exacerbation or reactivation of symptoms, then this is commonly reported in military cases (i.e., 38.2%) and sometimes seen in civilian cases (i.e., 15.3%).

To date, there has not been any systematic study of delayed-onset PTSD following mTBI. Conceptually, it is possible that sustaining an mTBI could contribute to delayed-onset PTSD in military personnel. Following combat-related psychological trauma and an mTBI that involves loss of consciousness and posttraumatic amnesia, many patients feel the need to understand the gap in knowledge of the event that affected them. There are case reports of patients with TBI confabulating events in order to make sense of what occurred to them during the loss of consciousness; patients tend to reconstruct events in a way that is consistent with their current mood state (Bryant, 1996). A civilian longitudinal study found that 40% of mTBI patients recalled aspects of their injury 2 years later, even though 1 month after the injury they were amnesic of these events (Harvey & Bryant, 2001). It is possible that some trauma-exposed service members who suffered a traumatic experience in the context of loss of consciousness and PTA may subsequently reconstruct events in a way that consolidates the trauma memory. Given that (1) PTSD can develop in civilians and military personnel who experience psychological trauma and an mTBI, (2) PTSD actually might be more common in civilians who experience polytrauma involving an mTBI (Bryant et al., 2010; Hoge et al., 2008), and (3) delayed-onset PTSD is more common in military than civilian settings (Andrews et al., 2007), military personnel may be more prone to delayed-onset PTSD because they tend to reconstruct their traumatic experiences over time after their deployment (see Verfaellie et al., Chapter 5, this volume, for further discussion of this issue). Understanding the trajectory of PTSD development, following deployment, in those with and without a history of mTBI would address this issue. The possibility that trauma memory reconstruction in the post-deployment period contributes to PTSD needs to be studied in military populations, and points to the potential importance of ensuring that adaptive, rather than maladaptive, reconstructions of events occur in the months after injury.

Causes of Long-Term Symptoms and Problems Following mTBI

There is currently much concern over the symptoms and problems arising from mTBI in military forces. Hundreds of millions of dollars are devoted to research and service delivery to manage the possible health consequences of deployment-related mTBI, but there is much controversy over the cause(s) of long-lasting symptoms and problems. In a large-scale survey of U.S. service members, health impairment was significantly higher in those individuals who screened positive for a prior mTBI, including reported poor general health, days off work, medical visits, and somatic and postconcussive symptoms. However, a history of deployment-related mTBI was not significantly related to the health problems and symptoms after analyses controlled for the effects of traumatic stress and depression (Hoge et al., 2008). This finding has been replicated in other large-scale military studies (Schneiderman et al., 2008). Similarly, a recent large-scale study of civilians with polytrauma found that impaired functioning was not increased by the presence of mTBI; however, there were significant deficits in functioning if a patient sustained a psychological disorder along with the mTBI (Bryant et al., 2010). Taken together, these studies suggest that physical, social, and occupational impairment might be more strongly related to psychological factors occurring after trauma exposure, such as PTSD and depression, rather than to a past mTBI.

Extrapolating from the scientific literature in athletes and civilians, it is likely that the large majority of military personnel and veterans who sustained an mTBI during deployment and were not medically evacuated recovered fully, or nearly fully, from this injury. Some service members and veterans report post-concussion-like symptoms long after their injuries. It is *possible*, of course, that some of these symptoms are due to the residual effects of an mTBI (see Bigler & Maxwell, Chapter 2, and Iverson, Chapter 3, this volume, for a review). However, reporting symptoms long after an injury does not mean the symptoms are caused by the remote injury. As illustrated in Figure 12.2, it is essential to appreciate that symptoms reported years after an mTBI might be wholly attributable in some individuals to *co-occurring conditions* (e.g., PTSD, anxiety, depression, chronic pain, sleep problems, substance abuse, social psychological factors, and contextual factors). These conditions are associated with symptoms that are virtually identical to postconcussive symptoms (Gasquoine, 2000; Gunstad & Suhr, 2004; Iverson & McCracken, 1997; Karzmark, Hall, & Englander, 1995; McCauley, Boake, Levin, Contant, & Song, 2001; Meares et al., 2008; Meares et al., 2011; Smith-Seemiller et al., 2003; Wilde et al., 2004). The comorbidity problem, and that these symptoms are nonspecific, presents nearly insurmountable challenges for precisely and accurately determining if a service member is experiencing long-term problems associated with one or more past mTBIs. The symptoms associated with these comorbid conditions can co-occur with subtle lingering effects of an mTBI but frequently mimic the long-term adverse effects of an mTBI. A biopsychosocial conceptualization of poor outcome from mTBI is presented by Iverson (Chapter 3, this volume).

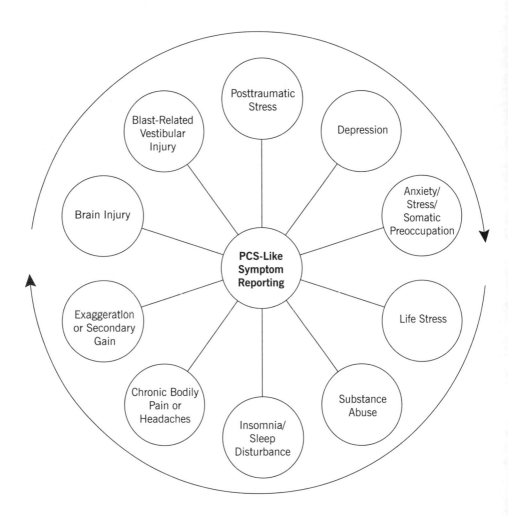

FIGURE 12.2. Factors that can influence post-concussion-like symptom reporting postacutely or long after an mTBI. From Iverson, Langlois, McCrea, and Kelly (2009). Copyright 2009 by Taylor & Francis. Reprinted by permission.

Avoiding Misattribution and Iatrogenesis

When dealing with mTBI, psychological health, and general medical problems in returning service members, there is a risk for misattribution and iatrogenesis (i.e., the condition is induced by the health care provider's manner, behavior, or activity). In this context, iatrogenesis can occur if a service member with mental health problems is convinced by a health care provider that he is permanently brain-damaged when, in fact, he is not.

At present, some service members who sustained an mTBI during deployment become convinced that a range of nonspecific postdeployment symptoms are caused solely by brain damage, when the cause of these symptoms might be multifactorial. This is unfortunate because it communicates a unitary cause with a poor prognosis. During the 1991 Gulf War, there was marked concern of chemical weapons, which might have contributed to presentations of medically unexplained symptoms (Clauw et al., 2003; Iversen, Chalder, & Wessely, 2007; Lee, Gabriel, Bolton, Bale, & Jackson, 2002). One viewpoint is that veterans attributed somatic symptoms and experiences to exposure to chemical agents, which resulted in significant concerns about their health. The attributional mechanism underpinning somatic responses has been well documented in some disorders, such as panic disorder, health anxiety, and hypochondriasis (Clark & Wells, 1997; Clauw et al., 2003; Engel, 2004). In these disorders, people tend to be hypervigilant to somatic cues because they believe they represent a threat to their physical well-being. For example, the patient with panic disorder may believe that an alteration in his respiration is a sign of imminent choking or that a slight pain in the chest is indicative of an approaching cardiac arrest. Similarly, a person with health anxiety may constantly search his or her body for any alterations in appearance of function to determine if there are signs of malignancy. Once the sensation or sign is detected (which is not difficult to do), the person may interpret the significance of the sensations in a negative manner, such that small somatic cues are perceived as indicative of dire outcomes.

Service members affected by traumatic stress are at risk for hypervigilance to threat and to physical, emotional, and cognitive symptoms. Fear network models of PTSD posit that these individuals preferentially allocate attention to stimuli of concern because of their fear of threat (Foa & Kozak, 1986). Consistent with this proposal, people with PTSD are hypervigilant to threat in emotional Stroop (Bryant & Harvey, 1995; McNally, Kaspi, Riemann, & Zeitlin, 1990), dot probe (Bryant & Harvey, 1997), and eye-tracking (Bryant, Harvey, Gordon, & Barry, 1995) paradigms. Further, people with PTSD not only overattend to perceived external threats (Ehlers & Clark, 2000), but they also overattend to somatic and physical symptoms (Smith & Bryant, 2000).

Therefore, there is a possibility that if somatic and emotional symptoms are overattributed to mTBI, then we might inadvertently encourage a postdeployment syndrome in which service members and veterans mistakenly attribute problems associated with mental health, chronic pain, and community integration to permanent brain injury. Some service members and veterans might then abandon hope for improvement. This scenario could lead to a reduction in the self-efficacy and expectancy of recovery that is known to be associated with better outcomes after difficult life events (Hobfoll et al., 2007).

Implications for Treatment

We have the responsibility to provide high-quality treatment and rehabilitation to service members who experience health and mental health problems arising from operational deployment. These services should be timely, evidence-based, and focused on improving health and general functioning.

Military personnel are at risk for combat-related and noncombat-related mTBIs. Some of these injuries, especially combat-related injuries, will occur in psychologically traumatic circumstances. In the days (and sometimes weeks) following these injuries, from an *operational perspective*, a service member might not be fit for duty due to mild cognitive compromise, slowed reaction time, diminished judgment, and modest physical limitations relating to vision and balance. From a *health and welfare perspective*, there is a need postdeployment for evidence-based specialized assessment, treatment, and rehabilitation services. Two broad recommendations for providing services to military personnel are provided below.

First, attempts should be made to facilitate early identification of mTBI in-theater and to encourage medical evaluation, immediate rest, and, if necessary, stress-related debriefing following injury. It is also important to promote the expectation of recovery. Acute symptoms and problems are typically time-limited and are likely to resolve spontaneously. There are several published studies with civilians showing that providing education and reassurance is associated with better recovery (Minderhoud, Boelens, Huizenga, & Saan, 1980; Relander, Troupp, & Af Bjorkesten, 1972). Educational brochures or sessions usually provide information regarding common symptoms, the likely time course of recovery, reassurance of recovery, and suggested coping strategies following mTBI (e.g., Mittenberg, Tremont, Zielinski, Fichera, & Rayls, 1996; Paniak, Toller-Lobe, Reynolds, Melnyk, & Nagy, 2000; Ponsford et al., 2002; Wade, King, Wenden, Crawford, & Caldwell, 1998). It will take time and additional research to determine optimal in-theater acute management and early intervention strategies.

Second, it is essential to appreciate that service members and veterans with a history of mTBI frequently have chronic comorbid conditions and problems. Traumatic stress, depression, chronic pain, insomnia, substance abuse, life stress, and marital and family distress, singly or in combination, can cause a diverse range of "post-concussion-like" symptoms. For example, problems with sleep are commonly reported postdeployment (Zeitzer et al., 2009), and chronic pain is a common problem in veterans (Gironda, Clark, Massengale, & Walker, 2006). All of these problems can mimic, or obscure, the lingering effects of a brain injury. This supports treatment approaches that emphasize *treating what is treatable* to try to reduce suffering and improve functioning (Brenner, Vanderploeg, & Terrio, 2009; Iverson et al., 2007). Systematically treating certain problems (e.g., sleep disturbance, depression, or anxiety) may have concomitant benefits in other areas (e.g., headaches and cognition) in service members.

Psychological treatments are effective for reducing symptoms and improving functioning in patients with PTSD (Bisson & Andrew, 2007). There is some evidence that psychological treatment can reduce symptoms in patients with comorbid mTBI and anxiety problems (Soo & Tate, 2007). Psychological and behavioral treatments can also improve sleep and reduce psychological distress in people with insomnia (Zeitzer et al., 2009). There is also evidence that cognitive-behavioral therapy (CBT) is effective in reducing PTSD symptoms shortly after mTBI (Bryant, Moulds, Guthrie, & Nixon, 2003). This study randomly allocated patients who sustained mTBIs 2 weeks after injury to either CBT or supportive counseling. The CBT involved psychoeducation, imaginal and *in vivo* exposure, and cognitive restructuring; the imaginal exposure focused on whatever memories the patients had either prior to or following loss of consciousness and PTA. Moreover, other studies of panic disorder and health anxiety have shown that correcting patients' maladaptive appraisals about somatic sensations is effective for reducing their attention to, and anxieties about, these conditions (Barlow, 1988). Taken together, it seems logical that providing interventions that aim to reduce traumatic stress and encourage appraisals relating to multifactorial underpinnings of common post-concussion-like symptoms would help reduce symptom burden and improve functioning. It needs to be emphasized, however, that there is currently no evidence pertaining to the effects of trauma-focused therapy on post-concussion-like symptoms following mTBI.

Physical conditioning and supervised exercise programs might also be useful as adjunctive treatment and of appeal to a group of men and women accustomed to physical training. Moderate-intensity aerobic exercise has been associated with positive effects on mood and self-esteem (Ekeland, Heian, Hagen, Abbott, & Nordheim, 2004), and it promotes a general sense of well-being. Exercise is associated with changes in neurotransmitter systems of the brain. The glutamatergic, dopaminergic, noradrenergic, and serotonergic systems demonstrate particular benefits (Chaouloff, 1989; Molteni, Ying, & Gomez-Pinilla, 2002), which in turn contribute to improved mood and to a general sense of well-being (Callaghan, 2004; Conn, 2010; Duman, 2005). In adults, exercise can be an effective treatment for mild and even more severe depression (Babyak et al., 2000; Daley, 2008; Dunn, Trivedi, Kampert, Clark, & Chambliss, 2005; Lawlor & Hopker, 2001; Mead et al., 2008, 2009; Penninx et al., 2002; Rethorst, Wipfli, & Landers, 2009). It has also been shown to have substantial beneficial effects on anxiety (Broman-Fulks & Storey, 2008; Merom et al., 2008; Smits et al., 2008). Exercise is associated with improved sleep quality (Youngstedt, 2005) and reduced pain and disability in patients with chronic low back pain (Bell & Burnett, 2009; Henchoz & Kai-Lik So, 2008), and it has been studied for its beneficial effects on the treatment of migraines and other types of headaches. Regular long-term aerobic exercise reduces migraine frequency, severity, and duration (Koseoglu, Akboyraz, Soyuer, & Ersoy, 2003; Lockett & Campbell, 1992). Moreover, researchers are beginning to use exercise as a treatment modality for people who are slow to recover from an mTBI (Gagnon, Galli, Friedman, Grilli, & Iverson, 2009; Leddy et al., 2010).

Conclusions

Military service members are at risk for sustaining an mTBI. There were 30,703 medically verified brain injuries coded in the entire DoD Health Care System in 2010 (as of February 2011; see Table 12.1). Of these injuries, 81% were classified as mild. mTBIs can result in serious short-term physical, emotional, and cognitive symptoms. The most serious forms of this injury can result in long-term changes in functioning. Isolated mTBIs, on the mild end of the mild injury spectrum, carry an excellent prognosis for rapid recovery and return to duty. However, many service members experience a combination of physical injuries, psychological trauma, and an mTBI. An mTBI and traumatic stress reaction can occur as a result of the same event, or separate events.

Service members who are wounded in combat are also at increased risk for PTSD, depression, and/or chronic pain. These comorbidities make it challenging to determine if a service member does or does not suffer from residual symptoms associated with the mTBI. Traumatic stress, life stress, depression, insomnia, chronic pain, marital and family distress, and substance abuse, singly or in combination, can be the proximate cause for post-concussion-like symptoms. As such, emphasizing a single explanation for symptoms, such as brain injury, carries a risk of iatrogenesis. Moreover, emphasizing brain injury as an explanation might hinder treatment efforts in some cases. We believe that it is important to aggressively *treat what is treatable* to try to reduce suffering and improve functioning among service members and military veterans. Psychological, physical, and cognitive symptoms can have multifactorial causation; systematically treating specific chief complaints (e.g., sleep disturbance and anxiety) might result in concomitant benefits in other areas (e.g., headaches and cognition) in some service members. If we focus our efforts to treat what we can treat, we will reduce suffering and improve functioning and quality of life for military service members and veterans.

Author Note

The views expressed in this chapter are those of the authors and do not reflect the official policy of the Department of Defense, U.S. Army, or the United States Government.

References

Andrews, B., Brewin, C. R., Philpott, R., & Stewart, L. (2007). Delayed-onset posttraumatic stress disorder: A systematic review of the evidence. *American Journal of Psychiatry, 164*(9), 1319–1326.

Babyak, M., Blumenthal, J. A., Herman, S., Khatri, P., Doraiswamy, M., Moore, K., et al. (2000). Exercise treatment for major depression: Maintenance of therapeutic benefit at 10 months. *Psychosomatic Medicine, 62*, 633–638.

Barkhoudarian, G., Hovda, D. A., & Giza, C. C. (2011). The molecular pathophysiology of concussive brain injury. *Clinical Sports Medicine, 30*(1), 33–48, vii–iii.

Barlow, D. H. (1988). *Anxiety and its disorders: The nature and treatment of anxiety and panic.* New York: Guilford Press.

Barr, W. B., & McCrea, M. (2001). Sensitivity and specificity of standardized neurocognitive testing immediately following sports concussion. *Journal of the International Neuropsychological Society, 7*, 693–702.

Bell, J. A., & Burnett, A. (2009). Exercise for the primary, secondary and tertiary prevention of low back pain in the workplace: A systematic review. *Journal of Occupational Rehabilitation, 19*(1), 8–24.

Birmes, P., Brunet, A., Carreras, D., Ducasse, J. L., Charlet, J. P., Lauque, D., et al. (2003). The predictive power of peritraumatic dissociation and acute stress symptoms for posttraumatic stress symptoms: A three-month prospective study. *American Journal of Psychiatry, 160*(7), 1337–1339.

Bisson, J., & Andrew, M. (2007). Psychological treatment of post-traumatic stress disorder (PTSD). *Cochrane Database of Systematic Reviews, 3*, CD003388.

Bombardier, C. H., Fann, J. R., Temkin, N., Esselman, P. C., Pelzer, E., Keough, M., et al. (2006). Posttraumatic stress disorder symptoms during the first six months after traumatic brain injury. *Journal of Neuropsychiatry and Clinical Neurosciences, 18*(4), 501–508.

Brenner, L. A., Vanderploeg, R. D., & Terrio, H. (2009). Assessment and diagnosis of mild traumatic brain injury, posttraumatic stress disorder, and other polytrauma conditions: Burden of adversity hypothesis. *Rehabilitation Psychology, 54*(3), 239–246.

Broman-Fulks, J. J., & Storey, K. M. (2008). Evaluation of a brief aerobic exercise intervention for high anxiety sensitivity. *Anxiety, Stress, and Coping, 21*(2), 117–128.

Bryant, R. A. (1996). Posttraumatic stress disorder, flashbacks, and pseudomemories in closed head injury. *Journal of Traumatic Stress, 9*(3), 621–629.

Bryant, R. A., & Harvey, A. G. (1995). Processing threatening information in posttraumatic stress disorder. *Journal of Abnormal Psychology, 104*(3), 537–541.

Bryant, R. A., & Harvey, A. G. (1997). Attentional bias in posttraumatic stress disorder. *Journal of Traumatic Stress, 10*(4), 635–644.

Bryant, R. A., Harvey, A. G., Gordon, E., & Barry, R. J. (1995). Eye movement and electrodermal responses to threat stimuli in post-traumatic stress disorder. *International Journal of Psychophysiology, 20*(3), 209–213.

Bryant, R. A., Moulds, M., Guthrie, R., & Nixon, R. D. (2003). Treating acute stress disorder following mild traumatic brain injury. *American Journal of Psychiatry, 160,* 585–587.

Bryant, R. A., O'Donnell, M. L., Creamer, M., McFarlane, A. C., Clark, C. R., & Silove, D. (2010). The psychiatric sequelae of traumatic injury. *American Journal of Psychiatry, 167*(3), 312–320.

Callaghan, P. (2004). Exercise: A neglected intervention in mental health care? *Journal of Psychiatry and Mental Health Nursing, 11*(4), 476–483.

Cardena, E., & Spiegel, D. (1993). Dissociative reactions to the San Francisco Bay Area earthquake of 1989. *American Journal of Psychiatry, 150*(3), 474–478.

Chaouloff, F. (1989). Physical exercise and brain monoamines: A review. *Acta Physiologica Scandinavia, 137,* 1–13.

Clark, D. M., & Wells, A. (1997). Cognitive therapy for anxiety disorders. In L. J. Dickstein, M. B. Riba, & J. M. Oldham (Eds.), *Cognitive therapy* (pp. 9–43). Washington, DC.: American Psychiatric Press.

Clauw, D. J., Engel, C. C. Jr., Aronowitz, R., Jones, E., Kipen, H. M., Kroenke, K., et al. (2003). Unexplained symptoms after terrorism and war: An expert consensus statement. *Journal of Occupational and Environmental Medicine, 45*(10), 1040–1048.

Coldren, R. L., Kelly, M. P., Parish, R. V., Dretsch, M., & Russell, M. L. (2010). Evaluation of the Military Acute Concussion Evaluation for use in combat operations more than 12 hours after injury. *Military Medicine, 175*(7), 477–481.

Conn, V. S. (2010). Depressive symptom outcomes of physical activity interventions: Meta-analysis findings. *Annals of Behavioral Medicine, 39*(2), 128–138.

Daley, A. (2008). Exercise and depression: A review of reviews. *Journal of Clinical Psychology in Medical Settings, 15*(2), 140–147.

Dobscha, S. K., Clark, M. E., Morasco, B. J., Freeman, M., Campbell, R., &

Helfand, M. (2009). Systematic review of the literature on pain in patients with polytrauma including traumatic brain injury. *Pain Medicine, 10*(7), 1200–1217.

Duman, R. S. (2005). Neurotrophic factors and regulation of mood: Role of exercise, diet and metabolism. *Neurobiology of Aging, 26* (Suppl. 1), 88–93.

Dunn, A. L., Trivedi, M. H., Kampert, J. B., Clark, C. G., & Chambliss, H. O. (2005). Exercise treatment for depression: Efficacy and dose response. *American Journal of Preventative Medicine, 28*(1), 1–8.

Ehlers, A., & Clark, D. M. (2000). A cognitive model of posttraumatic stress disorder. *Behavior Research and Therapy, 38*(4), 319–345.

Ekeland, E., Heian, F., Hagen, K. B., Abbott, J., & Nordheim, L. (2004). Exercise to improve self-esteem in children and young people. *Cochrane Database of Systematic Reviews, 1*, CD003683.

Engdahl, B., Dikel, T. N., Eberly, R., & Blank, A. Jr. (1998). Comorbidity and course of psychiatric disorders in a community sample of former prisoners of war. *American Journal of Psychiatry, 155*(12), 1740–1745.

Engel, C. C. Jr. (2004). Post-war syndromes: Illustrating the impact of the social psyche on notions of risk, responsibility, reason, and remedy. *Journal of the American Academy of Psychoanalysis and Dynamic Psychiatry, 32*, 321–334.

Fann, J. R., Burington, B., Leonetti, A., Jaffe, K., Katon, W. J., & Thompson, R. S. (2004). Psychiatric illness following traumatic brain injury in an adult health maintenance organization population. *Archives of General Psychiatry, 61*(1), 53–61.

Foa, E. B., & Kozak, M. J. (1986). Emotional processing of fear: Exposure to corrective information. *Psychological Bulletin, 99*(1), 20–35.

Freinkel, A., Koopman, C., & Spiegel, D. (1994). Dissociative symptoms in media eyewitnesses of an execution. *American Journal of Psychiatry, 151*(9), 1335–1339.

Gagnon, I., Galli, C., Friedman, D., Grilli, L., & Iverson, G. L. (2009). Active rehabilitation for children who are slow to recover following sport-related concussion. *Brain Injury, 23*(12), 956–964.

Galetta, K. M., Barrett, J., Allen, M., Madda, F., Delicata, D., Tennant, A. T., et al. (2011). The King–Devick Test as a determinant of head trauma and concussion in boxers and MMA fighters. *Neurology, 76*(17), 1456–1462.

Gasquoine, P. G. (2000). Postconcussional symptoms in chronic back pain. *Applied Neuropsychology, 7*(2), 83–89.

Gil, S., Caspi, Y., Ben-Ari, I. Z., Koren, D., & Klein, E. (2005). Does memory of a traumatic event increase the risk for posttraumatic stress disorder in patients with traumatic brain injury?: A prospective study. *American Journal of Psychiatry, 162*(5), 963–969.

Gironda, R. J., Clark, M. E., Massengale, J. P., & Walker, R. L. (2006). Pain among veterans of Operations Enduring Freedom and Iraqi Freedom. *Pain Medicine, 7*(4), 339–343.

Giza, C. C., & Hovda, D. A. (2001). The neurometabolic cascade of concussion. *Journal of Athletic Training, 36*(3), 228–235.

Giza, C. C., & Hovda, D. A. (2004). The pathophysiology of traumatic brain injury. In M. R. Lovell, R. J. Echemendia, J. T. Barth, & M. W. Collins (Eds.), *Traumatic brain injury in sports* (pp. 45–70). Lisse, The Netherlands: Swets & Zeitlinger.

Glaesser, J., Neuner, F., Lutgehetmann, R., Schmidt, R., & Elbert, T. (2004). Posttraumatic stress disorder in patients with traumatic brain injury. *BMC Psychiatry, 4,* 5.

Golding, H., Bass, E., Percy, A., & Goldberg, M. (2009). Understanding recent estimates of PTSD and TBI from Operations Iraqi Freedom and Enduring Freedom. *Journal of Rehabilitation Research and Development, 46*(5), vii–xiv.

Grieger, T. A., Cozza, S. J., Ursano, R. J., Hoge, C., Martinez, P. E., Engel, C. C., et al. (2006). Posttraumatic stress disorder and depression in battle-injured soldiers. *American Journal of Psychiatry, 163*(10), 1777–1783; quiz, 1860.

Grossman, A. B., Levin, B. E., Katzen, H. L., & Lechner, S. (2004). PTSD symptoms and onset of neurologic disease in elderly trauma survivors. *Journal of Clinical and Experimental Neuropsychology, 26*(5), 698–705.

Gunstad, J., & Suhr, J. A. (2004). Cognitive factors in postconcussion syndrome symptom report. *Archives of Clinical Neuropsychology, 19*(3), 391–405.

Harvey, A. G., & Bryant, R. A. (1999). Dissociative symptoms in acute stress disorder. *Journal of Traumatic Stress, 12*(4), 673–680.

Harvey, A. G., & Bryant, R. A. (2000). Two-year prospective evaluation of the relationship between acute stress disorder and posttraumatic stress disorder following mild traumatic brain injury. *American Journal of Psychiatry, 157*(4), 626–628.

Harvey, A. G., & Bryant, R. A. (2001). Reconstructing trauma memories: A prospective study of "amnesic" trauma survivors. *Journal of Traumatic Stress, 14*(2), 277–282.

Henchoz, Y., & Kai-Lik So, A. (2008). Exercise and nonspecific low back pain: A literature review. *Joint Bone Spine, 75*(5), 533–539.

Hickling, E. J., Gillen, R., Blanchard, E. B., Buckley, T., & Taylor, A. (1998). Traumatic brain injury and posttraumatic stress disorder: A preliminary investigation of neuropsychological test results in PTSD secondary to motor vehicle accidents. *Brain Injury, 12*(4), 265–274.

Hobfoll, S. E., Watson, P., Bell, C. C., Brymer, M. J., Friedman, M. J., Friedman, M., et al. (2007). Five essential elements of immediate and mid-term mass trauma intervention: Empirical evidence. *Psychiatry: Interpersonal and Biological Processes, 70,* 283–315.

Hoge, C. W., Castro, C. A., Messer, S. C., McGurk, D., Cotting, D. I., & Koffman, R. L. (2004). Combat duty in Iraq and Afghanistan, mental health problems, and barriers to care. *New England Journal of Medicine, 351*(1), 13–22.

Hoge, C. W., Goldberg, H. M., & Castro, C. A. (2009). Care of war veterans with mild traumatic brain injury—flawed perspectives. *New England Journal of Medicine, 360*(16), 1588–1591.

Hoge, C. W., McGurk, D., Thomas, J. L., Cox, A. L., Engel, C. C., & Castro, C. A. (2008). Mild traumatic brain injury in U.S. soldiers returning from Iraq. *New England Journal of Medicine, 358*(5), 453–463.

Hoge, C. W., Terhakopian, A., Castro, C. A., Messer, S. C., & Engel, C. C. (2007). Association of posttraumatic stress disorder with somatic symptoms, health care visits, and absenteeism among Iraq war veterans. *American Journal of Psychiatry, 164*(1), 150–153.

Hudon, C., Belleville, S., & Gauthier, S. (2008). The association between depressive and cognitive symptoms in amnestic mild cognitive impairment. *International Psychogeriatrics, 20*(4), 710–723.

Iversen, A., Chalder, T., & Wessely, S. (2007). Gulf War illness: Lessons from medically unexplained symptoms. *Clinical Psychology Review, 27*(7), 842–854.

Iverson, G. L. (2005). Outcome from mild traumatic brain injury. *Current Opinion in Psychiatry, 18*, 301–317.

Iverson, G. L. (2006). Misdiagnosis of the persistent postconcussion syndrome in patients with depression. *Archives of Clinical Neuropsychology, 21*(4), 303–310.

Iverson, G. L. (2010). Clinical and methodological challenges with assessing mild traumatic brain injury in the military. *Journal of Head Trauma Rehabilitation, 25*(5), 313–319.

Iverson, G. L., Lange, R. T., Gaetz, M., & Zasler, N. D. (2007). Mild TBI. In N. D. Zasler, H. T. Katz, & R. D. Zafonte (Eds.), *Brain injury medicine: Principles and practice* (pp. 333–371). New York: Demos Medical Publishing.

Iverson, G. L., Langlois, J. A., McCrea, M. A., & Kelly, J. P. (2009). Challenges associated with post-deployment screening for mild traumatic brain injury in military personnel. *Clinical Neuropsychologist, 23*(8), 1299–1314.

Iverson, G. L., & McCracken, L. M. (1997). "Postconcussive" symptoms in persons with chronic pain. *Brain Injury, 11*(11), 783–790.

Kang, H. K., Natelson, B. H., Mahan, C. M., Lee, K. Y., & Murphy, F. M. (2003). Posttraumatic stress disorder and chronic fatigue syndrome-like illness among Gulf War veterans: A population-based survey of 30,000 veterans. *American Journal of Epidemiology, 157*(2), 141–148.

Karzmark, P., Hall, K., & Englander, J. (1995). Late-onset post-concussion symptoms after mild brain injury: The role of premorbid, injury-related, environmental, and personality factors. *Brain Injury, 9*(1), 21–26.

Koseoglu, E., Akboyraz, A., Soyuer, A., & Ersoy, A. O. (2003). Aerobic exercise and plasma beta endorphin levels in patients with migrainous headache without aura. *Cephalalgia, 23*, 972–976.

Lanius, R. A., Bluhm, R., Lanius, U., & Pain, C. (2006). A review of neuroimaging studies in PTSD: Heterogeneity of response to symptom provocation. *Journal of Psychiatric Research, 40*(8), 709–729.

Lawlor, D. A., & Hopker, S. W. (2001). The effectiveness of exercise as an intervention in the management of depression: Systematic review and meta-regression analysis of randomised controlled trials. *British Medical Journal, 322*(7289), 763–767.

Leddy, J. J., Kozlowski, K., Donnelly, J. P., Pendergast, D. R., Epstein, L. H., & Willer, B. (2010). A preliminary study of subsymptom threshold exercise training for refractory post-concussion syndrome. *Clinical Journal of Sport Medicine, 20*(1), 21–27.

Lee, H. A., Gabriel, R., Bolton, J. P., Bale, A. J., & Jackson, M. (2002). Health status and clinical diagnoses of 3000 UK Gulf War veterans. *Journal of the Royal Society of Medicine, 95*(10), 491–497.

Levin, H. S., Brown, S. A., Song, J. X., McCauley, S. R., Boake, C., Contant, C. F., et al. (2001). Depression and posttraumatic stress disorder at three months after mild to moderate traumatic brain injury. *Journal of Clinical and Experimental Neuropsychology, 23*(6), 754–769.

Lockett, D. M., & Campbell, J. F. (1992). The effects of aerobic exercise on migraine. *Headache, 32*, 50–54.

MacDonald, C. L., Johnson, A. M., Cooper, D., Nelson, E. C., Werner, N. J., Shimony, J. S., et al. (2011). Detection of blast-related traumatic brain injury in U.S. military personnel. *New England Journal of Medicine, 364*(22), 2091–2100.

Madakasira, S., & O'Brien, K. F. (1987). Acute posttraumatic stress disorder in victims of a natural disaster. *Journal of Nervous and Mental Disease, 175*(5), 286–290.

Mather, F. J., Tate, R. L., & Hannan, T. J. (2003). Post-traumatic stress disorder in children following road traffic accidents: A comparison of those with and without mild traumatic brain injury. *Brain Injury, 17*(12), 1077–1087.

Mayou, R. A., Black, J., & Bryant, B. (2000). Unconsciousness, amnesia and psychiatric symptoms following road traffic accident injury. *British Journal of Psychiatry, 177*, 540–545.

McCauley, S. R., Boake, C., Levin, H. S., Contant, C. F., & Song, J. X. (2001). Postconcussional disorder following mild to moderate traumatic brain injury: Anxiety, depression, and social support as risk factors and comorbidities. *Journal of Clinical and Experimental Neuropsychology, 23*(6), 792–808.

McNally, R. J., Kaspi, S. P., Riemann, B. C., & Zeitlin, S. B. (1990). Selective processing of threat cues in posttraumatic stress disorder. *Journal of Abnormal Psychology, 99*(4), 398–402.

Mead, G. E., Morley, W., Campbell, P., Greig, C. A., McMurdo, M., & Lawlor, D. A. (2009). Exercise for depression. *Cochrane Database of Systematic Reviews, 3*, CD004366.

Meares, S., Shores, E. A., Taylor, A. J., Batchelor, J., Bryant, R. A., Baguley, I. J., et al. (2008). Mild traumatic brain injury does not predict acute postconcussion syndrome. *Journal of Neurology, Neurosurgery and Psychiatry, 79*(3), 300–306.

Meares, S., Shores, E. A., Taylor, A. J., Batchelor, J., Bryant, R. A., Baguley, I. J., et al. (2011). The prospective course of postconcussion syndrome: The role of mild TBI. *Neuropsychology, 25*, 454–465.

Mental Health Advisory Team V. (2008). *Operation Iraqi Freedom 06–08: Iraq. Operation Enduring Freedom 8: Afghanistan, chartered by the Office of the Surgeon Multi-National Force-Iraq, the Office of the Command Surgeon and the Office of the Surgeon General United States Army Medical Command.* Available online at *www.armymedicine.army.mil/reports/mhat/mhat_v/ MHAT_V_OIFandOEF-Redacted.pdf.*

Merom, D., Phongsavan, P., Wagner, R., Chey, T., Marnane, C., Steel, Z., et al.

(2008). Promoting walking as an adjunct intervention to group cognitive behavioral therapy for anxiety disorders—A pilot group randomized trial. *Journal of Anxiety Disorders, 22*(6), 959–968.

Milad, M. R., Rauch, S. L., Pitman, R. K., & Quirk, G. J. (2006). Fear extinction in rats: Implications for human brain imaging and anxiety disorders. *Biological Psychology, 73*(1), 61–71.

Minderhoud, J. M., Boelens, M. E., Huizenga, J., & Saan, R. J. (1980). Treatment of minor head injuries. *Clinical Neurology and Neurosurgery, 82*(2), 127–140.

Mittenberg, W., Tremont, G., Zielinski, R. E., Fichera, S., & Rayls, K. R. (1996). Cognitive-behavioral prevention of postconcussion syndrome. *Archives of Clinical Neuropsychology, 11*(2), 139–145.

Molteni, R., Ying, Z., & Gomez-Pinilla, F. (2002). Differential effects of acute and chronic exercise on plasticity-related genes in the rat hippocampus revealed by microarray. *European Journal of Neuroscience, 16*(6), 1107–1116.

North, C. S. (2001). The course of post-traumatic stress disorder after the Oklahoma City bombing. *Military Medicine, 166*(Suppl. 12), 51–52.

North, C. S., Nixon, S. J., Shariat, S., Mallonee, S., McMillen, J. C., Spitznagel, E. L., et al. (1999). Psychiatric disorders among survivors of the Oklahoma City bombing. *Journal of the American Medical Association, 282*(8), 755–762.

North, C. S., Pfefferbaum, B., Tivis, L., Kawasaki, A., Reddy, C., & Spitznagel, E. L. (2004). The course of posttraumatic stress disorder in a follow-up study of survivors of the Oklahoma City bombing. *Annals of Clinical Psychiatry, 16*(4), 209–215.

Paniak, C., Toller-Lobe, G., Reynolds, S., Melnyk, A., & Nagy, J. (2000). A randomized trial of two treatments for mild traumatic brain injury: 1 year follow-up. *Brain Injury, 14*(3), 219–226.

Penninx, B. W., Rejeski, W. J., Pandya, J., Miller, M. E., Di Bari, M., Applegate, W. B., et al. (2002). Exercise and depressive symptoms: A comparison of aerobic and resistance exercise effects on emotional and physical function in older persons with high and low depressive symptomatology. *Journals of Gerontology: Series B, Psychological Sciences and Social Sciences, 57*(2), P124–P132.

Ponsford, J., Willmott, C., Rothwell, A., Cameron, P., Kelly, A. M., Nelms, R., et al. (2002). Impact of early intervention on outcome following mild head injury in adults. *Journal of Neurology, Neurosurgery and Psychiatry, 73*(3), 330–332.

Radanov, B. P., Dvorak, J., & Valach, L. (1992). Cognitive deficits in patients after soft tissue injury of the cervical spine. *Spine, 17*(2), 127–131.

Ramchand, R., Schell, T. L., Karney, B. R., Osilla, K. C., Burns, R. M., & Caldarone, L. B. (2010). Disparate prevalence estimates of PTSD among service members who served in Iraq and Afghanistan: Possible explanations. *Journal of Traumatic Stress, 23*(1), 59–68.

Rauch, S. L., Shin, L. M., & Phelps, E. A. (2006). Neurocircuitry models of post-traumatic stress disorder and extinction: Human neuroimaging research—past, present, and future. *Biological Psychiatry, 60*(4), 376–382.

Relander, M., Troupp, H., & Af Bjorkesten, G. (1972). Controlled trial of treatment for cerebral concussion. *British Medical Journal, 4*(843), 777–779.

Rethorst, C. D., Wipfli, B. M., & Landers, D. M. (2009). The antidepressive effects of exercise: A meta-analysis of randomized trials. *Sports Medicine, 39*(6), 491–511.

Rona, R. J., Hooper, R., Jones, M., Iversen, A. C., Hull, L., Murphy, D., et al. (2009). The contribution of prior psychological symptoms and combat exposure to post Iraq deployment mental health in the UK military. *Journal of Traumatic Stress, 22*, 11–19.

Ropper, A. (2011). Brain injuries from blasts. *New England Journal of Medicine, 364*(22), 2156–2157.

Ruzich, M. J., Looi, J. C., & Robertson, M. D. (2005). Delayed onset of posttraumatic stress disorder among male combat veterans: A case series. *American Journal of Geriatric Psychiatry, 13*(5), 424–427.

Sbordone, R. J., & Liter, J. C. (1995). Mild traumatic brain injury does not produce posttraumatic stress disorder. *Brain Injury, 9*, 405–412.

Schneiderman, A. I., Braver, E. R., & Kang, H. K. (2008). Understanding sequelae of injury mechanisms and mild traumatic brain injury incurred during the conflicts in Iraq and Afghanistan: Persistent postconcussive symptoms and posttraumatic stress disorder. *American Journal of Epidemiology, 167*(12), 1446–1452.

Schwab, K. A., Ivins, B., Cramer, G., Johnson, W., Sluss-Tiller, M., Kiley, K., et al. (2007). Screening for traumatic brain injury in troops returning from deployment in Afghanistan and Iraq: Initial investigation of the usefulness of a short screening tool for traumatic brain injury. *Journal of Head Trauma Rehabilitation, 22*(6), 377–389.

Shephard, B. (2001). *A war of nerves: Soldiers and psychiatrists in the twentieth century.* Cambridge, MA: Harvard University Press.

Smith, K., & Bryant, R. A. (2000). The generality of cognitive bias in acute stress disorder. *Behavior Research and Therapy, 38*(7), 709–715.

Smith-Seemiller, L., Fow, N. R., Kant, R., & Franzen, M. D. (2003). Presence of postconcussion syndrome symptoms in patients with chronic pain vs. mild traumatic brain injury. *Brain Injury, 17*(3), 199–206.

Smits, J. A., Berry, A. C., Rosenfield, D., Powers, M. B., Behar, E., & Otto, M. W. (2008). Reducing anxiety sensitivity with exercise. *Depression and Anxiety, 25*(8), 689–699.

Solomon, Z., Shklar, R., Singer, Y., & Mikulincer, M. (2006). Reactions to combat stress in Israeli veterans twenty years after the 1982 Lebanon war. *Journal of Nervous and Mental Disease, 194*(12), 935–939.

Soo, C., & Tate, R. (2007). Psychological treatment for anxiety in people with traumatic brain injury. *Cochrane Database of Systematic Reviews, 3*, CD005239.

Southwick, S. M., Morgan, C. A. 3rd, Darnell, A., Bremner, D., Nicolaou, A. L., Nagy, L. M., et al. (1995). Trauma-related symptoms in veterans of Operation Desert Storm: A 2-year follow-up. *American Journal of Psychiatry, 152*(8), 1150–1155.

Tanielian, T., & Jaycox, L. H. (Eds.). (2008). *Invisible wounds of war: Psychological and cognitive injuries, their consequences, and services to assist recovery.* Santa Monica, CA: Rand Corporation.

Terrio, H., Brenner, L. A., Ivins, B. J., Cho, J. M., Helmick, K., Schwab, K., et al. (2009). Traumatic brain injury screening: Preliminary findings in a U.S. Army brigade combat team. *Journal of Head Trauma Rehabilitation, 24*(1), 14–23.

Toomey, R., Kang, H. K., Karlinsky, J., Baker, D. G., Vasterling, J. J., Alpern, R., et al. (2007). Mental health of US Gulf War veterans 10 years after the war. *British Journal of Psychiatry, 190*, 385–393.

Vanderploeg, R. D., Belanger, H. G., & Curtiss, G. (2009). Mild traumatic brain injury and posttraumatic stress disorder and their associations with health symptoms. *Archives of Physical Medicine and Rehabilitation, 90*(7), 1084–1093.

Wade, D. T., King, N. S., Wenden, F. J., Crawford, S., & Caldwell, F. E. (1998). Routine follow up after head injury: A second randomised controlled trial. *Journal of Neurology, Neurosurgery and Psychiatry, 65*(2), 177–183.

Warden, D. L., & French, L. (2005). Traumatic brain injury in the war zone. *New England Journal of Medicine, 353*(6), 633–634.

Wilde, E. A., Bigler, E. D., Gandhi, P. V., Lowry, C. M., Blatter, D. D., Brooks, J., et al. (2004). Alcohol abuse and traumatic brain injury: Quantitative magnetic resonance imaging and neuropsychological outcome. *Journal of Neurotrauma, 21*(2), 137–147.

Youngstedt, S. D. (2005). Effects of exercise on sleep. *Clinical Sports Medicine, 24*(2), 355–365, xi.

Zeitzer, J. M., Friedman, L., & O'Hara, R. (2009). Insomnia in the context of traumatic brain injury. *Journal of Rehabilitation and Research Development, 46*, 827–836.

CHAPTER 13

Estimating the Costs of Care

Ann Hendricks, Maxine Krengel, Katherine M. Iverson,
Rachel Kimerling, Carlos Tun, Jomana Amara, and Henry L. Lew

Traumatic brain injury (TBI) is an important public health concern in the United States, particularly as service members return home from the combat operations in Afghanistan, Iraq, and other locations in service of Operations Enduring Freedom and Iraqi Freedom (OEF/OIF) and Operation New Dawn (OND). According to the U.S. House Committee on Veterans' Affairs, more than 2 million service members have served at least one tour of duty in service of OEF/OIF and hundreds of thousands have served more than one tour (U.S. House Committee on Veterans' Affairs, March 18, 2010). Longer deployments and more redeployments place considerable strain on health care systems in terms of care for military personnel with mild TBI (mTBI), as well as posttraumatic stress disorder (PTSD).

Indeed, PTSD is a substantial problem among OEF/OIF veterans in its own right and it commonly co-occurs with TBI (Carlson et al., 2010; Hoge & Castro, 2006; Hoge et al., 2008). For example, between 64 and 67% of OEF/OIF Veterans Health Administration (VHA) patients with confirmed TBI also have a diagnosis of PTSD (Carlson et al., 2010; Iverson, Hendricks, Kimerling, Krengel, Meterko, Stolzman, et al., 2011). Non-treatment-seeking samples likewise have shown high rates of the comorbidity, with just over one-third of those screening positive for TBI also screening positive for PTSD (Tanielian & Jaycox, 2008). Although the occurrence of both TBI and PTSD is receiving unprecedented attention in the clinical literature, little is known about the economic toll resulting from these problems and their treatment costs in the long run. To shape health care policy to meet the clinical needs of individuals with TBI and/or PTSD, clinicians and researchers can draw on economic information to inform their work.

For the nonveteran population, more emphasis is now placed on the lasting effects and costs associated with civilian head injuries, including sports concussion. For example, the Centers for Disease Control and Prevention, National Center for Injury Prevention and Control has created guidelines and produced "toolkits" for infants, youth sports, the elderly, and physicians' private practices (Centers for Disease Control and Prevention, 2011). As with military TBI, psychiatric disorders often emerge with civilian mTBI. A recent prospective study of Australian civilians with mTBI indicated that during the 12 months following the injury, over 7% had developed new onset PTSD, 6% had developed generalized anxiety disorder, 7% had developed agoraphobia, and 7% had developed depression (Bryant et al., 2010). A comprehensive overview of the costs associated with TBI resulting from civilian injuries (e.g., motor vehicle accidents, interpersonal violence, falls, sports-related concussions) is beyond the scope of this review despite the increased importance of the large costs related to emergency response teams, emergency room visits, lengthy hospital stays, exploratory medical testing, and follow-up care. Therefore, this chapter centers on the costs of treating mTBI and PTSD in military veterans, but connections are drawn to civilian injuries where possible.

For clinicians, understanding health care costs is important for comprehending how to best address patient needs. This review does not provide extensive treatment implications, but it is noteworthy that, as with other conditions, the length of treatment may increase (and costs rise) as a direct result of insufficient initial diagnosis and care (Baldessarini, 1989; Hall, 1994; Wells et al., 1989). If patients are not provided with appropriate treatment avenues, they may become disillusioned with the medical community and as such require longer treatment or further support from family members. In addition, without proper assessment and treatment, exacerbations in physical and mental health symptoms may occur (McCarthy et al., 2006). This chapter is intended to help the clinician gain knowledge of the direct and indirect costs relevant to initiatives designed to optimize treatment outcomes for patients with mTBI and/or PTSD.

In addition to direct clinical care costs, this chapter discusses the financial burden placed on OEF/OIF patients and civilians suffering from mTBI and PTSD, on caregivers, and on society at large. Given the average age (about 32 years) and earning potential of the relatively young veterans in this OEF/OIF cohort, and that very young children (ages 0–4) and adolescents are disproportionately represented among civilian TBIs (Faul, Xu, Wald, & Coronado, 2010), these indirect costs are especially important. Financial burdens include the length of time the individual will be absent from gainful employment, will require assistive services to remain in school or at work, and will have an impact on the type and amount of treatment many individuals will choose to obtain. Financial considerations also affect clinicians' ability to provide treatment initiatives in traditional care facilities.

This chapter is not intended as a complete review of the literature on health care costs associated with PTSD and mTBI in the acute and chronic stages. Such reviews already exist (e.g., McGarry et al., 2002; Schootman, Buchman, & Lewis, 2003) and have pointed out the shortcomings in current understanding of the direct costs of care for mTBI and PTSD. Instead, our overview summarizes treatment information in four parts. Specifically, we provide (1) estimates of the incremental direct medical costs of treating both mTBI and PTSD rather than either condition alone; (2) estimates of costs associated with different models of care (i.e., outpatient vs. inpatient care); (3) long-term direct and indirect costs that may result from not treating the conditions effectively; and (4) clinical implications of the relative costs, including long-term costs and those borne by the patient compared to the health care system paying for the care.

We take a societal perspective on costs (Gold, Siegel, Russell, & Weinstein, 1996). If costs in one part of the system decline because services (and therefore costs) in another part of the system increase, the impact on the whole (whether a net increase or decrease) is taken into account. We base our direct medical cost estimates of treating one condition (mTBI only or PTSD only) versus two conditions (mTBI plus PTSD) on Department of Veterans Affairs (VA) benefits, which covers medical and psychiatric conditions related to military service at 100% (i.e., no patient payment) for up to 5 years following separation from the military (and longer if the conditions are disabling). Thus, our estimates of medical costs are not restricted to the limited perspective of a hospital, nursing home, or clinical practice.

A societal perspective also incorporates the impact on the individual and his or her family and friends. Some types of treatment place a greater burden and cost on these individuals than do other treatments. For example, outpatient visits tend to be much less costly to the medical system (e.g., the insurer or the system like the VHA that provides the care) than an equal number of inpatient days of care, but the former may require significantly more expense for travel to and from the outpatient clinics compared to an inpatient stay. Indirect costs of treatment, such as travel or lost workdays, which are borne directly by the patient (or perhaps his or her parents in the case of youth injuries), may affect whether the patient misses appointments, delays treatment, or requires additional appointments, all of which may increase waiting times for other individuals and result in lost work productivity for clinicians with high rates of "no shows." Attendance at care may also influence the extent to which patients can and do recover from these conditions.

Incremental Cost of Treating One versus Both Conditions

In this section, we first present VHA costs from our study of patients who were deployed at some time since 2002 to OEF/OIF and were screened within the VHA for mTBI during fiscal year (FY) 2008 or the first half of FY 2009 (October 1, 2007, through March, 2009; Hendricks et al. 2011). We then briefly list the types of direct costs incurred by patients and families, without attaching monetary values to these cost categories. Finally, we present a listing of some of the major components of evidence-based treatments such as psychotherapies, rehabilitation therapies, and medications for mTBI and PTSD, with estimates of minimal payments based on publicly available Medicare payment rates for the therapies and examinations plus prescription medication prices at Costco (a publicly available price list for a low-cost pharmacy retailer).

Annual Costs to VHA by Condition for FY 2008

Table 13.1 displays annual total costs to the VHA for patients with mTBI or PTSD (or both) and compares them with the costs for patients with neither condition. The mTBI designation comes from VHA's national TBI screening system. VHA administers a national four-part TBI screen as part of its electronic medical records system for clinical reminders to all veterans who report OEF/OIF deployment (Department of Veterans Affairs, 2009). Veterans who respond positively to one or more problem in each of the four sections of the TBI screen are considered to screen positive for TBI; the clinician is then instructed to discuss the results with the veteran and offer a referral for a comprehensive TBI evaluation. The determination of a TBI diagnosis is made by the clinical evaluator who uses a defined protocol, as part of a comprehensive TBI evaluation, to collect information about the origin of the injury, assess symptoms, confirm or rule out mTBI, and list possible follow-up care in a treatment plan. The PTSD diagnosis for Table 13.1 is from VHA utilization data for face-to-face visits with clinicians who listed the diagnosis as a reason for the visit. For patients with only the PTSD diagnosis, we distinguish between those who initially screened negative for mTBI and those who screened positive but had TBI ruled out in the comprehensive TBI evaluation. Patients in all of these categories can and often do have other diagnoses, both medical and psychiatric. Thus, it is important to recognize that costs of patients with positive screens who had TBI ruled out likely reflect other comorbidities being evaluated or treated.

Table 13.1 also presents mean costs for VHA inpatient and outpatient care (excluding outpatient medications). For the inpatient costs, we calculated the means for care provided in the medical/surgical wards or bed sections of the VHA and contrasted them with the means for care provided in psychiatric and long-term care wards (nonmedical/surgical care). These distinctions underscore important cost differences for these patient groups.

First, the variation in annual costs within each cell depicted within Table 13.1 is large, especially for inpatient costs (as indicated by standard deviations that are many times the mean values). Given the variation, the differences in acute medical/surgical inpatient care across diagnostic groups are not statistically significant except for patients with mTBI only, who had medical/surgical costs significantly lower than those for any other patient group in this table. However, nonmedical/surgical inpatient costs (reflecting psychiatric, rehabilitation, and long-term care stays) are significantly different across the diagnostic groups.

TABLE 13.1. Mean (*SD*) Annual Costs per Patient in Dollars of VHA Services by Diagnoses (Columns A–E) and Type of Cost, FY 2008

			PTSD only[b]			
			Negative	Positive		
		TBI only[a]	TBI	TBI	Both TBI	
	Neither	(CTE)	screen	screen	and PTSD	
	A	B	C	D	E	Statistical significance
Number	126,457	1,592	54,761	3,371	5,093	
Inpatient medical/ surgical	193 (3,738)	146 (1,639)	268 (3,196)	286 (3,110)	273 (2,342)	$p < .001$ for Column B vs. any other column; else NS
Inpatient nonmedical/ surgical[c]	286 (7,368)	724 (9,673)	1,282 (8,941)	1,755 (10,326)	2,673 (12,110)	$p < .05$ for Column B vs. C; else $p < .001$
Outpatient	1,993 (2,851)	3,976 (3,864)	4,503 (5,448)	5,710 (5,413)	7,010 (6,435)	All possible pairwise comparisons between columns $p < .001$
Total	2,472 (9,415)	4,846 (10,953)	6,053 (12,473)	7,750 (13,610)	9,957 (15,980)	All possible pairwise comparisons between columns $p < .001$

Note. Standard deviations are reported in parentheses following the mean annual costs.
[a] TBI designations generally identify patients with mild severity although a small, unidentified subset have moderate severity.
[b] For the "PTSD Only" category, we identified two groups of patients for FY 2008: those who also had a negative screen for TBI and those with a positive screen for TBI who later had the diagnosis ruled out in a comprehensive TBI evaluation (CTE). The costs for these subgroups are shown separately.
[c] Nonmedical/surgical care includes psychiatric and long-term care.

Second, the average costs of three of the care categories (i.e., nonmedical/surgical inpatient, outpatient, and total costs) increase across the rows of Table 13.1 from patients with neither diagnosis (lowest costs) to those with mTBI only, PTSD only, and both mTBI and PTSD diagnoses (highest costs). Further, these differences are all statistically significant except for that in nonmedical/surgical inpatient care for patients with TBI only compared to PTSD only (column B vs. C). This direct relationship between inpatient costs for psychiatric or long-term care bed sections across the diagnosis groups reflects that patients with both conditions tend to receive more care in VHA and therefore incur higher costs.

Third, the incremental annual cost of having both diagnoses compared to only one is roughly $4,000 to $5,000 ($9,957-$6,053 = $3,904; $9,957-$4,846 = $5,111). This difference is significantly greater than the difference between the costs for either diagnosis alone compared to patients with neither diagnosis ($2,472). This may be due, in part, to increased costs associated with other common comorbidities, especially psychiatric conditions (e.g., depression), which are common among patients with both mTBI and PTSD (see Iverson, Chapter 3, this volume). In addition, these average VHA costs are for the first year in which these war-zone veterans were routinely screened for mTBI in VHA; therefore, the higher costs may reflect additional evaluations and consults to determine the causes of other symptoms uncovered during the mTBI screening process and to provide treatment for them. The expectation is that in general these cost differences would diminish over time as conditions are effectively treated and thus alleviated.

The higher outpatient costs for patients with PTSD may be due to various factors. One such factor may be poorer physical health among veterans with PTSD as there is now strong evidence linking PTSD to poor health, including increased rates of health conditions that may become chronic (Schnurr, Green, & Kaltman, 2007), even among OEF/OIF veterans, whose trauma exposure was relatively recent (Seal, Bertenthal, Miner, Sen, & Marmar, 2007). Another factor may relate to differences in the clinical guidelines for the treatment of PTSD relative to mTBI. VHA clinical guidelines indicate that PTSD patients can be referred for psychotherapy and medications (e.g., Institute of Medicine, 2008), whereas the treatment guidelines are not as clear for the treatment of mTBI. For example, prolonged exposure (PE) and cognitive processing therapy (CPT) are recommended as the first-line treatments for PTSD (Veterans Health Administration, 2003), with nationwide clinician training efforts underway making these treatments available to all veterans with PTSD being treated in VHA. These clear treatment guidelines may lead to an increase in the availability and utilization of the treatments for patients with mTBI and PTSD, which lead to higher costs in the short term. However, as stated previously, as individuals' symptoms diminish, they require reduced amounts of care and hence lower overall costs.

Differences in costs for veterans with mTBI and/or PTSD underscore the importance of ascertaining psychiatric problems for civilians with mTBI (Kamm, 2005). PTSD may be somewhat less common among civilians who experience some types of non-war-related mTBIs (e.g., sports injuries) because the threat to life will be absent; however, other civilian TBI sources (e.g., motor vehicle accidents, interpersonal violence) are associated with life threat and may be more likely to be associated with PTSD, as demonstrated by high rates of comorbid PTSD and mTBI in trauma centers (Bryant et al., 2010). In addition to the potential for PTSD comorbidity, civilian mTBIs may be associated with other conditions. For example, motor vehicle accidents are often associated with depression and/or anxiety (Mayou, Bryant, & Ehlers, 2001). Sports concussion injuries, especially in young athletes, may result in depression, although at lower rates than with other sports injuries (Mainwaring, Hutchison, Bisschop, Comper, & Richards, 2010). Physical accidents in the elderly resulting in mTBI are relatively common and correlate with mood changes, such as depression and anxiety (Goldstein, Levin, Goldman, Clark, & Altonen, 2001). These are just a few of the many attributes that the clinician needs to take into account when developing treatment plans. Treatment of physical ailments may be delayed or prolonged because of fatigue and irritability associated with patients' mental issues, which must be treated along with the more physical outcomes of the brain injury.

Direct Costs to Patients and Families

The costs described above are for medical and psychiatric treatment provided by VHA for veterans and is typically paid through health insurance for nonveterans. However, patients may still have medical and psychiatric expenses that are not covered by VHA or health insurance (e.g., over-the-counter medications, copays). In addition, patients and families bear other costs related to the care summarized above. Table 13.2 lists just a few major cost categories to the private-sector patient (including veterans who do not qualify for VHA services who must seek care in the private sector) and family for direct medical care for symptoms related to mTBI. Although these costs may appear small to a health care provider when weighed against the average direct medical costs reflected in VHA's experience with these patients, the costs may be large enough to prevent some patients from starting or continuing treatment for their mTBI and/or PTSD. This disincentive may be particularly strong for the nonmedical costs (e.g., for travel, child care, lost wages) that increase in direct proportion to the number of days that the patient comes to a provider's office for treatment.

TABLE 13.2. Costs to the Patient and Family

- Out-of-pocket medical expenditures
  - With insurance
    - —Over-the-counter medicines
    - —Deductibles
    - —Copayments
    - —Self-help materials
  - If items not covered by insurance
    - —Glasses
    - —Hearing aids

- Travel costs
  - Gas
  - Tolls
  - Parking

- Child care

- Lost wages if time is taken from work

There are also potential intangible costs, many of which cannot easily be valued in dollar terms, if at all. A major intangible cost is the potential stigma at work or in the community if the service member seeks care for deployment-related conditions. Fear of stigma may cause some service members to try to "tough it out" instead of seeking help. This delay of care can result in cognitive, physical, and psychological problems getting worse (Brenner, Vanderploeg, & Terrio, 2009), which may be associated with increased health care costs when the patient does seek help. Additionally, the very symptoms of the conditions themselves may interfere with receiving care. For instance, Pietrzak, Johnson, Goldstein, Malley, and Southwick (2009) found that PTSD mediated the relationship between mTBI and perceived barriers to receiving mental health care. For some civilians with mTBI (e.g., athletes), the same value to "tough it out" may lead them to deny the extent of their symptoms and avoid treatment.

Components of Evidence-Based Treatments for mTBI and PTSD

Table 13.3 highlights some of the more common types of treatment that clinicians offer patients with mild/moderate TBI and PTSD along with a summary of the most common types of symptoms that are treated. Costs depend on who the payer is; therefore, the cost estimates in Table 13.3 should be viewed as illustrative of low-cost alternatives. We have been conservative in our estimates and used the lowest estimates for 2011 that were readily accessible and can be replicated by other health care economists. We used Medicare nonfacility (i.e., not in a hospital) professional fees for

TABLE 13.3. Outpatient Treatment Modalities for mTBI and PTSD with Estimates of Costs

Symptom	Treatment	Resources	Cost estimate
Mild TBI			
	Education	Printed material on symptoms/ recovery	$15
		Single session	$35/individual
Headaches	Evaluation	Appointment	$100–150
	Medications	Sumatriptan 100 mg orally every day for 1–2 months	$125
Sleep disorders	Medications for 3–6 months at bedtime	Ambien 5 mg	$752/3 months 5 mg
		Zolpidem	$23/3 months 5 mg
		Prazosin	$22/3 months 1 mg
Visual problems	Evaluation	Appointment	$100
	Sunglasses	Prescription if needed	$100
Hearing problems	Evaluation	Appointment	$100–150
	Hearing aid	Prescription if needed	$1,500–2,000
Depression	Medications for 2–6 months	Sertraline 100–200 mg/day	$24–88
		Citalopram 20 mg/day	$14–42
Other emotional symptoms (e.g., irritability)	Evaluation Therapy	Appointment	$75 or more per session
Neurocognitive dysfunction	Therapy with psychologist	1 outpatient session/ week for 6–8 weeks	$150 per session
		Total of 6–8 sessions	$900–1,200
Speech problems	Therapy	Varies with problem	Varies with treatments
Vestibular problems (e.g., balance problem, dizziness)	Vestibular rehabilitation	2 sessions/week for 6–10 weeks	$75 per session $900–1,500

(cont.)

TABIE 13.3. *(cont.)*

Symptom	Treatment	Resources	Cost estimate
Pain	Physical therapy for low back pain	2 visits/week for 2 months (10–15 visits)	$750–1,125
	Medications	Ibuprofen 600 mg three times a day for 30 days	$8/100
		Naproxen 500 mg/day	$8/100
		Tramadol 50 mg/day	$13/100
		Percocet 1 tablet three times a day for 2–3 months	$40/30 online/not available at Costco
		Epidural steroid injection	Varies by site (e.g., lumbar) and number of visits required
PTSD	Education	Printed material on symptoms/recovery	$15
		Single session	$35/individual
	Psychotherapy:		
	• CBT / CPT	Individual: 12 50-minute sessions	$120/session = $1,440
	• PET	Individual: 12–15 90-minute sessions	$156/session = $1,875
	• SIT	Individual: 8–15 50-minute sessions	$120/session = $960–1,800
	• EMDR	Individual: 12 50-minute sessions	$1,440
Anxiety, depression, flashbacks, nightmares	SSRIs: • 12 weeks to assess initial response • Medication management • Medication indefinitely if PTSD is chronic • HEDIS quality measure > 6-month treatment period	• Sertraline 50–100 mg/day • Citalopram 20–60 mg/day • Paroxetine 20–60 mg/day • Fluoxetine 20–60 mg/day	Annual costs: $92–88 (100 mg is less) $38–114 $110–240 $38–114

(cont.)

TABLE 13.3. *(cont.)*

Symptom	Treatment	Resources	Cost estimate
	Antidepressants	TCAs:	
		• Clomipramine 50 mg	$28/100
		• Amitriptyline 100 mg	$10/100
		• Desipramine 10 mg	$105/100
		• Nortriptyline 50 mg	$16/100
		• Doxepin 100 mg	$11/100
		• Imipramine 50 mg	$39/100
		MAOIs:	
		• Zelapar	$1,051/120
		• Parnate 10 mg	$173/100
		• Nardil 15 mg	$173/180
	For nightmares	• Prazosin 1 mg	$22/3 months

Note. CBT, cognitive-behavioral therapy; CPT, cognitive processing therapy; PET, prolonged exposure therapy; SIT, stress inoculation therapy; EMDR, eye movement densitization and reprocessing; SSRIs, selective serotonin reuptake inhibitors; TCAs, tricyclic antidepressants; MAOIs, monoamine oxidase inhibitors; HEDIS, Healthcare Effectiveness Data and Information Set.

various evaluations and treatments for either condition, and the prices for medications charged by Costco, a low-cost retailer that makes its prices publicly available on the Internet (at *www.costco.com/Pharmacy*).

The cost estimates in Table 13.3 are not intended as an explanation for differences in the average costs presented in Table 13.1. Table 13.1 includes all care provided by VHA, much of which may not relate directly to either mTBI or PTSD. The VHA patients may have many comorbidities, both physical and emotional. In addition, the service-specific expenditures by VHA for its services in FY 2008 will also differ from those listed in Table 13.3, which illustrate psychosocial treatments and medications in 2011.

Several points are worth noting when evaluating Table 13.3. First, most patients do not need every type of treatment listed in Table 13.3. Total treatment costs will not be the sum of all services listed in the table, but readers can begin to understand the relative costs for different types or combinations of treatment for mTBI and/or PTSD. Second, many services in Table 13.3 have low annual costs, but if a patient with a chronic problem requires services every year, the cumulative costs can be expensive. Third, some services may consist of one course of intensive treatment with booster or refresher treatments in the future. Fourth, additional stressors and medical circumstances a patient faces over a decade or more will vary widely and affect actual health care costs as well.

Costs Associated with Different Models of Care

The list of services in Table 13.3 sets the stage for considering the costs of different treatment models. We first give an estimate for an outpatient program to treat mTBI and compare that with an estimate for outpatient therapy for PTSD. We note where savings are possible from combining the two types of treatment. We then summarize the impact of providing care on an inpatient versus an outpatient basis.

Estimating Program Costs

mTBI

The VHA, Center for Disease Control and Prevention, and Department of Defense stress in their Clinical Practice Guidelines that the vast majority of patients who have sustained an mTBI improve with no lasting clinical sequelae, but, in a small minority of patients, symptoms may persist beyond 6 months to a year (Veterans Health Administration, 2003, p. 7). The guidelines state that early education of patients and their families is the best available treatment for mTBI and for preventing or reducing persistent symptoms, an important factor in understanding the increased costs with insufficient initial intervention (Veterans Health Administration, 2003, p. 31). Given that mTBI treatment options are presented by Ponsford (Chapter 10, this volume), we will not highlight specific types of treatment initiatives.

The guidelines list headache as the single most common symptom associated with mTBI, and assessment and management of headaches related to mTBI should be similar to those for other causes of headache. The guidelines further indicate that treatment of other symptoms (e.g., somatic complaints and psychiatric symptoms) should be tailored to the patient's "symptom presentation" (Veterans Health Administration, 2003, p. 8). Providing patient education and offering treatment for headaches and other pressing somatic symptoms are relatively inexpensive and their treatment should be integrated with any comprehensive evaluation of the patient's condition so that he or she leaves the encounter with the health care system with some immediate understanding of the condition(s) (Lew et al., 2008). Further, sometimes there is not a single course of treatment, but options for helping address the symptoms that patient and provider need to consider collaboratively.

The cost of a half-hour of one-on-one education might be lower than $50 in 2011 (Table 13.3). This cost estimate is based on distributing a book that discusses mTBI and its treatment and a nonphysician educator reviewing the material with the patient and answering questions. The book, such as those currently available at retail for $15, might have to be purchased by the patient if the insurer does not cover it as a separate benefit, but providers can undoubtedly make educational materials available at a lower cost than this estimate. Of course, the cost to the provider and the payment from the insurer (or the patient) would also be less if the educational session included several patients in a group.

The most costly treatments for symptoms associated with mTBI for veterans and other concussion patients alike include therapy for neurocognitive dysfunction, psychosocial treatments, family therapy, vocational counseling, and brand-name drugs for depression. As discussed by Ponsford (Chapter 10, this volume), instruction on compensatory strategies to work around attention and memory impairment may be necessary to assure that patients are able to maintain focus and learn in their other treatment episodes, including those for PTSD and depression. In many instances, the cognitive rehabilitation and psychoeducational approaches that may enhance continued gains in the postacute stages (McCrae, 2008) are not readily available to all patients (e.g., to students through school systems).

Costs are also affected by a patient's preference for specific medications and the specific clinical complaints. Although many generic drugs may be used for treatment of symptoms of depression, anxiety disorders, and PTSD, veterans may choose drugs not available through the VA pharmacy. This will increase health care costs as they are specially ordered through the pharmacy (for VHA patients). Newer drugs and alternative complementary medical treatments, such as acupuncture and yoga, traditionally not available within the VHA system (but provided in some medical centers) or covered by private health insurance are other unexpected costs to the health care system or to the patient and family.

PTSD

Initial treatment for PTSD is more costly than that for mTBI, because cognitive-behavioral approaches, such as cognitive processing therapy (CPT), prolonged exposure therapy (PET), and stress inoculation therapies, can require a few months or more to cover all the material and achieve results. Even at a minimal payment rate under the Medicare program, a course of CPT would likely cost around $2,000. In addition to therapist wages, costs also include CPT handouts and materials, which are provided to patients within VHA and presumably in private-sector programs. These are relatively low costs, however, primarily resulting from printing materials and photocopying.

Coordination of Care

Providers can realize savings from coordinating care for mTBI and PTSD (what economists refer to as "economies of scope") and avoiding duplication of certain types of care potentially required for both PTSD and mTBI (e.g., psychoeducation for the patient and family, treatment for sleep disorders, treatment/medications for depression, or polypharmacy more generally). This type of coordination of care is also key in reducing the costs borne by the patient and his or her family. Coordinated care reduces the total number of days required for receiving all of the treatments, reducing the time a patient has to take off work or away from family, cutting the costs of travel to and from the clinic, and decreasing costs for child care while the patient is away from home. These factors might increase the commitment and ability of some patients to participate fully in a treatment plan.

Inpatient versus Outpatient Programs

Another important difference in treatment models from a cost perspective is whether care is provided on an inpatient or an outpatient basis. The differences can be seen in both the costs covered by the payer and those borne directly by the patient and family. Inpatient care is more costly to the health care system than outpatient care because it requires coverage of room and board in addition to the treatment services and medications. Additionally, unlike outpatient services, inpatient care requires a proportion of the staff to be employed around the clock. The high costs associated with inpatient care contribute to insurers' policies of not covering inpatient care for some types of treatment. If the care is provided in a medical ward, room and board costs can be quite large, especially compared to the lower cost of having the patient stay at home and commute to the medical facility for care. However, special wards or units with less medical equipment and reduced medical supervision at night can reduce the room and board costs from more than $1,000 a night to less than $100 (even outside the VHA).

Long-Term Costs of Not Providing Treatment

If untreated, mTBI and/or PTSD may make future medical and psychiatric issues more likely (Brenner et al., 2009; Priebe et al. 2009), potentially adding to the costs of not treating the initial condition(s). For instance, a patient with untreated PTSD may turn to substance misuse as a way of managing his or her symptoms, which may evolve into substance abuse or substance dependence. Additionally, depression is common among individuals with mTBI and/or PTSD (Carlson et al., 2010; Tanielian & Jaycox, 2008). Both the initial mTBI and PTSD and the subsequent development of any additional, related disorders may affect physical health, which may lead to increased primary care and specialty care visits (Hoge et al., 2008; McCarthy et al., 2006; Schnurr & Green, 2004).

These conclusions are consistent with a longitudinal study of outpatient utilization and costs among veterans with TBI (Homaifar, Harwood, Wagner, & Brenner, 2009), in which about a quarter of the study population was classified as having sustained an mTBI. These patients had more primary care/internal medicine visits per year than those with moderate/severe TBI. For mild cases, the annual average cost increased with the time that had passed since the injury, but the analyses did not control for other conditions. Therefore, we do not know the long-term, direct medical costs associated with untreated mTBI. Additionally, we do not yet know the long-term effect of secondary impact syndrome when the brain is not given the time to recover between mTBIs. For PTSD, long-term costs are also not documented, but may well include repeated admissions for psychiatric or substance use disorders as well as exacerbations in chronic illness.

Occupational difficulties, including unemployment and few work hours, have been documented among individuals with mTBI (Dikmen et al., 1994) and PTSD (Smith, Schnurr, & Rosenheck, 2005). There is some evidence to suggest that untreated mTBI and/or PTSD symptoms contribute to familial and social difficulties (Milliken, Auchterlonie, & Hoge, 2007; Taft, Watkins, Stafford, Street, & Monson, 2011). Additionally, recent public health research has revealed that individuals from the OEF/OIF conflicts (with mTBI and PTSD and concurrent symptoms that reduce capabilities to maintain gainful employment) are more likely to become homeless and do so much sooner than individuals from prior conflicts (Gamache, Rosenheck, & Tessler, 2003).

The value of lost work productivity can be estimated in monetary terms from income flows by occupation, age, and education reported by the Census Bureau. The RAND simulations reported in Tanielian and Jaycox (2008) used wages and employment probabilities for veterans reported in the March 2007 Current Population Survey (p. 181) and reduced both measures for simulation subjects with PTSD and major depression based on the available literature, primarily Savoca and Rosenheck (2000). The impact of major depression was estimated to be about three times greater than for PTSD, reducing wages by over 45% compared to veterans without the condition.

There are currently no estimates of lost hours of work due to OEF/OIF or OND deployment-related injuries, although Hoge et al. (2008) reported that 23% of OEF/OIF military with mTBI missed 2 or more days of work due to illness in the prior month compared to 15% of those with other types of injuries and only 7% of those with no injuries. In a similar study, Hoge, Terhakopian, Castro, Messer, and Engel (2007) found that twice as many soldiers with PTSD missed 2 or more days of work due to illness in the prior month than those without PTSD (12% vs. 6.5%). Although the military might pay for the patient's retirement or the VHA might pay compensation for a disability, neither amount represents what the person had hoped to achieve and neither compensates society for the loss of the person's productivity during his or her lifetime.

To make the simulations more concrete, suppose that a 22-year-old patient might expect to be earning $30,000 a year in real estate or insurance sales. He or she might expect to earn $1.8 million during his or her working life. If chronic PTSD made it difficult to maintain full-time employment or work at more than a laborer's job, the loss in income could easily be over a quarter of a million dollars over a working lifetime of 40 years. That amount represents not only a loss to the patient and family, but also to society as a whole, which forgoes the differences in the services that the patient could have been producing if he or she were not disabled.

How Cost Issues Affect Individual Clinical Decision Making

The information presented in this chapter underscores that the costs of clinical treatment for mTBI and PTSD depend on the course of treatment(s) and the patient's personal circumstances. As highlighted in Table 13.3, there are many treatments that can help alleviate postconcussive (e.g., dizziness, sleep problems, hearing impairments) (French, Iverson, & Bryant, 2011) and PTSD (e.g., flashbacks, nightmares, numbing) (Iverson, Lester, & Resick, 2011) symptoms. Receiving these treatments can help prevent postconcussive and PTSD symptoms from becoming chronic or leading to other conditions that require hospitalization and further disability, which carry a heavy economic burden for health care systems and the patient.

The targeted outcomes of mTBI and PTSD treatment should include reintegration of the patient into his or her life in terms of successful job performance, ability to function in one's family and social relationships, and enjoyment of everyday life activities. Indeed, in research concerning patients primarily with severe TBI, return to work is a major outcome measure, reflecting this goal for treatment (Wehman et al., 2003). Poor clinical outcomes represent costs that are borne by families (both spouse and children) as well as the patient. If the treatment outcomes do not include successful reintegration into one's life, the course of treatment has not really altered the costs to the patient and society. Further, it is not enough to keep the patient out of the hospital or focus only on symptom remission. Reclaiming one's life includes restoring the patient's cognitive and emotional functioning, as closely as possible, to former levels to ensure a similar level of work productivity and enjoyment of a positive quality of life.

Another implication of recognizing the importance of reintegration of the patient into his or her life is the need for psychoeducation early in the process of treatment (French et al., 2011; Iverson et al., 2011). Psychoeducation includes providing information to the patient and his or her family members regarding the nature of mTBI and/or PTSD symptoms, and how such symptoms often occur on a spectrum. Not only is the patient helped by understanding what to expect, such information can help the patient understand and accept how he or she has changed as a result of the trauma(s), so that he or she can make informed decisions regarding treatment options that can help maximize functioning (Wilk & Hoge, 2010). Additionally, many family members desire family education (Sherman et al., 2009). Such programs can help family members feel less burdened and more effective in helping their loved ones, which can have a positive impact on their own health (Cuijpers & Stam, 2000; Hazel et al., 2004).

A health care system like VHA may realize some economies of scope in treating both conditions in an integrated manner, rather than sequentially. Improvements in emotional symptoms may be greater if physical or cognitive symptoms are addressed at the same time; likewise, physical conditions can improve with better mental health (Schnurr & Green, 2004). Dealing with both conditions will require the use of coordinators for the many types of care that the dually diagnosed mTBI/PTSD patients should be receiving. It has been suggested that coordinators for these patients can even be effective for arranging care across a variety of health needs, even those that are only indirectly related to mTBI or PTSD (Sayer et al., 2009). This effectiveness can come from cross-consultation and cross-education for providers in other care silos who may have less experience with these dually diagnosed patients.

Summary and Conclusions

Our overview of the health care costs associated with mTBI and/or PTSD clearly demonstrates the significant burden of these conditions on the health care system, the patient, and the family. Health care systems and individual providers should be mindful of how symptoms from one disorder can impact treatment for the other disorder. Additionally, health care systems and individual providers should take care to ensure that both conditions are addressed. For instance, individuals with mTBI often complain of difficulty with attention and short-term memory, skills presumably important for cognitively based treatments for many psychiatric conditions, including PTSD (Sayer et al., 2009). Therefore, psychoeducation about the impact of mTBI on cognitive functioning, cognitive rehabilitation, and early interventions for diminished attention and short-term memory may improve treatment directed at emotional and physical symptoms (McCrae, 2008; Ponsford et al., 2002; Whittaker, Kemp, & House, 2007). Military and VHA medical facilities offer treatment for these types of conditions, but the care may take place in separate clinics or departments, often with little coordination of care for individual patients (Sayer et al., 2009), which may lead to frustration on the part of the patient and maintenance of symptoms.

As noted earlier, the costs borne directly by the patient and family/ friends during treatment (travel costs, lost wages, child care, etc.) will make it difficult for the patient to accommodate treatment for all the aspects of both mTBI and PTSD in a short time span, yet prolonged treatment also increases the cost for the patient. In recommending treatments, it is likely beneficial for the clinician to be aware of the patient's work and home circumstances and try to balance the indirect costs to maximize the patient's ability and willingness to adhere to a treatment plan. Telehealth and web-based interventions can potentially reduce the number of trips to the office of providers and also improve treatment compliance. For example, there is promising data supporting the use of such interventions for PTSD (Greene et al., 2010; Lange et al., 2003; Litz, Engel, Bryant, & Papa, 2007). Clinicians will likely also find it helpful to inquire about potential treatment barriers and problem-solve these obstacles with the patient.

Clinical teams that can find ways to make treatment more easily available are likely to experience greater success with their patients and ultimately reduce the health care costs associated with mTBI and PTSD. For patients who work daytime jobs, evening or weekend clinics may substantially improve adherence to treatment and improve clinical outcomes, thereby reducing costs to the patient and the health care system. If a health care system cannot accommodate the patients' needs, the patients will be much less likely to come for care, resulting in larger long-term costs. With improvement in clinical guidelines, diagnostic procedures, and treatment initiatives, it is likely that health care costs related to mTBI, PTSD, and co-occurring disorders will decrease.

References

Baldessarini, R. J. (1989). Current status of antidepressants: Clinical pharmacology and therapy. *Journal of Clinical Psychiatry, 50,* 117–126.

Brenner, L. A., Vanderploeg, R. D., & Terrio, H. (2009). Assessment and diagnosis of mild traumatic brain injury, posttraumatic stress disorder, and other polytrauma conditions: Burden of adversity hypothesis. *Rehabilitation Psychology, 54,* 239–246.

Bryant, R. A., O'Donnell, M. L., Creamer, M., McFarlane, A. C., Clark, C. R., & Silove, D. (2010). The psychiatric sequelae of traumatic injury. *American Journal of Psychiatry, 167,* 312–320.

Carlson, K. F., Nelson, D., Orazem, R. J., Nugent, S., Cifu, D. X., & Sayer, N. A. (2010). Psychiatric diagnoses among Iraq and Afghanistan war veterans screened for deployment-related traumatic brain injury. *Journal of Traumatic Stress, 23*, 17–24.

Centers for Disease Control and Prevention. (2011). Injury prevention and control: Traumatic brain injury. Retrieved February 2, 2011, from *www.cdc.gov/Concussion*.

Cuijpers, P., & Stam, H. (2000). Burnout among relatives of psychiatric patients attending psychoeducational support groups. *Psychiatric Services, 51*, 375–379.

Department of Veterans Affairs and Department of Defense, Management of Concussion/mTBI Working Group. (2009). *VA/DoD clinical practice guideline for management of concussion/mild traumatic brain injury*. Washington, DC: Author.

Dikmen, S. S., Temkin, N. R., Machamer, J. E., Holubkov, A. L., Fraser, R. T., & Winn, H. R. (1994). Employment following traumatic head injuries. *Archives of Neurology, 51*, 177–186.

Faul, M., Xu, L., Wald, M. M. & Coronado, V. G. (2010). *Traumatic brain injury in the United States: Emergency department visits, hospitalizations, and deaths*. Atlanta, GA: Centers for Disease Control and Prevention, National Center for Injury Prevention and Control.

French, L. M., Iverson, G. L., & Bryant, R. A. (2011). Traumatic brain injury. In D. M. Benedek & G. H. Wynn (Eds.), *Clinical manual for the management of PTSD* (pp. 383–414). Washington, DC: American Psychiatric Publishing.

Gamache, G., Rosenheck, R., & Tessler, R. (2003). Overrepresentation of women veterans among homeless women. *American Journal of Public Health, 93*, 1132–1136.

Gold, M. R., Siegel, J. E., Russell, L. B., & Weinstein, M. C. (1996). *Cost-effectiveness in health and medicine*. New York: Oxford University Press.

Goldstein, F. C., Levin, H. S., Goldman, W. P., Clark, A. N., & Altonen, T. K., (2001). Cognitive and neurobehavioral functioning after mild versus moderate traumatic brain injury in older adults. *Journal of the International Neuropsychological Society, 7*, 373–383.

Greene, C. J., Morland, L. A., MacDonald, A., Frueh, B. C., Grubbs, K. M., & Rosen, C. S. (2010). How does tele-mental health affect group therapy process?: Secondary analysis of a noninferiority trial. *Journal of Consulting and Clinical Psychology, 78*, 746–750.

Hall, R. C. W. (1994). The clinical and financial burden of mood disorders cost and outcome. *Psychosomatics*. Retrieved October 6, 2010, from *www.drrichard-hall.com/Articles/mood.pdf*.

Hazel, N. A., McDonell, M. G., Short, R. A., Berry, C. M., Voss, W. D., Rodgers, M. L., et al. (2004). Impact of multiple-family groups for outpatients with schizophrenia on caregivers' distress and resources. *Psychiatric Services, 55*, 35–41.

Hendricks, A., Amara, J., Baker, E., Charns, M., Gardner, J. A., Iverson, K. M., et al. (2011). *Screening for mild traumatic brain injury in OEF-OIF deployed military: An empirical assessment of the VA experience*. Manuscript submitted for publication.

Hoge, C. W., & Castro, C. A. (2006). Post-traumatic stress disorder in UK and US forces deployed to Iraq. *Lancet, 368,* 837.

Hoge, C. W., McGurk, D., Thomas, J. L., Cox, A. L., Engel, C. C., & Castro, C. A. (2008). Mild traumatic brain injury in U.S. soldiers returning from Iraq. *New England Journal of Medicine, 358,* 453–463.

Hoge, C. W., Terhakopian, A., Castro, C. A., Messer, S. C., & Engel, C. C. (2007). Association of posttraumatic stress disorder with somatic symptoms, health care visits, and absenteeism among Iraq war veterans. *American Journal of Psychiatry, 164,* 150–153.

Homaifar, B. Y., Harwood, J. E., Wagner, T. H., & Brenner, L. A. (2009). Description of outpatient utilization and costs in group of veterans with traumatic brain injury. *Journal of Rehabilitation and Research Development, 46,* 1003–1010.

House Veterans' Affairs Committee. (2010, March 18). House Veterans' Affairs Committee holds roundtable discussion to identify specific reintegration issues facing veterans. Retrieved October 5, 2010, from *veterans.hourse.gov/news/PRArticle.aspx?NewsID=557.*

Institute of Medicine. (2008). *Treatment of posttraumatic stress disorder: An assessment of the evidence.* Washington, DC: National Academic Press.

Ishibe, N., Wlordarczyk, R. C., & Fulco, C. (2009). Overview of the Institute of Medicine's committee search strategy and review process for Gulf War and health: Long-term consequences of traumatic brain injury. *Journal of Head Trauma Rehabilitation, 24,* 424–429.

Iverson, K. M., Hendricks, A., M., Kimerling, R., Krengel, M., Meterko, M., Stolzmann, K. L., et al. (2011). Psychiatric diagnoses and neurobehavioral symptom severity among OEF/OIF VA patients with deployment-related traumatic brain injury: A gender comparison. *Women's Health Issues, 21*(45), S210–S217.

Iverson, K. M., Lester, K., & Resick, P. A. (2011). Psychosocial treatments. In D. M. Benedek & G. H. Wynn (Eds.), *Clinical manual for the management of PTSD* (pp. 157–203). Arlington, VA: American Psychiatric Press.

Kamm, R. L. (2005). Interviewing principles for the psychiatrically aware sports medicine physician. *Clinics in Sports Medicine, 24,* 745–769.

Lange, A., Rietdijk, D., Hudcovicova, M., van de Ven, J.-P., Schrieken, B., & Emmelkamp, P. M. G. (2003). Interapy: A randomized controlled trial of the standardized treatment of posttraumatic stress through the Internet. *Journal of Consulting and Clinical Psychology, 71,* 901–909.

Lew, H. L., Vanderploeg, R. D., Moore, D. F., Schwab, K., Friedman, L., Yesavage, J., et al. (2008). Overlap of mild TBI and mental health conditions in returning OIF/OEF service members and veterans. *Journal of Rehabilitation Research and Development, 45,* xi–xvi.

Litz, B. T., Engel, C. C., Bryant, R. A., & Papa, A. (2007). A randomized, controlled proof-of-concept trial of an Internet-based, therapist-assisted self-management treatment for posttraumatic stress disorder. *American Journal of Psychiatry, 164,* 1676–1683.

Mainwaring, L. M., Hutchison, M., Bisschop, S. M., Comper, P., & Richards, D.

W. (2010). Emotional response to sport concussion compared to ACL injury. *Brain Injury, 24,* 589–597.

Mayou, R., Bryant, B., & Ehlers, A. (2001). Prediction of psychological outcomes one year after a motor vehicle accident. *American Journal of Psychiatry, 158,* 1231–1238.

McCarthy, M. L., Dickmen, S. S., Langlois, J. A., Selassie, A. W., Gu, J. K., & Horner, M. D. (2006). Self-reported psychosocial health among adults with traumatic brain injury. *Archives of Physical Medicine and Rehabilitation, 87,* 953–961.

McCrae, M. A. (2008). *Mild traumatic brain injury and postconcussion syndrome.* Oxford UK: Oxford University Press.

McGarry, L. J., Thompson, D., Millham, F. H., Cowell, L., Snyder, P. J., Lenderking, W. R., et al. (2002). Outcomes and costs of acute treatment of traumatic brain injury. *Journal of Trauma: Injury, Infection, and Critical Care, 53,* 1152–1159.

Milliken, C. S., Auchterlonie, J. L., & Hoge, C. W. (2007). Longitudinal assessment of mental health problems among active and reserve component soldiers returning from the Iraq War. *The Journal of the American Medical Association, 298,* 2141–2148.

Pietrzak, R. H., Johnson, D. C., Goldstein, M. B., Malley, J. C., & Southwick, S. M. (2009). Posttraumatic stress disorder mediates the relationship between mild traumatic brain injury and health and psychosocial functioning in veterans of Operations Enduring Freedom and Iraqi Freedom. *Journal of Nervous and Mental Disease, 197,* 748–753.

Ponsford, J., Willmott, C., Rothwell, A., Cameron, P., Kelly, A. M., Nelms, R., et al. (2002). Impact of early intervention on outcome following mild head injury in adults. *Journal of Neurollogy, Neurosurgury, and Psychiatry, 73,* 330–332.

Priebe, S., Matanov, A., Jankovic Gavrilovic, J., McCrone, P., Ljubotina, D., Knezevic, G., et al. (2009). Consequences of untreated posttraumatic stress disorder following war in former Yugoslavia: Morbidity, subjective quality of life, and care costs. *Croatian Medical Journal, 50,* 465–475.

Savoca, E., & Rosenheck, R. (2000). The civilian labor market experiences of Vietnam-era veterans: The influence of psychiatric disorders. *Journal of Mental Health Policy and Economics, 3*(4), 199–207.

Sayer, N. A., Rettmann, N. A., Carlson, K. F., Bernardy, N., Sigford, B. J., Hamblen, J. L., et al. (2009). Veterans with history of mild traumatic brain injury and posttraumatic stress disorder: Challenges from provider perspective. *Journal of Rehabilitation Research and Development, 46,* 703–716.

Schnurr, P. P., & Green, B. L. (2004). *Trauma and health: Physical health consequences of exposure to extreme stress.* Washington, DC: American Psychological Association.

Schnurr, P. P., Green, B. L., & Kaltman, S. (2007). Trauma exposure and physical health. In M. J. Friedman, T. M. Keane & P. A. Resick (Eds.), *Handbook of PTSD: Science and practice* (pp. 406–424). New York: Guilford Press.

Schootman, M., Buchman, T. G., & Lewis, L. M. (2003). National estimates of hospitalization charges for the acute care of traumatic brain injuries. *Brain Injury, 17,* 983–990.

Seal, K. H., Bertenthal, D., Miner, C. R., Sen, S., & Marmar, C. (2007). Bringing the war back home: Mental health disorders among 103,788 US veterans returning from Iraq and Afghanistan seen at Department of Veterans Affairs facilities. *Archives of Internal Medicine, 167,* 476–482.

Sherman, M. D., Fischer, E., Bowling, U. B., Dixon, L., Ridener, L., & Harrison, D. (2009). A new engagement strategy in a VA-based family psychoeducation program. *Psychiatric Services, 60,* 254–257.

Smith, M. W., Schnurr, P. P., & Rosenheck, R. A. (2005). Employment outcomes and PTSD symptom severity. *Mental Health Services Research, 7,* 89–101.

Taft, C. T., Watkins, L. E., Stafford, J., Street, A. E., & Monson, C. M. (2011). Posttraumatic stress disorder and intimate relationship problems: A meta-analysis. *Journal of Consulting and Clinical Psychology, 79,* 22–33.

Tanielian, T., & Jaycox, L. H. (2008). *Invisible wounds of war: Psychological and cognitive injuries, their consequences, and services to assist recovery.* Santa Monica, CA: RAND Corp.

U.S. House Committee on Veterans' Affairs. (2010, March 18).

Veterans Health Administration Office of Quality and Performance, Department of Defense Clinical Practice Guideline Working Group. (2003). *Management of posttraumatic stress* (Publication #10Q-CPG/PTSD-04). Retrieved from *www.oqp.med.va.gov/cpg/PTSD/PTSD_Base.htm.*

Wehman, P., Kregel, J., Keyser-Marcus, L., Sherron-Targett, P., Campbell, L., West, M., et al. (2003). Supported employment for persons with traumatic brain injury: A preliminary investigation of long-term follow-up costs and program efficiency. *Archives of Physical Medicine and Rehabilitation, 84,* 192–196.

Wells, K. B., Hays, R. D., Burnam, M. A., Rogers, W., Greenfield, S., & Ware, J. E. (1989). Detection of depressive disorder for patients receiving prepaid or fee-for-service care. *Journal of the American Medical Association, 262,* 3298–3302.

Whittaker, R., Kemp, S., & House, A. (2007). Illness perceptions and outcome in mild head injury: A longitudinal study. *Journal of Neurology, Neurosurgery, and Psychiatry, 78,* 644–646.

Wilk, J. E., & Hoge, C. W. (2011). Military and veteran populations. In D. M. Benedek & G. H. Wynn (Eds.), *Clinical manual for the management of PTSD* (pp. 349–369). Washington DC: American Psychiatric Publishing.

PART V

CONCLUSIONS

CHAPTER 14

Understanding the Interface of Traumatic Stress and Mild Traumatic Brain Injury

Future Directions in Science and Clinical Practice

Jennifer J. Vasterling, Richard A. Bryant, and Terence M. Keane

As a result of modern warfare, posttraumatic stress disorder (PTSD) and mild traumatic brain injury (mTBI) co-occur with sufficient frequency to represent a major challenge to the health care systems charged with providing care to combat veterans (Sayer et al., 2009). The PTSD/mTBI comorbidity, however, is not limited to military populations. Certain civilian contexts (e.g., motor vehicle accidents, interpersonal violence) that are characterized by exposure to life threat confer risk of both PTSD and mTBI. Despite the frequency with which PTSD and mTBI occur concomitantly, neither the comorbidity nor its clinical management is well understood. In Chapter 1 (Vasterling, Bryant, & Keane), we posed four questions:

1. To what extent and via what mechanisms do PTSD and mTBI potentially complicate each other?
2. Which other factors complicate recovery from PTSD and mTBI?
3. What do we know about treatment of patients with comorbid PTSD/mTBI?
4. How should care of patients with PTSD and mTBI be optimally structured?

In this chapter, we return to these questions, addressing the first two questions within a broader discussion of mechanisms and the second two questions in a section devoted to the provision of care. We conclude with considerations of possible future directions in caring for patients with PTSD PTSD and mTBI.

Potential Mechanisms Underlying Comorbidity and Complicating Recovery

Neural and psychosocial factors influence both the development and course of PTSD and recovery from mTBI. As illustrated by Bigler and Maxwell (Chapter 2) and Iverson (Chapter 3), mTBI has a clear neurophysiological basis, but its recovery may be influenced by unresolved neuropathological features, subsequent neural insults (e.g., repeated exposures to blasts in military veterans and repetitive sports concussions in civilians), psychosocial factors such as depression and PTSD, symptom attributions, expectations for recovery, and contextual factors such as financial incentives, work status, family circumstances, and other stressors. As described by Hayes and Gilbertson (Chapter 4) and Verfaellie, Amick, and Vasterling (Chapter 5), the development and course of PTSD likewise is determined not just by the exposure to a psychologically traumatic event, but also by the availability of external (e.g., social support) and internal (e.g., adaptive coping strategies) resources, neural factors (e.g., brain and neurocognitive integrity), concurrent physical injury (including brain injury), and exposure to subsequent stressors (e.g., multiple military deployments, repetitive episodes of domestic violence). Thus, even when PTSD and mTBI are considered individually, recovery from psychological trauma and brain injury are typically determined by multiple factors. When PTSD and mTBI are considered in aggregate, the determinants of impairment arising from PTSD and mTBI will likely be even more complex.

The relationship between PTSD and mTBI is probably bidirectional: PTSD likely influences recovery from brain injury and mTBI likely influences recovery from psychological trauma. Importantly, although PTSD and mTBI are frequently comorbid, the relationship between PTSD severity and TBI severity cannot be fit, entirely, into a linear model. Some commentators suggest that, due to limited encoding of the trauma memory, PTSD cannot develop in response to a TBI event when the individual loses consciousness or cannot remember the event (Sbordone & Ruff, 2010). Although this view is not supported by studies demonstrating PTSD among patients with severe TBI (Bryant, Marosszeky, Crooks, & Gurka, 2000), the literature suggests that more severe TBIs are less likely than milder

TBIs to be associated with PTSD (Zatzick et al., 2010). Similarly, there is an inverse relationship between the extent of memory after the trauma and development of PTSD symptoms (Bryant et al., 2009; Gil, Caspi, Ben-Ari, Koren, & Klein, 2005). Once individuals with no brain injury are considered, however, the association between TBI and PTSD is no longer linear. As compared to no brain injury, the presence of TBI and, in particular mTBI, appears to confer additional risk of PTSD (Bryant et al., 2010; Hoge et al., 2008). Thus, a trauma-exposed person with a milder TBI is more likely to develop PTSD than a trauma-exposed person with no brain injury or a trauma-exposed person with a more severe TBI.

In considering why mTBI might lead to increased risk of PTSD and/ or exacerbation of PTSD symptoms, Verfaellie et al. (Chapter 5) discuss neurocognitive mechanisms associated with mTBI that potentially alter risk of PTSD, including neurocognitive deficits experienced in the acute phases of the injury. Bryant, Castro, and Iverson (Chapter 12) raise the corresponding possibility that neural networks implicated in the fear response following trauma are compromised by mTBI. Mild neurocognitive deficits may chronically interfere with successful coping in the small subset of mTBI patients who experience enduring TBI-related brain dysfunction. Of greater relevance to the larger group of mTBI patients whose deficits resolve over time, however, are acute TBI-related changes in brain functioning. These acute changes may influence the initial encoding of trauma memories and the processing of trauma-related emotions around the time of the injury. From a psychological perspective, this may be a critical period for the trauma-exposed person to integrate his or her affective responses with the traumatic experience and to form a cohesive and meaningful trauma narrative. Degradation of this process could be hypothesized to lead to unpredictable affective responses to reminders of the trauma, as well as uncontrolled retrieval of trauma memories (i.e., PTSD reexperiencing symptoms).

There are a number of other TBI-related factors that may exacerbate PTSD, including stress related to any functional impairment (e.g., occupational or social dysfunction) associated with the TBI. Further, physical injuries of any type (including TBI) often lead to poor psychological outcomes following trauma exposure (Blanchard et al., 1995; Sandweiss et al., 2011). As described by Otis, Fortier, and Keane (Chapter 6), even when mild, TBI may lead to physical discomfort such as headaches, which may in turn further exacerbate psychological distress.

PTSD and related psychiatric comorbidities may likewise impede recovery from mTBI and contribute to persistent postconcussive symptoms. Depression, for example, is commonly comorbid with PTSD. As discussed by Iverson (Chapter 3), there is significant evidence that both pre- and postinjury depression adversely affect recovery from mTBI. Similarly, as described by Najavits, Highley, Dolan, and Fee (Chapter 7), excessive substance use, a common PTSD comorbidity, may adversely affect TBI recovery via both direct neural mechanisms (e.g., alcohol neurotoxicity) and via psychosocial mechanisms (e.g., functional impairment, mood disturbance, reduced ability to benefit from psychoeducational and other cognitive rehabilitation strategies). PTSD may also impede recovery from mTBI by virtue of enhanced sensitivity to threat. As articulated by Bryant et al. (Chapter 12), PTSD-related hypervigilance to threat may extend not only to external stimuli but also to internal somatic sensations. In the case of mTBI, hypervigilance to physical symptoms associated with the injury may serve to perpetuate postconcussive symptoms and impede successful coping strategies such as the creation of positive expectancies.

Finally, postconcussive symptoms overlap with PTSD core and associated features. Areas of overlap include, for example, somatic symptoms, psychological symptoms (e.g., depression, irritability), sleep disturbance, and cognitive dysfunction (Stein & McAllister, 2009; Vasterling, Verfaellie, & Sullivan, 2009). Correspondingly, neural substrates (e.g., regions within the prefrontal cortex, hippocampus) underlying PTSD and mTBI overlap to some degree (Stein & McAllister, 2009; Vasterling et al., 2009). It is as yet unclear whether such overlap in underlying neuropathology and symptoms creates an additive effect in some patients that in turn challenges recovery from either or both conditions. The array of possible mechanisms underpinning the impairment secondary to PTSD and mTBI highlights the breadth that is needed in any framework that attempts to comprehensively understand mTBI. As proposed in the model described by Iverson (Chapter 3), there are multiple potential contributors to the phenomena known as mTBI. Iverson's chapter highlights that future research will benefit from a multidisciplinary approach that accommodates the important roles of memory, appraisals, social context, neuroimaging, genetics, and pain, to name just a few. Traditionally, the study of mTBI has occurred in silos of medical and psychological specialties with little communication between the disciplines. The emerging evidence highlights the need for a more inclusive and integrated approach to allow the full range of potential mechanisms to be studied in relation to each other.

Caring for Patients with PTSD and mTBI

PTSD and TBI, when occurring separately, are traditionally treated within different health care contexts. Care of PTSD is most often provided by mental health specialists (e.g., psychologists, psychiatrists, psychiatric social workers) within generalized mental health contexts and, in some settings (e.g., Veterans Healthcare Administration facilities), within specialized PTSD programs. Care of TBI is commonly the responsibility of rehabilitation specialists (e.g., physiatrists, rehabilitation psychologists, occupational therapists), neurologists, neuropsychologists and neuropsychiatrists. In certain settings (e.g., some military contexts), the portal of entry is most often primary care. Not surprisingly, there can be a certain amount of discomfort among providers when the comorbidity arises. PTSD care providers may not know what to expect in terms of recovery from TBI or how to best assess or care for it. Mental health providers may also be concerned that cognitive deficits associated with TBI will alter the effectiveness of psychosocial interventions for PTSD. Similarly, providers accustomed to treating TBI may be unfamiliar with the natural course and history of PTSD, PTSD assessment methods, and PTSD intervention options. There may be concern that psychological symptoms will render TBI interventions ineffective.

The complexity of managing comorbid PTSD and mTBI, however, extends beyond individual provider unfamiliarity with PTSD or mTBI. Accurate assessment is the foundation of subsequent care. As discussed by Ulloa et al. (Chapter 8), the significant symptom overlap between PTSD and postconcussive disorders can pose challenges in assessing comorbid PTSD and mTBI regardless of the provider's familiarity with the two conditions. Likewise, as described by Elhai et al. (Chapter 9), contextual factors such as litigation or compensation may threaten the validity of evaluations. It may be that, given the significant overlap in symptoms and underlying neural substrates, continued attempts to use psychological and neuropsychological test instruments to differentiate which symptoms are attributable to PTSD versus mTBI will yield limited gains in understanding how to best care for patients with the comorbidity. Instead, assessments may be more effectively used to identify problem areas that require intervention. For example, if a patient meets criteria for PTSD and exhibits cognitive deficits, both the PTSD and the cognitive deficits would serve as likely intervention targets, regardless of whether the cognitive deficits were caused primarily by PTSD or by the TBI. Likewise, when targeting alleviation of psychological distress and PTSD symptoms, it may not matter that psychological symptoms leading to a PTSD diagnosis were potentially exacerbated by TBI. Ultimately, these are all empirical questions awaiting scientific evidence to guide clinicians.

Regarding specific interventions for PTSD and mTBI, there is virtually no evidence addressing whether mTBI diminishes treatment response to PTSD interventions or whether PTSD adversely affects the effectiveness of mTBI interventions. Ponsford (Chapter 10) and Bryant and Litz (Chapter 11) describe interventions for mTBI and PTSD, respectively. Although there are clearly disorder-specific components inherent to mTBI and PTSD treatment strategies, both chapters highlight the importance of education, positive expectancies, and enhancement of coping skills, as well as the success of cognitive-behavioral interventions in alleviating emotional symptoms.

In addition to questions about how specific interventions might work in patients with comorbid PTSD and mTBI, how to best structure service delivery emerges as a critical question. Bryant, Castro, and Iverson (Chapter 12) discuss health care considerations specific to military TBI. In any setting, however, questions arise regarding the cost-effectiveness of the care, which contexts might be most appropriate to deliver the care, and how to best sequence various components of the care. Hendricks et al. (Chapter 13) use U.S. Veterans Health Administration data to describe the costs of providing care and to conversely estimate the considerable potential costs to society of not providing care. Given the various entry portals (e.g., rehabilitation settings, primary care, mental health settings) of patients with comorbid PTSD and mTBI, there is some danger of care becoming fragmented if not considered as part of interdisciplinary teams including both PTSD and TBI experts.

Even when multiple experts are part of a treatment team, however, one of the central questions regarding service delivery is whether integrated treatments that address both PTSD and TBI may be more effective than separate treatments, delivered either sequentially or concurrently. This question becomes even more salient when care of PTSD and mTBI are provided in separate contexts. Examples of integrated treatment models exist. For example, Otis et al. (Chapter 6) describe integrated treatment of PTSD and pain (a common TBI comorbidity). Similarly, Najavits et al. (Chapter 7) describe an integrated intervention for PTSD and substance use disorders. Although there are not yet published clinical trials examining integrated interventions for PTSD and TBI, the pain/PTSD, and substance abuse/PTSD interventions serve as potential models for the scientific study of treatments for PTSD/TBI.

Future Directions

To move forward in understanding how to best approach care of patients with comorbid PTSD and mTBI, there are several concepts raised by the various contributors to the volume that will likely help direct future work in this area. First, it is vital to recognize that neurophysiological and psychosocial mechanisms underlie both PTSD and mTBI. As a result, it may not be productive in clinical contexts to focus solely on making distinctions between symptoms caused by brain injury versus psychological factors. Patients may benefit from compensatory techniques regardless of the source of cognitive impairment; likewise, regardless of whether there is a brain injury or not, if PTSD is part of the clinical presentation, it is important to treat it.

There is currently a critical need for additional research that examines whether mTBI moderates treatment response for evidence-based PTSD interventions and likewise whether PTSD symptoms interfere with cognitive rehabilitation strategies among patients with enduring cognitive impairments following TBI. On one hand, there is evidence that cognitive-behavioral therapy may be delivered safely and effectively for patients with mTBI (Bryant, Moulds, Guthrie, & Nixon, 2003). On the other hand, preliminary evidence suggests that even natural variation in brain functioning may alter the response to cognitive-behavioral therapy for PTSD (Wild & Gur; Bryant, Felmingham, Kemp, et al., 2008a; Bryant, Felmingham, Whitford, et al., 2008b). In this regard, mTBI may be one (and perhaps not the most significant) of many sources of cognitive variation affecting treatment. Such research will help determine whether minor modifications or augmented cognitive rehabilitation strategies would enhance PTSD intervention in patients with certain cognitive deficits, regardless of the source of the deficits.

Second, we do not yet know how to best structure the delivery of care for patients with PTSD and mTBI. PTSD and brain injury are each frequently associated with complicating factors (e.g., pain, depression, substance abuse), features that may be compounded when PTSD and mTBI occur together. Thus, care of PTSD and mTBI will rarely be limited to PTSD and mTBI and will likely require a more comprehensive approach. Integrated care, whether at the level of a specific intervention or embedded within a system of care, may be beneficial. However, many questions remain regarding who, when, and where various aspects of care are most cost-effectively delivered. Ultimately, studies of service delivery models will assist us in understanding how complex patients possessing multiple comorbidities are best treated. Information available to date suggests that the greater we can integrate care, the more efficient that care will be in terms of limited burden to the patients, reduced costs to the system, and improved patient outcomes.

Third, if appropriately treated, the prognosis for either or both PTSD and mTBI can be good. However, if the symptoms of either PTSD or mTBI are considered to be a permanent condition attributed to immutable neurological factors, motivation and incentive may be compromised, and recovery impeded. There is much evidence that perception of self-efficacy and expectation of recovery play an important role in outcomes following posttraumatic stress (Hobfoll et al. 2007). This highlights the importance of defining not only PTSD, but also TBI, in a way that promotes recovery. Specifically, it is important to acknowledge that traumatic stress and mTBI are associated with reactions—whether emotional, cognitive, or somatic—that can often be effectively addressed with stress management and other psychosocial strategies (e.g., psychoeducation, cognitive-behavioral interventions, cognitive compensatory techniques) that are geared toward self-mastery and recovery from symptoms.

Numerous chapters in this volume have emphasized that the label of mTBI can have unintended, adverse effects by minimizing expectancy of recovery, and even facilitating hypervigilance to common sensations that can then be misinterpreted as signals of pathological neural processes. This can be especially problematic in cases of comorbid PTSD, where patients tend to be vigilant to bodily cues and overemphasize the potential adverse costs associated with these reactions (Smith & Bryant, 2000). It is critical, therefore, for policy statements and diagnostic manuals to accurately reflect what is known about the course and recovery from PTSD and mTBI when they occur separately and when they occur concomitantly.

The cascade of interest and research activity into the intersecting conditions of PTSD and mTBI is shedding new light on both conditions and how they may interact with each other. Instead of simply conceptualizing either disorder as a function of a single process (e.g., neurological, cognitive, emotion-based, attributional), a more comprehensive perspective recognizes that various mechanisms contribute to the symptoms of each disorder. A fundamental message that has emerged throughout this volume is the need to identify and manage *reactions* occurring in the wake of psychological trauma involving head injury rather than strictly labeling these responses as PTSD or mTBI. Overreliance on prescriptive diagnostic labels that understand each symptom as a function exclusively of PTSD or of mTBI may increase the risk of mistakenly attributing symptoms to a specific process; instead, we have learned that managing the responses with evidence-based strategies in ways that promote a sense of recovery will increase the likelihood of adaptation. There is no doubt that the recent surge in research activity into PTSD and mTBI will continue, and we can look forward to considerable insights in the near future about the risks, mechanisms, and treatments pertaining to each of these challenging disorders and their complex comorbidity.

References

Blanchard, E. B., Hickling, E. J., Mitnick, N., Taylor, A. E., Loos, W. R., & Buckley, T. C. (1995). The impact of severity of physical injury and perception of life threat in the development of post-traumatic stress disorder in motor vehicle accident victims. *Behaviour Research and Therapy, 33,* 529–534.
Bryant, R. A., Creamer, M., O'Donnell, M., Silove, D., Clark, C. R., & McFarlane,

A. C. (2009). Posttraumatic amnesia and the nature of posttraumatic stress disorder after mild traumatic brain injury. *Journal of the International Neuropsychological Society, 15*, 862–867.

Bryant, R. A., Felmingham, K. L., Kemp, A., Das, P., Hughes, G., Peduto, A., et al. (2008a). Amygdala and ventral anterior cingulate activation predicts treatment response to cognitive behaviour therapy for post-traumatic stress disorder. *Psychological Medicine, 38*, 555–561.

Bryant, R. A., Felmingham, K. L., Whitford, T., Kemp, A., Hughes, G., Peduto, A., et al. (2008b). Rostral anterior cingulate volume predicts treatment response to cognitive behavior therapy for posttraumatic stress disorder. *Journal of Psychiatry and Neuroscience, 33*, 142–146.

Bryant, R. A., Marosszeky, J. E., Crooks, J., & Gurka, J. A. (2000). Posttraumatic stress disorder following severe traumatic brain injury. *American Journal of Psychiatry, 157*, 629–631.

Bryant, R. A., Moulds, M., Guthrie, R., & Nixon, R. D. V. (2003). Treating acute stress disorder following mild traumatic brain injury. *American Journal of Psychiatry, 160*, 585–587.

Bryant, R. A., O'Donnell, M. L., Creamer, M., McFarlane, A. C., Clark, C. R., & Silove, D. (2010). The psychiatric sequelae of traumatic injury. *American Journal of Psychiatry, 167*, 312–320.

Gil, S., Caspi, Y., Ben-Ari, I. Z., Koren, D., & Klein, E. (2005). Does memory of a traumatic event increase the risk for posttraumatic stress disorder in patients with traumatic brain injury?: A prospective study. *American Journal of Psychiatry, 162*(5), 963–969.

Hobfall, S. E., Watson, P., Bell, C. C., Bryant, R. A., Brymer, M. J., Friedman, M. J., et al. (2007). Five essential elements of immediate and mid-term mass trauma intervention: Empirical evidence. *Psychiatry, 70*, 283–315.

Hoge, C. W., McGurk, D., Thomas, J. L., Cox, A. L., Engel, C. C., & Castro, C. A. (2008). Mild traumatic brain injury in U.S. soldiers returning from Iraq. *New England Journal of Medicine, 358*(5), 453–463.

Sandweiss, D. A., Slymen, D. J., Leardmann, C. A., Smith, B., White, M. R., Boyko, E. J., et al. (2011). Preinjury psychiatric status, injury severity, and postdeployment posttraumatic stress disorder. *Archives of General Psychiatry, 68*, 496–504.

Sayer, N. A., Rettmann, N. A., Carlson, K. E., Bernardy, N., Sigford, B. J., Hamblen, J. L., et al. (2009). Veterans with history of mild traumatic brain injury and posttraumatic stress disorder: Challenges from provider perspective. *Journal of Rehabilitation Research and Development, 46*, 703–716.

Sbordone, R. J., & Ruff, R. M. (2010). Re-examination of the controversial coexistence of traumatic brain injury and posttraumatic stress disorder: Misdiagnosis and self-reported measures. *Psychology Injury and Law, 3*, 63–76.

Smith, K., & Bryant, R.A. (2000). The generality of cognitive bias in acute stress disorder. *Behaviour Research and Therapy, 38*, 709–715.

Stein, M. B., & McAllister, T. W. (2009). Exploring the convergence of posttraumatic stress disorder and mild traumatic brain injury. *American Journal of Psychiatry, 166*, 768–776.

Vasterling, J. J., Verfaellie, M., & Sullivan, K. D. (2009). Mild traumatic brain injury and posttraumatic stress disorder in returning veterans: Perspectives from cognitive neuroscience. *Clinical Psychology Review, 29,* 674–684.

Wild, J., & Gur, R. C. (2008). Verbal memory and treatment response in post-traumatic stress disorder. *British Journal of Psychiatry, 193,* 254–255.

Zatzick, D. F., Rivara, F. P., Jurkovich, G. J., Hoge, C. W., Wang, J., Fan, M. Y., et al. (2010). Multisite investigation of traumatic brain injuries, posttraumatic stress disorder, and self-reported health and cognitive impairments. *Archives of General Psychiatry, 67,* 1291–1300.

Index

W

Warfare
  PTSD and traumatic brain injury and, 3
  TBI and, 16–17
White matter
  abnormalities after TBI, Plate 2.4
  changes in, 22
  DTI for assessing, 25, Plate 2.4
  in mTBI, 23–24, 27–28, 42, 42f, Plate 2.1
    selective damage to, 26

in pain syndromes, 113
strain effects to, 23–24
Wong–Baker Faces Scale, 117
Worker's compensation benefits,
    symptom exaggeration and,
    176
World Health Organization
  mTBI criteria of, 200
  mTBI definition of, 40–41
  mTBI guidelines of, 17
World Trade Center attacks, 17